Dr. Monica-Maria Stapelberg has been employed at various universities for many years as a lecturer in history of literature, as well as medieval languages, medieval history and cultural studies. Since retiring from academia, she has had three books published, aimed at the popular market. Monica lives on the east coast of Australia with her family.

THROUGH THE DARKNESS

GLIMPSES INTO THE HISTORY OF WESTERN MEDICINE

MONICA-MARIA STAPELBERG

CRUX
PUBLISHING

First published in the United Kingdom in 2015
by Crux Publishing Ltd.

ISBN: 978-1-909979-27-7

Also available as an ebook:
eISBN: 978-1-909979-28-4

Requests for permission to reproduce material from this work
should be sent to hello@cruxpublishing.co.uk

To Chris and Michael,
Shahina and Nita,
with love

CONTENTS

ACKNOWLEDGEMENTS

The ongoing research over the past five years, and consequent writing of this book on select aspects in the history of medicine, has been a source of rewarding discovery, mixed at times with incredulity, surprise, and great delight. Along the way, several people have actively supported the progression of this manuscript.

I would like to thank my husband Fred for his wholehearted encouragement, his counsel, and ever-patient understanding of my often-dogged preoccupation when researching the vast amount of material for this book.

My thanks go to my sons Chris and Michael – their medical careers, and further specialisation in different fields of medicine initially led me to delve into the fascinating history of the subject. Similarly, I sincerely wish to thank my daughter's-in-law Shahina and Nita for their continued support, love and friendship.

My appreciation also goes to my nieces Claudia and Candice, as well as to Marci and Mike, and my good friend Karin, for their enthusiastic interest in the subject matter.

Lastly, and by no means least, I wish to thank my publisher Christopher Lascelles from Crux Publishing for his invaluable, personable advice and guidance, his readiness to assist, and for initially recognising the book's possible potential.

Monica-Maria Stapelberg, December 2015

INTRODUCTION

Throughout history, medicine has undergone profound changes in its encounters with disease, death, and the enigmatic concept of illness. Today, medical practitioners have reached what is generally presumed to be a mature and enlightened stance on the theory and practice of medicine, backed by complex technological innovations that medical antecedents hundreds of years ago would have thought of as mysteriously magical or relegated to the realm of theology.

In this context, we can only contemplate with wry amusement how people centuries from now might regard our current science-based medical practices: they might be surprised and shocked at our propensity to poly-pharmacy; our overuse of antibiotics and therapeutic drugs; as well as the harshness and invasiveness of radiation therapy, chemotherapy, and radical surgery. Current practices that the medical establishment champions and holds in high esteem, might in future be found to be preposterous, and perhaps as appalling and outrageous as many of the past medical practices considered in this book.

When England's King Charles II lay dying in the year 1685, his twelve physicians fought for his life with unprecedented vigour, leaving no stone unturned in running through the whole gamut of cures known at the time. Over several days, the dying king was repeatedly bled from the jugular vein, purged, cupped, scarified and fed dozens of different concoctions, tinctures and powders. In addition to several enemas, strong emetics were administered to induce vomiting. The king's hair was shorn, pungent blistering agents were applied to the scalp, and he was seared with red-hot irons to further 'draw' out putrid humors. While pigeon excrement was diligently smeared on the soles of his feet, a tonic of liquorice and sweet almonds was used to calm him. When all this failed to sufficiently revive and strengthen him, he was given what physicians considered *the* most powerful medication at the time – forty drops of 'Spirit of Human Skull' – made specifically from the powdered skull of a man who had never been buried.

However, as the king continued to convulse more violently than before, the unanimous decision was reached to regularly administer the lavishly praised febrifuge Peruvian Bark – new to English medicine and only recently introduced to the *London Pharmacopoeia* at the time – today known as quinine. Although Charles looked his approaching death in the eyes with calm composure, his doctors tried to avert the inevitable by forcing additional potions down his throat: the famous Raleigh's Antidote, consisting of a multitude of herbs and animal extracts; powdered Goa Stone, artificially manufactured in Goa, India, made from clay, silt, shells, resin and musk; ammonium chloride; and lastly, oriental Bezoar Stone, found in the stomachs of deer, sheep and antilopes, consisting of a mixture of gallstones and animal hair.

But, all was to no avail and after several days of treatment the fifty-four year old king drew his last breath – he most probably died of chronic kidney disease. Although the various treatments administered to the dying monarch may seem bizzare to the modern reader, Charles's physicians clearly believed in the 'state-of-the-art' course of action they had taken in saving the life of the man, who was after all their most prominent client.[1]

It is in this vein that the tone of this book is set, containing facts that at times might amuse, astound, and on occasion might unfortunately repulse or even cause anger at the perceived ignorance of our learned forebears. From a modern 'armchair' perspective it is important not to lapse into what has been called 'the enormous condescension of posterity' by historians.[2] Nor should we judge the past by reference to the present as an inevitable progression towards 'best practice'. Just as medicine of the past was not a precursor to modern medicine, so medical practices and theories were not unsophisticated, nor were they primitive.

Past medical theories and practices simply approached illness and disease from a different viewpoint to that of modern doctors. Rooted in antiquity, in time-honoured traditions based on the irrefutable authority of Hippocrates (c.460-c.370 BCE) and Galen of Pergamum (129-c.200/216 CE), medicine for centuries relied on scholarly theories that made perfect sense when considering the actual knowledge and information physicians had at their disposal. Therefore, to qualify their practices as ignorant merely presumes our own knowledge as being ultimately superior. Hence, the goal of this book is to catalogue various medical practices in the past with equanimity, bearing in mind the censure our current medical technology might be subjected to in the future.

As the reader shall discover in the following chapters, the fascinating history of medicine in Europe is filled with curious, strange, alarming and gruesome cures, as well as virulent, confronting, torturous diseases. Many cures, although enthusiastically supported by physicians of the past, were all but useless, highly dangerous, and even lethal – doctors were as likely to maim or kill, as they were to cure. Even minor ailments could elicit life-threatening treatments, such as the repeated opening of veins, the amputation of limbs, and the cauterisation of wounds with red-hot iron or boiling hot oil.

In many cases the cure was far worse than the condition requiring it. On the other hand, physicians, surgeons and other medical practitioners worked under horrendous and difficult conditions, performing complicated, often delicate procedures on rough, blood-soaked wooden tables, and on writhing, screaming patients, without the aid of anaesthetics, drugs or proper hygiene. The study of anatomy was essentially performed on reeking, decomposing cadavers, by barehanded students or surgeons, their fingernails caked with dried blood and putrid flesh.

A specific aspect of medical history was played out tragically in the shadow of the gallows. In England especially, violent and bloody brawls between surgeons desperate to procure corpses for dissection, and the families of those condemned, are well documented and make morbidly fascinating reading. However, the relatively low number of corpses acquired in this manner from the gallows by medical schools led to another shocking chapter in the history of surgery and anatomy – a two hundred year period of body snatching – the procurement of fresh corpses from new graves.

Similarly, also connected to the scaffold, a little known part of medical history on the European continent concerned the executioners themselves. Highly skilled in anatomy as well as the use of medications, many executioners worked as renowned healers in several European countries. As hereditary healers, executioners occupied a sanctioned *niche* in the medical infrastructure of medieval and early modern towns, bringing them into contact with people of the highest social echelons, including aristocrats and even royalty.

Repulsive and disgusting examples of medications dominated medical directives right up to the eighteenth century. The practice of using excrement in prescriptions, generally referred to by medical historians as 'sewer pharmacology', was widespread in Europe. Orthodox medical practitioners also made abundant use of human flesh, blood, and bone in medications. 'Mummy', a medicinal preparation made from the remains of an embalmed, dried, or otherwise 'prepared body', as well as human cadaver parts and blood, were available in every pharmacy. Recipes of the times routinely included so-called 'corpse medicine'.

A further potent cure, considered especially effective in treating syphilis, involved treatments with mercury, which was in frequent use up until the twentieth century. Unfortunately, as part of the cure the patient died a slow death by mercury poisoning, racked with uncontrollable shaking spells, corrosion of the membranes in the mouth, teeth rattling loose in the gums, as well as a relentless deterioration of the bones.

Another part of medical history dealt with 'medical magic' or 'magical therapeutics', eagerly endorsed and propagated by physicians and other medical practitioners until the early eighteenth century. Through the once popular concepts of 'healing by transfer', as well as 'healing by sympathy', it was firmly believed that disease could not only be transferred and transplanted, but also transformed. Thus, the touch of the reigning monarch, the king's hand, was believed by all to be imbued with healing powers, transferred by his touch. While English and French monarchs healed by touch, alternate miraculous healing powers were attributed to the kings and queens of other European sovereign houses. Another form of 'medical magic' once widely advocated and used by physicians was the 'wound salve', 'weapon's salve', or 'powder of sympathy' – all fitting examples of healing by sympathy or at a distance.

Various chapters discuss different incurable epidemic diseases, prevalent during the Middle Ages and the early modern period: the Black Death or Great Mortality; Leprosy, known as the disease of the soul in ancient and medieval times; and syphilis the 'French Pox'. These are variously examined from a standpoint of social history, as well as contemporary medical treatments and failings, thereby creating the impetus for reassessment and reformation of medical practices.

Until the late eighteenth century, the internal workings of women's sexual organs were a mystery to physicians. From ancient times through to the Middle Ages and early modern period, the physiology of women, as well as the concepts of fertility, menstruation and childbirth, were shrouded in misconceptions that were firmly held by the orthodox medical establishment, endorsing amongst others, the notion of the 'wandering womb'. The idea that the womb was free to move from its normal position, thereby obstructing breathing, blocking passages and causing disease in women, continued amongst physicians for centuries.

A further important part of medical history concerned 'diagnosing' death. The fear of being buried alive is ancient, and hundreds of actual accounts of this having taken place are in existence. As putrefaction was once the only sure sign of death known to doctors, the inability to diagnose death lead to many bizarre devices and procedures – to protect the 'deceased' from coming alive in the coffin – including a system of 'waiting morgues' and 'safety coffins'.

Throughout this book there is an emphasis on social history relevant to the times as well as the medical aspects discussed. The material in the book pertains to western medicine and does not render a history of medicine or medical tradition. Instead, the different chapters offer random glimpses into this field, highlighting select, perhaps lesser-known aspects in the history of orthodox medical practices.

MEDICAL PRACTITIONERS OF THE PAST

Physicians – all theory, no practice

In modern times the term 'physician' refers to a specialist in internal medicine. In centuries past however, this term had a different connotation.

The medieval medical system was made up of several distinct divisions: physicians[1], surgeons and barber-surgeons. For centuries the term 'physician' referred to university-educated medical practitioners – they had theoretical knowledge and prescribed drugs. Their once less-distinguished colleagues, surgeons and barber-surgeons, were known as so-called 'empirics' – a term referring to non-university trained medical practitioners, some of whom were illiterate. Surgeons and barber-surgeons worked with their hands, typically with a knife and learned their skills by practical training.

Since ancient times, physicians formed the elite, the upper crust of the medical system – their position in society esteemed and prestigious. Galen of Pergamum (129-c.200/216 CE), personal doctor to two successive Roman Emperors[2] was a typical physician: he was scholarly and intelligent. However, he was also known for his arrogance and superciliousness. Not given to any pretence at modesty, Galen considered that he had consolidated and enlarged the sum of all medical knowledge of his time[3] and he had no hesitation in placing himself a few rungs above Hippocrates (c. 460 – c. 370 BCE), the Greek Father of Medicine. Unabashed, Galen proclaimed 'It is I, and I alone, who have revealed the true path of medicine. It must be admitted that Hippocrates already staked out this path…he prepared the way, but I have made it passable'.[4]

Galen's writing output was extraordinary and some 500 books are attributed to this renowned physician. With his overpowering verbosity and few opponents, his place in medical history was secure.[5] Incredibly, his ideas and teachings survived for more than one and a half millennia – some of his teachings were still in use in the eighteen hundreds – almost without adjustments and certainly without question.

Physicians have provoked mixed feelings in society since ancient times, probably due to their elevated status and assumed social superiority. Pompous physicians, more concerned with their purses than their patients, provided a favourite target for satirists. Proverbially 'the physician was more dangerous than the disease'.[6] In the same context, William Shakespeare (1564-1616), in *Timon of Athens* warned: 'Trust not the physician, his antidotes are poison'. Chaucer (1343-1400), the Father of English Literature, affirmed the frequent allegations, that physicians were greedily making money from the misery of others, by proclaiming 'for gold in physic is cordial, therefore he loved gold in special'.[7] Similarly, two hundred years later, Elizabethan satirist Thomas Dekker (1572-1632), declared that 'a good physician comes to thee in the shape of an Angel'[8] – a play on the word 'angel', which at the time was not only a divine messenger, but also an English gold coin.

Physicians distinguished themselves from other medical divisions through their university training. Universities, in the sense in which the term is generally understood, were specifically a creation of the Middle Ages – in spite of the fact that civilisations like the ancient Greeks and Romans, the Byzantine and other cultures, were familiar with forms of higher education. During the twelfth century, the first universities[9] were founded in Italy, France and England. All of these soon developed schools of medicine attracting students from across Europe. The Italian University of Bologna, the oldest in the world, began training physicians in 1219, with Oxford, the world's second-oldest university, following close behind.[10]

During the thirteenth century and beyond, a boy interested in medicine - girls were excluded from studying medicine - would have started his education at a grammar school at the age of eight or nine, focusing on the Seven Liberal Arts: geometry, arithmetic, astronomy, dialectic, rhetoric, grammar and music. Providing he could pay the required high fees, he would then enter university between the age of fifteen and eighteen and spend at least five to seven more years studying the Seven Liberal Arts, eventually specialising in one of the seven – doctors of those times were accomplished polymaths. Upon passing his examinations he would be awarded a baccalaureate degree and it was at this point that his medical education would begin, an education, which required several years.

The medical corpus studied at the time was classical in origin – in other words it dated back to at least the fifth century BCE – but medieval in format.[11] Up until the sixteenth century the orthodox medical texts of Hippocrates, Galen and their Islamic interpreters Avicenna (c. 980-1037)[12] and Rhazes (854-925), were rigidly upheld by European universities. Galen's assertion that physicians should understand philosophy had been construed as a call for book learning and the teaching of medicine in terms of set texts.

In order to become a better physician the classic teachers and their books had to be studied and discussed in depth, with an emphasis on logical disputation, arguing both sides of a point, examining an argument and coming to new conclusions. But *all* new proposals and suggestions were based on rehashing the old Hippocratic or Galenic texts with their notions founded on humoral balance. In other words, there was no discussion on real-life observations or research. Debate simply focused on theories put forward over a thousand years ago at that time. Any dissent was considered medical heresy and brought about definite consequences.

In the fifteenth century, when it was discovered that thirteenth century physician Mondino de Luzzi's (1270-1326) great anatomical textbook *Anathomia* contradicted Galen in some point of detail, the book was suppressed at various universities. Similarly, 'when John Geynes of the London College of physicians criticised Galen in 1559, he was condemned by his colleagues and forced to sign a document of recantation. [...] Vesalius voiced his disagreements with Galen only in a nervous and timid fashion'.[13] To question Galen's authority during the Middle Ages, was synonymous with medical blasphemy and certainly not favourable for any motivated student to pass an exam.

Specialists in diverse medical fields were unknown in medieval times. Medical writers would acknowledge proficiency in all illnesses – many of which they knew nothing about – rather than just one specific disease. The facade of learnedness and wisdom could be achieved by 'calling upon the authority of tradition, citing authorities or copying from authorities without citing them'.[14] Hence in *Canterbury Tales*, Chaucer indicates the physician's respected standing simply by listing the medical sages known to him: 'Well knew he the olde Esculapius, and Descorides, and eek Rufus, olde Ypocras, Haly, and Galyen, Serapion, Razis'[15] – Chaucer's listing of medical authorities goes on and on. As a result of their training, physicians were theoreticians, learned paragons, their expertise confined to words – worlds apart from those who physically tended the sick.

Few in numbers, physicians lived mainly in the cities, and as highly respected members of society, their services were expensive and generally affordable only to the wealthy. They went about their business dressed in the most splendid attire: impressive wigs, buckled shoes and ornate velvet coats – not to be soiled by contact with their patients. Customarily, university trained physicians did not have much physical contact with their patients, preferring to diagnose through verbal interchange. As they made no physical examinations – apart from taking the pulse – physicians knew 'very little about most internal diseases of heart, lungs, liver, and gastrointestinal tract'.[16] They considered it beneath their dignity to 'handle' those under their care – an unwillingness that was partly vindicated by the Hippocratic Oath, requiring physicians to never use a knife on a patient.

In fact, at the University of Paris, sixteenth century medical graduates had to swear that they would never engage in 'manual surgery'.[17] Another point in context is that many who undertook academic medical training and became physicians, had initially been churchmen. However, they were forbidden from practising surgery on religious grounds, as the bull *Ecclesia Abhorret a Sanguine* – the Church abhors blood – issued by Council of Tours in 1163, forbade priests and monks from spilling blood. This is why the Inquisition generally burnt heretics and witches – to avoid bloodshed.

If a physician considered an operation necessary, he would use his education in astrology to determine the most favourable time for the procedure with the help of astrological tables, and then leave the bloody business of cutting and slicing to an untutored, often illiterate, surgeon or barber. It should perhaps be mentioned that medieval medicine was intricately linked to astrology.

Physicians of the seventeenth century still combined their learning in physiology and anatomy with religious and astrological philosophy, in diagnosis and treatment. In other words, it was held that someone's physical constitution was determined at birth by the various positions of the planets. The great Renaissance physician Paracelsus (1493-1541) firmly asserted[18] that 'the physician who does not understand astronomy cannot be a complete physician because more than half of all diseases are governed by the heavens'.[19] All planetary bodies were thought to influence humans and nature through the emission of vapours – some of them detrimental, causing sickness and disease.

Following tradition, the essence of the physician's profession was to consider symptoms, scrutinise patients and their various excreta, examine the patient's pulse – Galen had theorised and written extensively on various pulse phenomena – and then pronounce on diagnosis and treatment in line with current theory. Typically, physicians followed Galen's emphasis on urinalysis, thereby establishing a diagnosis through uroscopy, which meant that it was not necessary to physically examine the patient. It was firmly held for centuries that all humoral imbalances could be identified through the examination of a patient's urine with the naked eye.[20]

Uroscopy evaluated the quality and the quantity of the urine, with reference to the concentration, smell, transparency, and the occurrence of sediment, foam or blood. This complex doctrine was given its final form during the thirteenth century, 'when it became a cunning system of unrealistic, fantastic subtleties',[21] especially if the evaluation was to involve proposed surgery – a painful, dangerous process at the time. During the sixteenth century – medical evaluation had not changed from practices of the thirteenth century – the ever-blunt Paracelsus commented about his fellow physicians in this context: 'All they can do is to gaze at piss'.[22]

After the examination of urine and various other excreta, physicians would suggest treatment. This generally involved explicit changes to diet; advice on respite, sleep and exercise; therapeutic baths and drugs, which were compounds of herbs, roots, various forms of excrement, human body parts, and numerous other 'exotic' ingredients (See Chapters on Corpse Medicine and Sewer Pharmacology). Considering some of the harsh treatments administered, it may be assumed that 'many patients must have suffered from the administration of emetics, purgatives and expectorants. Not a few must have died of water and salt depletion occasioned by these remedies'.[23]

Surgeons – always hands-on

While physicians ranked supreme in medical hierarchy, surgeons stood second, and whereas physicians generally avoided physical contact with their patients, surgeons were always 'hands on'. In fact, the term 'surgery', derived from the Latin term *chirurgia*, means 'working or done by hand'.[24] This separation of medicine into theory and practice was questioned over the centuries by various eminent surgeons and physicians: the distinguished surgeon Henri de Mondeville (1260-1316) commented that 'it is impossible to be a good surgeon if one is not familiar with the foundations and general rules of medicine and it is impossible for anyone to be a good physician who is absolutely ignorant of the art of surgery'.[25]

The same sentiment was echoed more than two hundred years later by Paracelsus, the one-man revolution, who publicly burnt the books of Galen and Avicenna in protest, and upset the medical profession and everyone else with his '...unorthodox ideas, monumental ego, and insistence on writing in German rather than "popish" Latin'.[26] He firmly believed that the division of medicine into the two separate fields of theory and practice was absurd and detrimental. According to Paracelsus, 'there can be no surgeon who is not also a physician' and 'where the physician is not also a surgeon he is an idol that is nothing but a painted monkey'.[27] However, the separation of theory and practice remained for several centuries.

Surgeons treated syphilis, abscesses, fistulas, rashes and other skin diseases, closed wounds, excised tumours, and performed phlebotomies (blood-letting), amputations, cauteries and bone settings. Intricate and impressive procedures dealing with anal fistulas, abdominal injuries, bladder stones and cataracts, set the surgical elite apart. Surgeons also performed trepanation, which meant drilling holes in patients' skulls, an operation relating to the 'extraction' of practically all ailments concerning the head. Such 'disorders' included inflammations, headaches, vertigo, and deafness. Astoundingly, considering that trepanation was generally performed while the patient was fully conscious, many of those operated on seem to have lived to tell the tale – and on numerous people the procedure was even performed more than once.

It should also be mentioned that until the late eighteen hundreds, hand washing was not customary before performing medical procedures and operations – the causes of sepsis were still unknown. Therefore, infections – often deadly – were a common result of all surgical interventions. Especially, since the general notion prevalent amongst most surgeons was to stuff incisions and wounds with whatever wadding was at hand, thereby almost guaranteeing the swift onset of infection.

In various European countries such as Italy and Germany, surgeons may have had some university training, but generally guild-apprenticeships were more common. On the whole, surgeons' medical knowledge was for centuries based on experience only. Surgeons were stationed in all towns and cities and some delivered their services mainly at markets and fairs, often travelling from one to the next. While onlookers joked and cajoled, the poor unfortunate patients subjected to the surgeons' knife endured wart cuttings, tooth extractions, and bloodletting. The fact that they would be on the move and far away if any complications set in, was afterwards, clearly to the surgeons' advantage!

Another group of surgeons perpetually travelled with campaigning armies, and picked up their wide-ranging experiences on the battlefield – the proverbial school of surgery.[28] In ancient times, Hippocrates had advised that 'he who wishes to be a surgeon should go to war'.[29] Army-surgeons were familiar with trauma surgery such as the treatment of fractures by splinting; the resetting of bones; and the application of cautery to wounds to stem bleeding. During the sixteenth century, the increased use of gunpowder in battle had aggravated the injuries facing surgeons. As opposed to wounds inflicted by swords or arrows, those caused by cannonball shrapnel and gunshots were more traumatic and prone to infection.[30] Cautery was applied to gunshot wounds, because gunpowder was widely held to be poisonous.

Surgeons also performed amputation of limbs – all without anaesthetic. Standard procedure at the time was to cauterise the open end of the amputated appendage with boiling oil or red hot metal, to seal off blood vessels and stop haemorrhaging. The additional pain caused by such procedures must have been unbearably excruciating. Renowned French army surgeon, Ambroise Paré (1510-1590), revived the ancient Greek method of tying off blood vessels instead of subjecting patients to the added pain of cautery. He also found it far more effective to treat wounds with a mixture of egg yolk, oil of roses and turpentine – the anti-septic properties of turpentine probably aiding the healing process.[31] Paré's famous saying was: 'I dressed him, God healed him'.[32]

The surgeons' tasks were definitely not for the fainthearted and are graphically described by Thomas Ross, warden of the London Fellowship of Surgeons in 1519: '…staunching blood, searing wounds with irons and other instruments, […] cutting the skull in due proportion to the pellicles[33] of the brain with instruments of iron, couching cataracts, taking out bones, sewing the flesh, lancing boils, cutting apostums, burning cancers and other like, setting in joints and binding them with ligatures'.[34] In addition, surgeons repaired hernias in the groin, cut through the perineum to remove stones from the bladder, and performed operations on the eyes, 'including one for cataract in which the lens was pushed down with a needle inserted into the eyeball'.[35]

In spite of great progress in the field of medicine, surgery-methods during the early nineteenth century, had changed little over the centuries, and 'without anaesthesia or antiseptics, operations were generally crude, frequently agonising and often deadly'.[36] Surgical methods and procedures – always performed barehanded – must have differed from gruelling torture only in motivation, and must have been akin to the torments of hell, not only for the patient but also for those observing and performing the operation. Although endeavours were sometimes made to use pain relief, these could be fatal, as they often included poisons such as hemlock, opium, mandrake, or deadly nightshade. Generally, surgery was performed on fully alert, screaming patients – held or tied down if necessary – by surgeons with dirty implements and dirty hands, while the operating table was a wooden slab, with grooves to allow blood to drip onto the sawdust below.

A lithotomy, the removal of bladder stones, was such a torment that sufferers would only undergo the agonizingly painful operation when the throbbing from the stone pressing against the bladder became intolerable. Bladder stones were very common at the time, even amongst children, which may have been diet-related. Bladder stones may have been attributable to the fact that drinking water in cities and towns, was generally polluted and invariably dangerous, leaving ale, beer, and wine as the main beverages of choice for all ages – in other words no one really drank water. The procedure to remove such stones was not only risky but also distressingly painful.

The standard practice for a lithotomy was to truss the patient up like a chicken, ankles tied to the hands, buttocks exposed, and to then pass large unyielding instruments up the urethra. Alternately, the surgeon would insert a finger into the hapless patient's rectum, feel for the stone, and press it outwards. Then cuts were made through the perineum, between the genitals and anus, to draw the stone out – all without the benefit of anaesthetic. No wonder that many chose to rather suffer the illness than any attempt at a cure! However, it must be added that those brave enough to undergo the procedure were generally successfully relieved of their varying calculi.

During the first half of the eighteenth century, those surgeons who received any training at all would begin learning their craft at the age of fourteen and fifteen. Paying high fees, these adolescent boys – girls were excluded from this elite world – were apprenticed to a master surgeon for up to seven years. During this time, they were bound by strict rules, having to live in their master's house, work all hours without remuneration or holiday, and prohibited from marrying, drinking, theatre going, or gambling.

The study of anatomy was not a given. If apprentices were lucky and could afford it, they would perhaps spend a few months at anatomy lectures in Edinburgh or Paris. Alternately, they might attend one of the brief courses offered in London. After the long apprenticeship with a modicum of anatomy, the typical trainee would enrol as the pupil of an established surgeon for up to a year, henceforth walking the wards of a London hospital – a privilege that again demanded a hefty fee.

Then the would-be surgeon could take the examination at Surgeons' Hall to qualify for a diploma allowing him officially to practice. 'Finally he could start as a junior surgeon on the first rung of the hospital career ladder. [...] As in all realms of life in Georgian Britain, nepotism was the surest route to advancement in London's voluntary hospitals; the tradition of fathers recruiting sons, and uncles handing over to nephews, would persist throughout the century. Once set up in a hospital job, it was a steady if protracted path to a lifelong position as a senior surgeon with a lucrative private clientele. [...] ...in the unregulated shambolic medical world of the eighteenth century, innumerable surgeons attained status and fortune despite bucking the system.[...] Many young men [...] became successful surgeons with scant experience or training: they skipped the apprenticeship between anatomy lessons, spent at most a few months walking the wards and walked into practice without ever securing a diploma'.[37]

By the mid-eighteen hundreds, surgical sutures were still made of catgut, 'sharpened with spit' and 'surgeons walked around with scalpels in their pockets. If a tool fell onto the blood-soiled floor, it was dusted off and inserted back into the pocket – or into the body of the patient on the operating table'.[38] By and large however, the English surgical elite had more in common with physicians than with their inferior competitors, the barber-surgeons.

Barber-surgeons – a hybrid-occupation

In England and the German states, barber-surgeons formed part of the medical hierarchy. But it was different in other European countries. For instance, in the southern in the southern European countries of Italy, Spain, and southern France, the hybrid-occupation of barber-surgeons never gained any standing.

In England barber-surgeons were distinct from surgeons and made no affectation of being elite. They made up the third medical division. Most of them were illiterate with no formal education, and their training came solely through practical experience. Barbers performed minor 'surgical' tasks such as phlebotomy, cautery, and tooth extractions; as well as basic procedures, such as cupping, setting simple fractures, and applying poultices. Their great attraction with the general populace was the low fee they charged. Generally barber-surgeons only pursued their medical obligations on a part-time basis, while their main income was from cutting and trimming hair, and shaving their clients.

The traditional barber pole, once associated with the service of phlebotomy, and bloodletting through leeches, became emblematic of the barber-surgeon profession.[39] The red and white stripes on the pole symbolised the bandages used during the practice of bloodletting: red for bloodstained and white for clean bandages. Originally, these bindings were suspended on the pole to dry, and as they blew in the breeze they would twist to form the coiled pattern still found on modern day barber poles.

Guilds, apprenticeships and colleges

Many studies have recorded the rivalry among physicians, surgeons and barber-surgeons, and the most noteworthy aspect of that rivalry was the general detachment of physicians from clinical medicine. Physicians theorised and high-handedly set the trend in medicine, but had no practical experience whatsoever. For example, professor of medicine at Montpellier and Paris, Jean Astruc (1684-1766), wrote a manual on obstetrics without ever delivering a single baby. Another eminent Paris physician, Philippe Hecquet (1661-1737), wrote his *Traité de la Peste* in 1722 without having had contact with any victims of the plague.[40] Many such examples are extant, with physicians commanding most of the literature, thus leaving surgeons and physicians pitted against each.

In order to understand such rivalries, it is important to appreciate the whole system of guilds and apprenticeships, prevalent in the medical system for centuries. During thirteenth century Europe, as population numbers increased, trade blossomed, and cities became more and more complex, medicine 'needed to organize itself'[41] – something, which initially took place in Italy with medical guilds taking accountability for the examination of their candidates, as well as apprenticeships.

In southern Europe the gulf between physicians and surgeons was not prevalent, and surgery was deemed a desirable skill for physicians to acquire. Here, during the thirteenth century a license to practice medicine could be obtained after only five years of study, which included surgery[42] – hence the professional animosity between physicians and surgeons was avoided. Not so however in some European countries, where surgery was not included in the academic medical curriculum.

In France, even when surgery was eventually added to the curriculum, this discipline was always under direction from physicians, while surgeons performed the actual knife-work – in other words, got their hands bloody. But, in 1687, surgery in this country experienced a serendipitous upsurge in status as a result of a much-publicised operation on King Louis XIV (1638-1715) for an anal fistula.[43] The operation on the king was successful, although this is not surprising 'when it is appreciated that the surgeons involved had spent a year practising on less prestigious mortals with the same complaint'.[44] Almost forty years later, in 1724, King Louis XV, endowed Paris University with no less than five chairs of surgery, despite loud protestations from angry physicians who until then had held the monopoly in teaching theory of surgery – without ever having touched a scalpel. From this time on, surgeons who now filled these positions at University were authorized to teach both anatomy and surgery. The *Académie Royale de Chirugerie* was founded in 1731 – conferring international prestige on the Paris schools for anatomy and surgery.

In England the path to independence in surgery took a while longer. The Guild of Surgeons (founded in 1368) and the Guild of Barbers (founded in 1376) merged in 1540 [45] by an act of parliament, to form the Barber Surgeons Company.[46] Henceforth, surgeons were to carry out all surgical procedures, as well as treat all skin diseases, abscesses, wounds, tumours, and set bones. Barbers on the other hand were forthwith limited to bloodletting, tooth drawing, cauterisation, haircutting and shaving.[47] Several subsequent acts were passed laying the foundations for a medical system 'overrun with anomalies and riven with rivalries. It was a mess that got messier with every successive attempt to rationalise it'.[48]

The unrelenting endeavour to improve their social standing was a long uphill battle for surgeons in England. Until the early eighteenth century, they continued to play second fiddle to physicians, because surgery was still taught through apprenticeship and organised into guilds. But, in 1745 surgeons finally succeeded in severing their connection with barbers; the split finally indicating surgery as a craft in its own right. In 1800, the Company of Surgeons was granted royal licence to become the Royal College of Surgeons.

However, rivalries between physicians and surgeons continued – in fact, a remnant of such rivalries is covertly expressed to this day: in modern times it is still customary in England and select Commonwealth countries, not to address members of the Royal College of Surgeons as 'Doctor'. This dates back to when the College of Surgeons received its royal charter in 1800 and the subsequent insistence by the Royal College of Physicians that all surgical contenders should have a medical degree first and foremost. Therefore, aspiring surgeons initially studied medicine to receive the title 'Doctor', after which they would undergo training to obtain the Diploma of Fellowship from the Royal College of Surgeons. Thereafter, surgical fellows would revert back to the title 'Mr', 'Miss' or 'Mrs' as a snub to the Royal College of Physicians.

But what of the governing body regulating physicians in England? Soon after the succession of Henry VIII (1491-1547), an act was passed by the British parliament in 1511, with regard to the 'Science and Cunning of Physic and Surgery', which was reputedly being practiced by a 'multitude of ignorant persons, of whom the greater part have no insight in the same, nor in any other kind of learning'.[49] Weavers, smiths, cunning women and other untrained persons were causing grievous bodily harm to the 'King's people' with their varying attempts at cures.

The act passed in 1511 therefore ruled that anyone wanting to practice 'physic', or medicine, was to subject himself to assessment by bishops or other ecclesiastical authorities who could grant a license to practice medicine – at the time it was still widely held that the Church was in charge of the welfare of the soul as well as the physical body. Seven years after the passing of this act, the relatively small number of physicians in London petitioned to be incorporated as a college. However, before the founding of the College of Physicians of London in 1518, Henry VIII – ever defiant of the Church – issued a ruling stripping the Church of its power to regulate medicine. Forthwith, the new body known as the 'College of Physicians', would make all relevant medical decisions, issue licenses to those qualified and skilled sufficiently to practice 'physic', as well as punish malpractice and '…by inference have undefined authority over apothecaries'[50] – thereby provoking the ire and heated protest of this medical division, and unleashing rivalries, between apothecaries and physicians, which were to last for centuries.

After its initial establishment, the 'College of Physicians' did not fit too well into the contemporary London social setting. At the time, all forms of business and trade activities were regulated by guilds, which supervised the apprentice systems responsible for training new candidates for each trade. Bound to a particular 'master', traineeships typically lasted for many years until the obligatory standard of skill had been attained. Once training had been completed, candidates were considered 'free' to practice their craft autonomously.

In addition to the apprentice system, each guild was also involved in political and social goings-on, as well as status and attire of its members – each guild having its own colours and uniforms. Guilds fought fiercely amongst each other over matters of superiority. They continuously jockeyed for a preferred position on the official list of the twelve principal companies, from whose membership the Lord Mayor of London was chosen annually. The most powerful guild was the Company of Mercers or cloth merchants, followed by the Grocers, to which apothecaries belonged, the Drapers, the Fishmongers, the Goldsmiths and so on.[51]

As the College of Physicians had a very small membership – thirty-one by the end of the sixteenth century[52] – compared to the large Companies sporting thousands of members, it did not fit comfortably into this care-fully arranged system. But, in spite of a small membership, the College had huge influence, with many of its fellows personally attending the monarch. At the time the College was a mere 'gentlemen's club',[53] restricting membership to graduates from Oxford and Cambridge, as well as adherents of the Church of England, thereby weakening the originally intended formal regulation of the medical profession.

In manners and traditions, the College conformed to academic ways. In fact, the College of Physicians was then a very rare organisation – it was a professional body. But, unlike other major European cities, London housed neither a university nor a medical faculty. Hence, the College, in its early form, had no connection with teaching or training, despite the fact that it directed control of medical practice and set the standard for medications through the preparation and publication of the *London Pharmacopoeia* or *Pharmacopoeia Londinensis*, as it was known. When the first edition was published in 1618, a royal proclamation made its use compulsory for the whole of England and Wales.[54,55] Various fines imposed on those practicing without a licence, financed the College. Gradually, during the seventeenth century, the College of Physicians became known as the 'Royal College of Physicians of London'.

Critics saw the Royal College of Physicians as a conformist and protectionist body, which did not always grasp opportunities to lead the broader medical profession. In addition, the Royal College of Physicians was unable to restrict medical practices, as its jurisdiction did not stretch beyond London. Predictably, the large number of surgeons and apothecaries increasingly felt that they had the prerogative to treat the rapidly expanding population of London without restrictions from physicians.

Apothecaries or herbalists

Apothecaries are difficult to place in the medieval medical hierarchy, as their public role was difficult to distinguish from physicians at the time. Not only did apothecaries make up prescriptions or recipes, but they also prescribed drugs and treated the poor with herbs and various concoctions. However, they lacked knowledge and understanding of the human body, and any training they may have had was as herbalists. Until the mid-thirteenth century it was difficult to distinguish apothecaries from grocers – in fact, they formed part of the Company of Grocers. This was owing to the fact that apothecaries often doubled up as merchants of the rare, exotic powders and ingredients such as mummy and various cadaver parts, which they mixed into their medicines. Many of these were imported, costing prohibitive amounts, and by the fifteenth century apothecaries had a worse reputation amongst the common people than physicians.

People were often desperate for remedies, but there was no way of ascertaining what these contained, and there were many accusations and assertions of mouldy drugs and rotten, stale medications. The suspicion was always rife that a little sawdust, flour, powdered stone or dried grass, had been included in the medication to add volume – no one could prove otherwise. The distrust of dispensers of medicines is clearly stated in the following fifteenth century text: 'The apothecary's craft is the most full of deceit of all crafts in the world, for the apothecaries lack no deceit in weighing their spice, for either the balance is not right or else the beam is not equal or else they will hold the tongue of the balance still in the hollow with their finger when they are weighing. They care nothing for the wealth of their soul in order that they may be rich'.[56]

On the whole however, apothecaries provided a necessary and invaluable service. They eventually broke free from the Company of Grocers in 1617, receiving royal license by James I, and henceforth the Society of Apothecaries authoritatively regulated pharmacy in London. But, outside the capital, unorthodox practitioners and quacks flourished, as there were no regulations applicable to pharmacists and druggists [57] – or any other medical practitioners for that matter. Soon after receipt of their royal charter, members of the Society of Apothecaries began confronting the College of Physicians' for control in practising medicine.

One of the fiercest voices for medical reform was herbalist Nicholas Culpeper (1616-1654). He radically attacked the elitist attitude of medical practitioners, their greed and the exorbitant prices they charged, as opposed to the universal availability of nature's medicine. Culpeper attempted to make medical treatments more accessible to the poor by educating them about maintaining their health. His ambition was to reform the system of medicine by questioning traditional methods and knowledge, and exploring new solutions for ill health.

Culpeper especially angered the College of Physicians by translating the Latin *Pharmacopoeia Londinensis* into English in 1649. This outraged physicians countrywide as it threatened their monopoly. The exclusive use of Latin by physicians maintained their tight grip on the healing 'mysteries'. As all medical texts were written in Latin at the time, it rendered medical knowledge elitist, a 'closed book' to the uneducated. But Culpeper changed this *status quo* by demystifying medicine for ordinary people. In 1653, his groundbreaking publication the *English Physician* – still in print and known as *Culpeper's Herbal* in modern times – became one of the most popular and enduring books in British history. The book was sold at an affordable price and incorporated instructions on how to use the various cures contained therein. Culpeper recommended generally familiar herbs, which could be picked by the general populace and used to treat various ailments at home. Half a century later, apothecaries were officially granted the right to practice medicine.

Non-professional practitioners

Last, but not least in the medieval medical hierarchy, were unlicensed, non-professional practitioners. Scant proof of their sphere of work survives. They charged the lowest rates and probably did a bit of everything. As women were barred from practicing formal medicine,[58] they were forced into this non-professional category, functioning as so-called 'cunning' women and midwives. In the eighteenth century 'cunning women' were still very much a part of rural villages in England, and were consulted to treat various illnesses and diseases '…promising with remarkable assurance that they could heal a variety of ailments using a combination of magical rituals and semi-religious invocations or spells'.[59] Procedures included burning or burying animals alive, or dragging them through bushes, thereby seemingly transferring the disease; or immersing patients in water flowing in a particular direction, or touching them with a magical charms.

In the mid-eighteenth century Britain still had no uniform system of medical education and no regional system of medical licensing [60] – basically, anyone, qualified, or not, could practice as a physician or any other type of medical practitioner outside of London. Almost a century later, formal regulation of medical practice began with the establishment of the British Medical Association in 1832. Thereafter, with the founding of the General Medical Council in 1858, a system of professional regulation and a standard for qualified and unqualified doctors was officially set.

II

HUMORAL BODIES –
A HEALTHY BALANCE

From Greco-Roman antiquity onwards, supernatural explanations in medicine were steadily replaced by theories addressing a natural basis for disease and treatment. In other words, medicine and religion were becoming detached. Hippocratic medicine emphasised the connection between healthy human bodies and harmony in nature – the relationship between microcosm and macrocosm. Medicine was placed on a structured and rational footing, and physicians increasingly viewed the physical body as integral to law-governed elements.[1]

Humoral theory – a fourfold pattern

Out of such perceptions grew humoral theory and its widespread and lasting impact dominated medicine and its understanding of the human body, for millennia. This probably occurred because there were few diseases and symptoms for which humoral theory could not provide some sort of easy rationalisation. But it put a brake on medical investigation and progress. Although practically worthless, the theory of humors was 'believed and acted upon by the medical profession and others for nearly two thousand years without being recognised as mumbo-jumbo and arrant nonsense'.[2]

'The theory of the four humors arose out of Hellenic philosophy in an attempt to relate all things to universal laws'.[3] Humoral theory was based on the perception that all matter in the universe – including the human body – comprised of the four elements of fire, air, water and earth. The notion of four basic elements[4] to connect the material world was first proposed by the Greek pre-Socratic philosopher Empedocles (c. 490–430 BCE). This fourfold pattern was of course greatly adaptable to much of humankind's environs: to the seasons, the winds, the elements, as well as the directions in the heavens. Closely connected to this system of belief was the idea, generally attributed to Hippocrates, that the human body contained the four essential elements in the form of humors. It was a notion offering a collective rationalisation, in which human personality, disposition, as well as all diseases, could find justification – all illnesses and diseases could be ascribed to an imbalance of the four humors.

During a time when the ancient Greeks were preoccupied with fluid mechanics and hydraulics – waterwheels, valves, chambers and pistons – this preoccupation also affected Greek medicine and pathology.[5] 'To explain illness, Hippocrates fashioned an elaborate doctrine based on fluids and volumes' – four cardinal fluids, 'each with a unique colour, viscosity and essential character'.[6] Hippocrates had observed that blood, once removed from the body, separated into four parts: a black substance that settled at the bottom; a deep red liquid; a red liquid speckled with some white material; and a yellowish liquid on top. Ancient physicians categorised these different liquids as the four principle body fluids; black bile, blood, phlegm[7] and yellow bile.[8] This makes more sense when it is recognised that the word humor is derived from the Latin term *umorem*, meaning 'fluid'.

Subsequently, the four humors were grouped with the four elements according to their perceived shared qualities: black bile was perceived as cold and dry, therefore corresponding to earth; blood was hot and moist, corresponding to air; phlegm was cold and moist, corresponding to water; and yellow bile was hot and dry, corresponding to fire.

Galen followed Hippocrates in his theory of the four humors, but then expounded on the concept to include the various temperaments and specific complexions of people. In addition, each humor was also linked to the organ of its formation, as well as a specific season. For example, black bile was linked to the spleen, to autumn, and to a melancholic state of mind. This resulted in sadness, depression and worry, as well as guile and cowardice. In appearance, melancholics were thought to be dark in skin and hair tone. Such complex categorisations applied to all four humors.[9] In modern times a remnant of humoral theory remains when we use the terms 'melancholy', 'sanguine', 'phlegmatic' and 'choleric', to describe various temperaments, and still refer to a person being of 'good or ill humor'.

To further complicate matters, it was believed that the various humors ebbed and flowed in conjunction with the four seasons. Each humor was thought to predominate in a particular season.[10] For instance, it was thought that during the icy winter months an over-abundance of phlegm predominated, hence causing lung problems and the coughing up of this fluid. This constituted a fitting explanation for the observation of increased colds during the icy northern winters. In spring, when the blood-part of body humors was thought to predominate, especially among young energetic people, safety measures against excess in the 'blood' humor would be taken, 'either by eliminating blood-rich foods like red meat, or by blood-letting, to purge excess'.[11]

In addition, astrology was tied in with the system of humors. In the same way that the signs of the zodiac were coupled with certain elements, so they were linked to the four humors and to all the various body parts and organs. For example, a person born under the sign of Gemini was thought prone to lung problems. This was attributed to the association of Gemini with water; water in turn was linked to phlegm, which was connected to the lungs. Therefore, as mentioned in the previous chapter, in order to effectively treat patients, every medieval physician had to be able to cast a patient's horoscope and was generally well versed in astrology.

The theory of humors also applied to the sexes. During the seventeenth century, the fundamental physical difference between men and women, as defined by physicians, was still thought to lie in their humoral natures. The elements of water and phlegm – cold and moist qualities – were held to be far more dominant in women than in men. Generally, medical texts stressed the belief that women were weaker and wetter versions of men, and therefore more disposed to specific illnesses. Therefore the sex of the patient was of utmost importance when diagnosing various ailments. On the other hand, the discharging of excess blood during menstruation was also thought to spare women various diseases.

Considering that physicians had to weigh up these numerous, different, and varying factors regarding humoral theory in order to make a diagnosis, the sheer complexity of facts must have been challenging to say the least.

'Cooking' – the origin of humors

But how did the humors originate in humans? Galen distinguished three 'faculties' in the body, namely the nutritive faculty of the liver; the vital faculty of the heart; and the logical faculty of the brain. The most outstanding figure of speech used in Galenic medicine was 'cooking', or Greek *pepsis*. It was theorised that whatever the body ingested was changed to different fluids through diverse stages of 'cooking', while each of the three vital organs also permeated the fluids with a specific 'spirit', or Greek *pneuma*.[12]

During the digestive process, food was broken down in the stomach into the semi-refined form of blood called chyle.[13] This was then passed through the portal vein to the liver where it was 'cooked' – in other words, the liver produced blood from chyle. Yellow bile and black bile were seen as by-products of the process by which the liver converted chyle into blood.[14] During this process 'natural spirit' was added to produce the four humors. From the liver, 'venous blood' – Galenic physicians were not familiar with the circulatory system – went to certain parts of the body to nourish them.

But some 'venous blood' travelled by way of the vena cava to the heart to undergo a further stage of 'cooking', whereby 'vital spirit' was added. The blood then became lighter and thinner, and was called 'arterial blood'. This blood could be measured through the pulse, and would travel to various parts of the body producing sensation and warmth by seeping rather than circulating or pulsing through the body. Similarly, blood was thought to pass between the heart's 'three' ventricles – the belief in the three-ventricled human heart was a legacy of Galen's animal dissection – through invisible pores in the septum. The heart's pumping was believed to cause an ebb and flow in the blood vessels and nerves – Galen perceived nerves as hollow tubes originating in the liver. At the base of the brain, vital blood was further transformed through the addition of 'animal spirit' or 'soul'. This blood, carried through the 'hollow' nerves enabled sensation and movement.[15]

Originating in the liver, humors were processed four times over; once for each humor, and each stage of the 'cooking' process produced waste products or by-products – so-called 'superfluities'. These superfluities, if not excreted, were thought to build up in the body and produce 'corrupt' or 'evil'[16] humors, thus making the body more susceptible to disease and illness.[17] Therefore, especially in times of plagues, physicians advised all foods which were deemed difficult to digest, and hence prone to producing 'superfluities', to be avoided. These theories held sway for many centuries, continuing the strong emphasis on purges and emetics in order to rapidly expel 'superfluities'.

Humoral balance equals health

The fundamental concept in humoral theory was that health equated balance. Humors nourished the body and were held to provide the material for sperm and for the fetus during pregnancy. An unhealthy body signified imbalance, which could be identified through a specific change on the exterior of the body. This change could be in complexion, temperament, pulse, or temperature, or regarding an excreted fluid such as urine. 'Thus a flow (defluxion) of humors to the feet would produce gout, or catarrh (defluxion of phlegm from the head to the lungs) would be the cause of coughing'.[18] The physician's task in the treatment of all diseases therefore involved the rebalancing of humors.

To establish the degree of humoral imbalance and health of the liver, which was after all the generator of humors, physicians followed Galen's emphasis on examination of the pulse – Galen had theorised and written extensively on pulse phenomena – and on urinalysis. Urine, examined with the naked eye, was evaluated with reference to quality, quantity, concentration, smell, transparency, and the occurrence of sediment, foam or blood.

Once a physician had established, which humor was at fault, it could then be rebalanced either through diet, or by eliminating the perceived surplus humor. Elimination was achieved through purging, bloodletting, laxative medications and emetics, and through bodily wastes such as urine, faeces, pus and sweat.

Humoral balance achieved through diet, would generally use a treatment of opposites. For example, if an overabundance of cold and moist phlegm was diagnosed, the patient would be assigned remedies associated with hot and dry foods, herbs and potions. Pepper, mustard, or spicy herbs would 'heat' up the body from the inside and have a drying effect. In addition, bleeding the patient was invariably recommended.

Another method of balancing the humors was to cause a persistent inflammatory reaction, giving rise to so-called 'laudable pus'. Pus was erroneously thought to be a good sign of healing – a premise stemming from Hippocrates' theory on the treatment of wounds, which remained influential for centuries. He theorised that pus was derived from polluted blood. Hence, the phrase 'laudable pus', as the festering of wounds was essential for healing to take place, 'conveying poisoned blood out of the body'.[19] This was still regarded as paramount to wound healing in the eighteenth century. To produce as much pus as possible in order to drain fluids from the body in a persistent, controlled method, harsh blistering agents would be applied.[20]

Alternately, physicians would use cautery by applying a red-hot instrument to the skin, to produce blisters, which then released fluids. Once a blister had become visible, it could be maintained for as long as was considered necessary, by constant irritation. Especially in cases of asthma or paralysis, blistering was very popular.

As stated at the beginning of this chapter, humoral theory held sway amongst physicians and medical scholars for almost two millennia. However, cracks began to appear in humoral theory in 1543 with the publication of Andreas Vesalius' (1514-1564) *De Humani Corporis Fabrica*. Apart from physical anomalies, varying with conventional long held views regarding the human body, no matter how diligently anatomist Vesalius looked, he could not find Galen's black bile, one of the four mainstays of humoral theory. 'The lymphatic system carried a pale, watery fluid; the blood vessels were filled, as expected, with blood. Yellow bile was in the liver. But black bile – Galen's oozing carrier of cancer and depression – could not be found anywhere'.[21] Thinking he was at fault and not Galen, Vesalius at first prevaricated about his discovery, heaping 'even more praise on the long-dead Galen. However, an empiricist to the core, Vesalius left his drawings just as he saw them, leaving others to draw their own conclusions. There was no black bile'.[22] Further doubts regarding Galenic concepts continued to emerge over the coming centuries. It was time to throw off the 'deadweight' of the past, the unquestioning homage to antiquity.

But, it was not until the late nineteenth century with the concrete establishment of the germ theory of disease by French microbiologist Louis Pasteur (1822-1895) and German physician Robert Koch (1843-1910) that the role of microscopic pathogens in causing disease was fully understood. Similarly, the growing fields of psychology and psychiatry during that century progressively replaced the notion of complexion or temperament being a part of humoral medicine. As a result, humoral medicine declined. However, certain aspects of Galenic humoral theory endured in medical practice until well into the nineteenth century, often with unfortunate results...

III

PHLEBOTOMY, PURGES AND OTHER MEDICAL MARVELS

Therapeutic bleeding – a medical mainstay

For millennia, humankind's diverse beliefs about blood[1] have allegorically 'flowed' through the veins of history. From remote antiquity, physicians used phlebotomy, or bloodletting, as a standard therapeutic procedure. Then, during classical times, this procedure attained definition to conform to the humoral doctrine of disease at the hands of Hippocrates and his interpreter Galen. Although blood has always been associated with the life force, it was also observed as being naturally expelled from the body through bodily functions such as menstruation or nosebleeds. This type of 'natural evacuation suggested the practice of blood-letting, [...] serving for centuries as a therapeutic mainstay'.[2]

Galen was convinced that nature prevented disease by discharging excess blood – after all, did not menstruation spare women from many diseases?[3] Therefore, humoral balance of the body had to be maintained throughout. Because blood was perceived as containing all four humors, remedial bleeding was deemed to restore such balance. Therapeutic bleeding or phlebotomy[4] was performed via the lancet – a procedure known as venesection – or the gentler forms of blood letting, via leeches or cupping.

Galen recommended and performed phlebotomy for practically every illness. Surprisingly, even in cases of haemorrhages from blood vessels, wounds, and other forms of blood loss, bleeding was still deemed necessary and proper[5] – as long as careful consideration was given to where and when the blood was let, and how much of it was drained. For serious medical conditions, Galen advised phlebotomy twice a day. The first bleeding was to be stopped before the patient fainted,[6] but the second time a physician could bleed 'as far as loss of consciousness'.[7]

Galen encouraged physicians to persevere with this practice by stressing: 'I have seen some of them from the chilling that invariably accompanies fainting, sweat from the whole body and passing faeces, after which they quickly recover from their disease [...] however, pay attention to the diminution of the pulse, feeling it while the blood is still flowing [...] so that you will never cause your patient death instead of loss of consciousness'.[8] In other words, physicians would knowingly endeavour to bleed a patient to the point of syncope or temporary loss of consciousness – a tricky procedure that could ultimately lead to shock and death.

In addition, there was the danger of infection and the even greater hazard of accidentally cutting a nerve or an artery instead of a vein, leading to unstoppable bleeding. Almost certainly, through the centuries '...bloodletting based on a totally erroneous idea, must have weakened or killed, directly or indirectly, many thousands of people, all with the best intentions'.[9]

Because the practice was regarded as a surgical procedure, beneath the dignity of university-trained physicians, in the course of time it came to be performed almost entirely by barber-surgeons, even though physicians prescribed it. One or even two veins would be manually perforated and occasionally further shallow cuts would be made, to cause additional blood flow. Even the very young were subjected to phlebotomy – cupping, leeching, and venesection. However, as an early nineteenth century account emphasized, children had to be 'watched' carefully during the procedure for signs of 'exhaustion'.[10]

It was not sufficient for a patient to simply be bled – bleeding had to occur from the appropriate vessel. As each organ was associated with a particular vein, a specific 'corrupt' humor could be 'drained' from the organ by tapping into the perceived connecting vein. For example, a choleric individual, having too much yellow bile, needed draining from the vein that 'led' to the gall bladder.[11] However, which specific veins supplied which organs, in support of this theory, had not been clearly established. Anatomy, until the sixteenth century, was based strictly on Galen's teachings. Galen never dissected humans – this was prohibited during his time and only Barbary apes, goats and pigs were dissected, the assumption being that animals were anatomically identical to humans. In addition, the circulatory system was unknown up until the first half of the seventeenth century.

As mentioned in the previous chapter, physicians were well versed in astrology. The right time and appropriate body site for bloodletting was determined through use of the zodiac and birth charts. These were medieval charts that indicated the planetary influences over the various organs of the body and the different ailments that could overwhelm them. For example, diseases of the neck and throat were controlled, and also cured, by the constellation of Taurus; Scorpio controlled and cured the genitals; Capricorn the knees; Pisces the feet... and so on.[12] Any curative proposals by physicians therefore included astrological projections.

Bleeding by derivation and revulsion

In order to be successful, phlebotomy had to be performed in two specific ways: first, by derivation, which referred to phlebotomy close to the affected area. Second, by revulsion, which meant that blood was drawn at the furthest point from the affected area. If a patient was to be bled prophylactically – in other words to prevent disease – then bleeding was to be carried out as far from the disease site as possible, to divert corrupt humors from it. But, if the patient was being bled therapeutically to cure an existing disease or illness, then the bleeding had to be performed from the nearest blood vessels to the site.

In 1514 a dispute arose in Paris among physicians regarding this very question. Namely, whether one should incise a vein on the affected side of the body or on the opposite side. In view of the universal application of remedial phlebotomy this controversy became ruthless and widespread amongst various learned physicians. In the 'whole history of medicine there is no more extensive and polemical a literature than that which revolved around this question'.[13] The underlying reason for the dispute was that the Hippocratic practice of phlebotomy had become corrupted during medieval times under the influence of Arabic medicine. However, it was not until the Renaissance at the beginning of the sixteenth century with the recovery of classical learning, that it became apparent just how far traditional methods of phlebotomy had diverged from the original teachings of Hippocrates.

In the same year, a well-documented dispute in France represented the Hippocratic and Arabic views on phlebotomy.[14] The true Hippocratic and Galenical technique [15] of bloodletting required phlebotomy close to the site of the ailment and the removal of a 'sensible' quantity of blood – enough to make the patient pass out. The Arabic phlebotomy procedure on the other hand, was to bleed the patient from a point as far away from the region of the ailment as possible. In addition, only a token amount of blood was to be removed. Renowned anatomist Vesalius' contribution to the argument, published in his *Venesection Letter* in 1539, was highly significant because he introduced into the thus far unproductive controversy an entirely new element – the findings of direct observation. Eventually this led to the discovery of the venous valves, which later provided William Harvey (1578-1657) with the key to unlock the secret of the circulatory system.

Famous 'bleedings'

Various famous 'bleedings' have been recorded for posterity. In his book *The Last Days of Charles II*, Raymond Crawfurd gives a detailed account of best practice medical ministrations of the times to the dying king. One morning, when Charles II (1630–1685) suffered severe convulsions while being shaved – his mouth foaming, and eyes rolling back – his personal physician, Edmund King (1629-1709), bled the monarch without delay, extracting a pint[16] of blood from a vein in his right arm 'with immediate good effect'.[17] Urgent messages were at once dispatched to the king's numerous personal physicians, summoning them to the king's bedside.

Soon twelve medical specialists arrived at his bedside. After hurried consultation, another eight ounces[18] of royal blood were drawn by scarification of the shoulders and subsequent cupping. Then a strong 'antimonial' emetic was administered, as well as a full dose of 'sulphate of zinc'[19] to make sure that vomiting would be speedily induced. In addition, strong purgatives and several enemas were given. The king's hair was then shorn, pungent blistering agents were applied to the scalp, and he was seared with red-hot irons – to further 'draw' out putrid humors. The bleeding, purging, as well as numerous other 'aggressive' treatments continued for several days, until the fifty-four year old king drew his last breath.

Doubtless, bloodletting often went too far. Although not numerous, various records of unfortunate outcomes resulting from excessive phlebotomy on distinguished personages have been documented. Detailed accounts and payments attest to Mary Stuart, Queen of Scots (1542-1587) being subjected to therapeutic bloodletting on many occasions. On one occasion however, the ineptitude of a physician probably saved the Queen from the fate of mortal blood loss. Clear signs that the Queen had a recurring stomach ulcer emerged at Perth, in Scotland in 1561. But, this was no simple stomach ulcer. Mary had vomited blood on several occasions to the point where she was in a state of shock from loss of blood. Fortunately on this occasion, in 1661, 'the only doctor available, a certain Arnault, was not familiar with the age's fashion of bloodletting. If he had been it would have probably resulted in therapeutic murder'.[20]

A specific example of such therapeutic murder is the well-known case of Italian king, Victor Emmanuel II (1820-1878). As was customary at the time, doctors bled him for five days in order to treat his pneumonia, in addition to attaching to him numerous bloodthirsty leeches.[21] Unfortunately the king died of 'complications', which may very well have resulted from extreme blood loss. This is possibly what French playwright Jean-Baptiste Molière (1622-1673) was referring to two hundred years earlier, when he stated that 'One should never say a person died of pneumonia. What ought to be said is that he died of four doctors and two druggists'.[22]

When the first president of the United States of America, George Washington (1732-1799), was suffering from acute laryngitis, his condition was initially treated with a medicinal mixture of molasses, vinegar, and butter,[23] as well as vinegar gargles. In addition, blister of cantharides, made from a preparation of dried beetles,[24] was placed against his throat. His three attending physicians administered several doses of Calomel – a mercury compound – and repeated 'vapours of vinegar'. Vomiting agents and laxatives were also recurrently administered.

In addition, the president was heavily bled several times. He was himself an ardent advocate of phlebotomy, 'having used it successfully to cure various maladies affecting his Negro slaves'.[25] Modern historians and medical authorities estimate the total amount of blood removed from the president 'amounted to 3.75 litres, drawn over a period of nine to ten hours', which, considering his stature and weight would have amounted to more than half of his blood volume being extracted in a short period of time.[26] The president's exterior calm before his death inevitably would have been due to 'profound hypotension and shock',[27] induced by an excessive loss of blood.

Phlebotomy remains the cure-all

Half a century later, these measures were still regarded as most powerful and effective. Although cracks had already appeared in Galenic medicine during the sixteenth and seventeenth centuries, phlebotomy and purging were still widely advocated medical measures used by physicians during the mid-nineteenth century in Europe and America. Bloodletting was especially recommended for bone disease, pneumonia, kidney disease, all inflammatory disorders, as well as 'irritation of the brain, the chest and abdomen'.[28]

In 1830 American physician Marshall Hall (1790-1857) wrote the widely acclaimed book on *The Morbid and Curative Effects of the Loss of Blood*. He advocated that bloodletting until the 'appearance of syncope'[29] or collapse, was almost always called for and that 'scarcely a case of acute or indeed of chronic disease occurs, in which it does not become necessary to consider the propriety of having recourse to the lancet'.[30] Medical opinion at the time espoused the notion that 'the diseases which most require the use of the lancet, are precisely those which best bear the loss of blood'.[31] Hall stated categorically that 'as long as bloodletting is required, it can be borne; and as long as it can be borne, it is required'.[32] In addition, he emphasised that the earlier the use of the lancet was applied in the development of an illness, the better the outcome, especially in the case of fevers or inflammations. Similarly, in pleuritis and pneumonia 'one early bloodletting to syncope'[33] was thought to subdue the disease entirely. In addition to phlebotomy, Hall also advised the application of leeches – in some cases thirty to fifty at a time – followed by blistering.[34]

In the 1850's, notes on procedures at the New York General Hospital included treating post-surgical infections by opening large orifices in each arm of the patient and cutting 'both temporal arteries' to let blood flow freely from these, 'all at the same time' in order to bleed the patient until convulsions ceased.[35] Another set of doctor's notes, prescribing a remedy for lung cancer, stated that 'small bleedings give temporary relief, although, of course, they cannot often be repeated'.[36]

Leeching and cupping

As previously mentioned, gentler forms of bloodletting using leeches or cupping, were also used on patients. Leeching[37] was already an established bloodletting practice in ancient times.[38] In English the term 'leech' derives from the Anglo-Saxon word *laece*, meaning to heal, and *leech* was the collective old English word for 'medical practitioners' – those who practiced all forms of healing.[39]

Often physicians would recommend leeching or cupping to be applied concurrently with venesection. Barber-surgeons, who supplied the leeches – attaching between twenty and fifty of the bloodsuckers at a time – performed all these procedures. Leeching, although repulsive, required little skill. However, treatments were not without problems. Firstly, leeches would not always bite and tended to crawl out of reach. Secondly, their bites would leave tiny wounds, which continued to bleed and ooze for days. In spite of this, they were popularly used and the slimy, cold, little suckers could be used for various complaints, in places, which were inaccessible to phlebotomy or cupping. For instance, inside the mouth, the nose, ears, anus or vagina – one can only shudder with revulsion.

In therapeutic cupping, a cup especially made for this procedure was heated by burning something inside it. Then the scorching cup was immediately placed over those body parts deemed to necessitate bloodletting – body parts which had been incised or greased beforehand. Suction from the hot cup would cause it to fill with blood. Alternately, if the skin had not been cut, the suction would produce a blood blister instead. Generally, cups were applied for ten to fifteen minutes at a time. This was thought to draw corrupt humors to the surface, away from those organs perceived to be affected by illness.

Purges and emetics to restore well-being.

Although bloodletting was the prevailing form of medical treatment, cleansing the bowels was deemed equally important and both treatments were often implemented concurrently. The first medieval illustrations of enema equipment consist of a tube attached to a pump action bulb made of a dried pig's bladder. After the seventeenth century, enema apparatus' were mainly designed for self-administration.

During the Middle Ages and centuries later, the enema jug formed an important part of every household – daily enemas were still considered essential. Because constipation was regarded as a disease rather than a symptom, purgatives or cathartics were regularly prescribed – even to treat diarrhoea. This was thought to help remove noxious humors. King Louis XIV of France is rumoured to have had at least two hundred enemas and as many purges during the last year of his life,[40] which explains the more than two hundred and sixty four *chaises nécessaires* or 'conveniences' at Versailles at the time. Naturally, when the monarch set the 'enema' example, who were the courtiers, and everyone else for that matter, not to follow suit?

Apart from bleeding, powerful laxatives, and enemas, to purge the bowels, emetics to induce vomiting were equally important. In this regard, there was one particularly popular substance that 'did the job' so to speak. One of the most widely prescribed, highly effective laxatives and diuretics used by physicians was a mercury compound, known as Calomel. This white, powdery compound of mercury and chlorine, also known as mercurous chloride, prescribed to be taken internally, was however highly toxic. Nevertheless, Calomel was widely used for centuries. Another highly poisonous substance, a violent irritant to stomach and bowels, was white Hellabore – extracted from the flower of the same name. Hellabore was commonly prescribed as an emetic and a purge, resulting in severe vomiting and diarrhoea – such purging thought to restore general wellbeing.

The 'king of purges', may well have been British pseudo-physician James Morison (1770–1840), who suffered from various ailments – real or imagined – for many years. Eventually, he decided to take matters into his own hands by developing a concoction, which he named 'Vegetable Universal Compound' – a very powerful laxative made from various herbs. Firmly believing that all diseases were caused by impurities in the blood, the compound's laxative effect was thought to 'purify' the blood. After some time, the compound became so popular that he fashioned it into pills, which became widely known as 'Morison's Pills'.

In 1828 he set up the 'British College of Health' in King's Cross London, where he trained other practitioners in the art of purging. After a series of fatalities, which were attributed to overuse of his pills – some people took as many as 50 at a time – Morison left England to escape numerous court cases in 1834 and moved to Paris. However, nothing impeded the popularity of the 'Vegetable Universal Compound', and not surprisingly, he left a considerable fortune to his decedents.[41]

One may question why the therapeutic practices of purging and bloodletting persisted for so long, especially when certain aspects of Galenic medicine were already queried during the sixteenth and seventeenth centuries, with the uncovering by Vesalius, of significant errors in anatomy and physiology. Although Spanish physician and theologian Michael Servetus (c. 1509-1553) had already correctly described pulmonary circulation in 1533 – he was burnt at the stake for heresy twenty years later – it was William Harvey who discovered the blood circulation in 1616. When he made public his findings in

1618, his announcement raised major questions regarding therapeutic and prophylactic bloodletting. Up until then, phlebotomy had been based on the assumption that blood seeped rather than circulated or pulsed through the body. In addition, it was fundamental to Galen's physiology that the veins in the human body originated in the liver – Harvey's dissections clearly refuted this. But, he was distinctly hesitant in revealing his findings.

According to Harvey, this part of Galenic medicine – the circulatory system – was an 'error held now for two thousand years'; he went on apologetically 'because it is so ancient and accepted by such great men',[42] how could he possibly refute it. Apart from committing what could be termed 'medical heresy' the public announcement of his controversial findings was also dangerous. The year 1618 was just three years after the Catholic Inquisition had formally declared Nicolaus Copernicus (1473-1543) a heretic and eighteen years after Giordano Bruno (1548-1600) had been burnt at the stake for 'suggesting, among other speculations that the blood must go round the body as the planets go round the sun'.[43] However, in spite of Harvey's discovery, the practice of phlebotomy continued for more than two hundred years – perhaps, as one researcher put it, because the continued practice 'resulted from the dynamic interaction of social, economic, and intellectual pressures'[44] in medical circles.

However, due to new treatments and technologies the old traditions were being increasingly questioned by prominent physicians in various European countries from the mid-nineteenth century onwards. At the Edinburgh School of Medicine, John Hughes Bennett (1812–1875) promoted new methods of pathology and physiology, supported by the microscope and the stethoscope. Through observation of the improved outcome in pneumonia patients, who had not been subjected to bloodletting, Bennett subsequently derided this practice as a dangerous therapy. He based his rejection of bloodletting on scientific verification, 'on pathologic concepts of inflammation and pneumonia derived from microscopic studies of inflamed tissues'.[45]

Similar studies on the efficacy of bloodletting, were conducted in Paris by physician Pierre Louis (1787–1872). Although his conclusions did not condemn bloodletting, he believed that its efficacy had been enduringly overvalued.[46] In addition, as mentioned in the previous chapter, studies by Pasteur, Koch and many others underlined the validity of the new scientific approach. In modern times, bloodletting remains conventional therapy for a very small number of conditions.

The following chapters offer a glimpse into the history of anatomy and dissection, a history that was at times filled with great social tragedy.

IV

OPENING UP THE DEAD –
A DISMEMBERED HISTORY

The history of dissection[1] follows an erratic path leading back to the ancient Greeks. Although Aristotle (384-322 BCE) had dissected animals in his time, human dissection was considered *taboo* – beyond all culturally accepted limits – in ancient Greece and amongst the Romans. However, during the early third century BCE, two Greek physicians, Erasistratus (c. 304-250 BCE) and Herophilus (335-280 BCE), despite breaching deeply entrenched beliefs and cultural mores at the time, conducted the first methodical explorations of the human body.

Although it could be said that the ancient Egyptians were quite familiar in 'finding their way' through the human body during the elaborate mummification processes of their dead – not only did they slice corpses open, but they also dissected out specific organs, which were separately preserved – the differences between religious mummification and systematic dissection are extensive. For example, while Egyptian embalmers, scraped and drained out the brain little by little through the nostrils of a corpse, Herophilus 'dissected the brain and the head meticulously enough to distinguish the ventricles of the brain to discover and describe seven pairs of cranial nerves'.[2] In addition he noted several other specific cranial features, and distinguished the cornea, iris, retina, and choroid coat of the eye. These are astonishing discoveries and a far cry from what was learnt through ancient embalming methods.

When considering the sacred laws of the ancient Greeks with regard to the human corpse,[3] as well as firmly held beliefs in connection with human skin[4] at the time, it is amazing that these two Greek physicians had the courage and temerity to violate established principles and carry out their empirical enquiry into the human body. After the death of Erasistratus and Herophilus, human dissection, which had so advanced the internal study of the human body, abruptly ceased. This period, during the early third century BCE, was 'not only the first but also the last time, in the roughly thousand years of ancient Greek science, that human cadavers were systematically dissected. It was not until the fourteenth century that systematic human dissection was resumed'. [5]

By the fourteenth century, Europe had six leading medical schools, located in Bologna, Salerno, Padua, Montpellier, Paris and Oxford. It was in Bologna at the beginning of this century that the serious study of anatomy through dissection is believed to have originated. Bologna medical school was distinctive in that it stressed above all the importance of surgery – a subject not even on the *curriculum* of other medical schools at the time.[6]

Mos Teutonicus – dismemberment of the corpse

Before discussing the study of human anatomy through dissection however, it should perhaps be mentioned that 'interference' with human corpses was a well-known practice during medieval times. This stemmed from the desire to bring dead Crusaders[7] back from the Holy Land for burial. It was not deemed desirable for kings and nobles, killed in battle or dying of natural causes, to be buried in Muslim territory. Another reason for burial on 'home soil' was that kings and nobles always maintained close ties to the religious orders, churches or abbeys that they had lavishly supported during their lifetime. Consequently it was considered of utmost importance that they be buried in these hallowed places, where the devout could pray for the salvation of their souls.

For those dying on foreign soil – and this included death in various European countries – transportation of their corpses, often over long distances, back to their European homeland, were prohibitive due to putrefaction, accelerated by warmer climates. Hence the custom of *mos Teutonicus* – literally meaning 'the German custom', as especially German aristocrats wanted to be buried in 'home soil' – was devised. This funerary process involved the removal of all flesh from the corpse. After dismemberment – often the heart was separately removed and kept airtight – the body parts were boiled for many hours, thereby separating the flesh from the bones and eventually leaving a completely clean skeleton. In this way the bones and the heart of the deceased could be easily transported from distant lands back to the homeland for proper burial. The boiled flesh and entrails would either be buried in foreign soil or dried and preserved in salt for transportation.

Although the Church generally accepted this practice, Pope Boniface VIII (1230-1303) in particular expressed his revulsion of the 'savage'[8] *mos Teutonicus*. His bull *De Sepulturis*, issued in 1299, expressly forbade the practice[9] – a ban that in fact proved ineffective, as the custom continued.[10] Unfortunately though, the Bull led to the widely held misinterpretation of prohibiting human dissection, thereby perhaps at times impeding investigation by anatomists fearing reprisals. In truth however, no general prohibition on dissection or autopsy of the human body applied in Christian Europe.

The beginnings of public dissection

The first recorded public dissection, performed by surgeon Mondino de' Luzzi, renowned author of the *Anatomia mundini*, took place in Bologna around 1315. Numerous illustrations of anatomy classes give us an idea of dissection proceedings during the fourteenth century: the cadaver, stretched out on a table, surrounded by enquiring, jostling students; the physician, magnificently attired in academic robes, standing high on a lectern, or seated on a raised dais above the proceedings, intoning the ancient knowledge of Galen or Avicenna from a book; the surgeon, knife in hand, providing the 'hands-on-illustration' to the reading, while a teaching assistant points out noteworthy characteristics. We do not know whether the illustrations of dissection scenes found in anatomical texts depict what 'really' happened within the anatomy theatre. However, it is certain that the whole demonstration was not 'used as a vehicle for novel observation',[11] but rather to confirm or underline what was being read from the old texts.

Because of the complexity of Galen's and other old texts, simplified anatomy guides were needed. Therefore, Mondino de' Luzzi's concise and practical *Anatomia mundini*, was exactly what was required, and became the standard dissectors' manual of the time. However, Galenic influence was still so entrenched that the *Anatomia mundini,* in spite of physical findings to the contrary, perpetuated ancient notions originally derived from animal dissection.

Galen, who may be counted among the first ancient anatomists, had firmly advocated that practical observation was central to the study of medicine. But, always mindful of avoiding contemporary taboos on human dissection, he had, almost on a daily basis, performed his dissections on Barbary apes, pigs and other animals. In this way, Galen achieved great milestones in the understanding of the nervous system, the mechanics of breathing, the heart and other organs. Unfortunately though, he analogised too closely between animal and human anatomy, which led to numerous serious misconceptions perpetuated for more than a thousand years: his anatomy of the womb was that of a dog, the positioning of the kidneys was based on the pig, and his understanding of the brain founded on cows.[12] Similarly, the ancient concept of the five-lobed liver and the three-ventricled heart persisted in medical circles for centuries, demonstrating how difficult it can be to shake off ideas and observations from the past. Hence, at the beginning of the fourteenth century anatomy was pure ancient knowledge – it had to wait for many, many decades before it became applied.

From Bologna, the practice of human dissection spread to other Italian medical schools and to the main universities of Europe,[13] during the fifteenth century. However, towards the end of that century, dissection for educational purposes took on a new purpose, thereby changing the process from a lecture entirely dedicated to training future medical practitioners, into an extravagant spectacle attracting a broad audience. In Italy and other European countries, these public anatomy lessons developed into ritualised ceremonies held in elaborate anatomy theatres specifically built to house these events.

The 'grand function'

The first such elaborate anatomy theatre was built, in 1563, at the University of Bologna, or the 'Studium' as the University was first known.[14] The anatomy theatre, the *Palazzo dell' Archiginnasio*, of Bologna University was a 'sumptuous and lordly anatomy theatre, one of the most renowned constructions in Italy',[15] and a source of constant amazement to visiting foreigners – the Bologna theatre could hold several hundred people. It was in this building, which still stands today [16] that the 'grand function' of public anatomy was held up until 1800, during carnival time.

Carnival time, traditionally celebrated in February, was the season best suited for dissection, not only to slow the putrefaction of cadavers during the cold month of Febuary, but also to enable the carnival maskers and revellers to participate as audience members. Similar to Bologna, public anatomy lessons at Pisa and other Italian universities were held during the carnival.[17]

Anatomy was definitely not a summer activity, and always took place in winter, as the icy cold in the northern hemisphere slowed putrefaction. In addition to being held in winter, the whole process of dissection was designed around the decomposition of the three main body cavities. According to Mondino's *Order of Dissection* the lower abdomen for obvious reasons was dissected first – a body part that would rapidly decompose, emanating the foulest odours – followed by the thorax and lastly the skull.[18] Many centuries later, in one of his *Reveries,* French philosopher Jean-Jacques Rousseau (1712-1778) vividly describes the sights and smells of public dissection: 'What a frightful display an anatomy amphitheatre provides: reeking cadavers, slobbering livid flesh, blood, disgusting intestines, ghastly skeletons, pestilential vapours'.[19]

The 'grand function' at Bologna, and other public anatomy theatres, was not a theoretical anatomy lesson or a dissection carried out by a teacher to educate his students. Rather, the 'grand function' was a complex ceremonial observance, lasting for fifteen days, attended by numerous dignitaries, eminent city authorities, scholars, students of anatomy, as well as curious carnival revellers. For this occasion the anatomy theatre was sumptuously decorated, the walls hung with damask, candlesticks illuminating the room, and two large torches placed on either end of the cadaver, displayed on the dissecting table in the middle of the theatre.

Before proceedings commenced, the Papal writ allowing dissection was formally read out. Thereafter, the dissection began, carried out by a medically trained person, while the professor initiated discussion among the audience, and occasionally approached the cadaver to indicate various displayed parts during the lesson. 'Meanwhile, in a nearby chapel, and at the expense of the anatomy professor, masses were said for the souls of those dissected'.[20]

Public anatomy was not confined to Italy, but found at all major European universities. In London, dignitary Samuel Pepys (1633-1703), Member of Parliament, and Chief Secretary to the Admiralty under King Charles II, was one of the first spectators to witness and describe a public dissection at Surgeons Hall. Generally – as was traditional in other European countries – such demonstrations lasted for several days, with lectures and discussions on the different body parts displayed in each lesson and sumptuous daily banquets to follow. 'After Pepys had listened to a lecture on the structure of the kidneys, demonstrated on the body of a recently hanged man in the elegant Inigo Jones Theatre on 27 February 1663, he enjoyed a fine dinner in the company's hall'.[21] Once dinner had been concluded numerous surgeons again closely inspected the mutilated body – clinical detachment or callousness?

Regardless at which European university public anatomy lessons were held, public dissections were a grisly spectacle. Public anatomies during the Renaissance period[22] were solemn, as well as festive occasions, which always attracted an audience of spectators not themselves engaged in the practice of medicine. When Vesalius, who was already famous at that time, was invited to Bologna to perform a public dissection in 1540, he declared that especially huge crowds attended his dissections of the genital organs.[23] The prospect of a gruesome display could be guaranteed to draw 'leering crowds of idle, curious and ghoulish gawpers'.[24]

In considering some of the characteristics of these public 'ceremonies' – the paid entrance ticket, as well as the recital of music to entertain the audience – their similarity to theatrical performances becomes apparent. But, what took place within Renaissance anatomy theatres was closely linked to events that had occurred on the outside, before the corpse was placed on the dissection table. The spectacle of public anatomy and that of capital punishment were intimately connected by various similarities, but especially so by one common element: the corpse of the executed offender. Approaching from opposite ends, both physician and executioner were linked as it were, by the outstretched corpse.

Numerous engravings and illustration of public executions show the carnival aspect of these events – noisy, rowdy occasions – with literally thousands of excited spectators attending, milling around the gallows vying for a view of the cruel spectacle. For renowned felons, the mob could swell to fifty thousand or more.[25] However, although the violent brawls between anatomists and spectators at public executions in England did not occur on the Continent, public sentiment about dissection nevertheless ran deep in most European countries.

It was only once the disorderly, public exhibition of execution had been separated from the more methodical display of public dissection during the late eighteenth century, that serious anatomical exploration and study began to take place. Prior to that, there was an all too close connection between execution and anatomy. During the sixteenth and seventeenth centuries, in England and other European countries, the criminal, the executioner, the anatomist, and their assistants all played a carefully coordinated role in the 'spectacle, which constituted the culture of dissection'.[26], [27]

Anatomy students from around Europe travelled to Italy to further their knowledge in this discipline. William Harvey, a colossus of the medical world,[28] and personal physician to King James I and King Charles I, studied anatomy in Padua for two years. Looking into the central sunken area from one of the concentrically raised wooden oval terraces, which made up the antomy theatre, Harvey 'gazed into that blood-spattered pit on many anatomical, and in particular venereal marvels, that he would later memorably recall in his lectures, including syphilitic ulcers that had gnawed into the stomach of a prostitute, a boy whose genitals had been bitten off by a dog and a man without a penis, who was apparently still capable of sex.'[29]

Anatomy lessons in Bologna and Padua were very popular with Italian and foreign students, as anatomy theatres were more readily available in

Italy than in other countries and there were sufficient corpses available for dissection in Bologna, and Padua. The corpses of hanged felons, generally middle-aged and in good health, were particularly sought after. However, not only the bodies of the executed were set aside for anatomy, but also the poor who died in hospital and would have had to be buried free of charge.

But, even though there was a seemingly abundant supply of cadavers, the 'function' could at times be delayed due to a lack of corpses, in which case students would 'roam' the city in search of someone who had 'suddenly died'.[30] On at least one documented occasion, the unavailability of a corpse for public dissection, led to immensely tragic circumstances: on 30 January 1681 the executed Antonio Bagnoli da Bagni di Lucca, was made available for anatomical dissection to a crowd of waiting students and onlookers. But sadly, the poor man had not been condemned to death, but to life imprisonment. However, in order to satisfy the demands of the Bolognaise anatomy school, 'the cardinal legate overruled the decree of life imprisonment, and had him condemned to death instead.[31]

While interest for the 'spectacular' aspect of the 'function' was extensive, its educational value during the sixteenth and seventeenth centuries was generally questioned. In the decades before William Harvey, public dissection was not calculated to reveal the particulars of physiology to a professional gathering. Rather, public dissection demonstrated the greatness and wisdom of the Creator and the intricacies of Creation through the displayed human body.

During these times, medical exploration at private dissections, as well as at many scientific academies, already focused on physiology, pathological anatomy, and the anatomy of various systems, such as the lymph and circulatory systems. Therefore, a display of the body's principal organs, as was conducted in public anatomy, was not considered of great educational value. The various other types of anatomical investigations were far more educational than public anatomy lessons because students were able to observe the specimens at a closer range, 'use magnifying glasses or microscopes, and to soak the specimens or to inject them with various substances'.[32]

The role of Renaissance artists in dissection

In examining the history of anatomical dissection, the role played by Renaissance artists in the growth and development of this discipline warrants lengthy discussion. Artists and medical men were in fact undergoing parallel development in the study of the human body during this time. Especially in Italy, where the serious study of anatomy first began, the influence of artists on the practice of dissection was enormous. Captivated by the human form, its bodily movements and proportions, artists developed naturalistic techniques to accurately represent the human body and its surroundings – their art was a true and faithful representation of natural phenomena.

In pursuit of understanding muscles and other physical structures of the human body more accurately, numerous Renaissance painters and sculptors turned to dissection, performing these 'when and where they could'.[33] Prominent painters like Leonardo da Vinci (1452-1519), Michelangelo (1475-1564), Albrecht Dürer (1471-1528), Titian (c. 1488-1576) and many others, are known to have actively participated in this practice. In fact, 'historical evidence indicates that between 1400 and 1543, more antomies were probably made by artists than by anatomists, although both worked together when they could'.[34]

Renaissance artist Leonardo da Vinci was a serious contributor to the knowledge of anatomy. Already at an early age, Leonardo is said to have passed many long night hours in the gruesome company of quartered or flayed corpses[35] – those from which the skin had been totally removed, laying open the superficial strands of muscles. In 1516, three years before his death, Leonardo is said to have remarked that he had dissected more than one hundred human bodies.[36]

Although dissections performed by artists were usually accomplished by Papal endorsement, Leonardo during the last years of his life, encountered opposition from Pope Leo X (1475-1521), who denied him access to the city's hospitals.[37] In fact, access to, and the attainment of corpses must have been an ever present need for artists. Michelangelo is said to have refused certain commissioned sculptures for the 'Church of the Holy Ghost' in Florence, unless he was 'paid' in cadavers sourced from cemeteries. 'There is thus evidence that the practice of resurrecting human bodies [...] occurred in Italy during the first part of the 16th century, and that dissection was done surreptitiously behind closed doors with the approval of the Church'.[38] It is therefore plausible that renowned artists had less trouble procuring corpses for dissection than the medical establishment, who were dependent mostly on the bodies of executed felons.

Leonardo made an in-depth study of the muscles, nerves, and the vascular, respiratory and genital systems, and completed more than 750 detailed anatomical drawings, remarkably accurate in their representation. But, in spite of Leonardo's study of human anatomy, his outlook remained traditional. He often followed convention rather than his anatomy-experienced eye, accepting, for example, the standard five-lobed liver and the Galenic doctrine of blood passing between the ventricles of the heart through 'invisible pores in the septum'.[39] Similarly, his 'drawings of the embryo were set within a traditional womb'.[40]

In all probability, Leonardo da Vinci began his anatomical examinations in pursuit of better pictorial representations, but soon his insatiable curiosity led him into scientific enquiry. Unfortunately, the textbook he had planned in association with anatomist Marcantonio della Torre (1481-1511) was never completed. However, had it been published, it would have revolutionised the sciences of anatomy and physiology.[41] Instead, the artists' magnificent sketches lay hidden for many centuries,[42] 'finally to be uncovered as a monument to the greatest mind of the Renaissance. But the influence of Leonardo was not entirely lost. His was the intellectual climate which made the work of Vesalius possible'.[43]

A milestone for medicine

A tremendous milestone and a monument for medicine, was the publication in 1543 of *De Humani Corporis Fabrica – On the Fabric of the Human Body* – by Belgian anatomist Andreas Vesalius. His greatest contribution lay in creating a solid foundation for anatomical study based on observed facts. But how did Vesalius attain his anatomical knowledge? Vesalius was admitted to the University of Paris at the age of eighteen. But what Vesalius desired most from his medical studies in Paris, '...dissection and instruction at the dissecting table',[44] was not readily available at the time. Vesalius himself stated that there was 'a great lack of the assistance of teachers in this part of medicine'.[45] Although the medical school of Paris had obtained its own building in 1477, no provision had been made for the teaching of anatomy by means of dissection. By 1493 occasional dissections were held in the basement of the hospital Hôtel Dieu. By 1526 anatomical demonstrations were still comparatively infrequent and, 'it is to be doubted that Vesalius witnessed three or four during his stay in Paris'.[46]

But, by his own initiative he attained considerable knowledge of anatomy. In order to obtain osteological (bone) specimens he became a constant frequenter of Montfaucon and the Cemetery of the Innocents. Montfaucon was a 'mound' outside the northern wall of Paris where a gibbet had been erected as early as the twelfth century. During Vesalius' time Montfaucon was occupied by the most imposing gallows in France – an enormous charnel house crowned by a colonnade of sixteen stone pillars thirty feet high, connected by wooden beams. The bodies of all felons executed at other sites within the city were brought to this sinister location.

Here they were suspended from the high beams until total decomposition warranted dumping their remains in the charnel house[47] below. Montfaucon was frequented by crows, rats and stray dogs, but provided outstanding riches for the avid anatomist. On his way to Montfaucon, Vesalius would also pass the Cemetery of the Innocents, where hundreds of victims of the plague had been buried. However, as victims had been hastily and shallowly buried, many skeletons had become disinterred over time, providing an abundant supply of bones for Vesalius and his fellow students to study.

Vesalius had come from a tradition steeped in Galenic scholarship; he had 'studied, edited and re-published Galen's books'.[48] But suddenly, through careful personal observations of the human body, the ancient authorities, in the eyes of Vesalius, lost their unquestioned authority – he in fact highlighted hundreds of anatomical errors introduced by Galen. For example, to name but a few, Vesalius realised that the lower jaw of humans consisted of only one bone – the mandible – not two as Galen had stated; he discovered that the human heart had four chambers, not three; that there were no pores between the ventricles of the heart as previously thought; and that major blood vessels had their origins in the heart, not the liver, as Galen had claimed.

However, Vesalius never challenged Galenical anatomy, and his perceived anti-Galenism has been over-exaggerated.[49] Rather, he accepted that Galen had based his work on animal dissections and hence he offered to 'correct' but not criticise Galen's anatomical descriptions whenever they were found not to agree with observation. Respectfully Vesalius declared: 'I, who yield to none in my devotion and reverence to Galen, neither can, nor should enjoy any greater pleasure than praising him'.[50]

In 1538, working with artists in Titan's studio, Vesalius published his detailed drawings – produced on the new printing press invented by Gutenberg – of complicated illustrations mapping the courses of arteries and veins, nerves and lymph nodes, and other structures of the human body. Together with an increasing awareness of how the various organs are interconnected came, 'a heightened interest in their functions. Physiology which had slept almost undisturbed since the days of Herophilus and Erasistratus, awakened to new life'.[51]

Heavily criticised by the church, Vesalius' most strident critics were Galenic anatomists. They maintained that if Galen's anatomy texts differed from that which was observed and written about by Vesalius, it was simply because the human body had physically changed in the intervening centuries. For example, sixteenth century anatomist Jacob Sylvius (1478-1555) a resolute adherent of Galenic anatomy – as were most physicians and surgeons at the time – vowed that Galen was in no way incorrect. Whenever his anatomy students revealed distinct physical disparities between Galen's texts and the dissected corpses in front of them, Sylvius' customary reply was that humans had clearly changed over the preceeding one thousand four hundred years.

A foul and mucky occupation

By the nineteenth century not much had changed on the Continent and in England for anatomy students: 'After handling human remains all day without wearing gloves – although they probably donned protective aprons and sleeve covers – the only washing facilities for their blood stained hands, the fingernails clogged with putrid flesh, would be a bucket of water pumped directly from the foul Thames. Some students combining anatomy instructions with a spell on the wards, would go on to pass deadly bacteria to their unfortunate patients'.[52] Similarly, numerous photos, in books on dissection relating to the late nineteenth and early twentieth centuries, still display barehanded [53] students at blood-soaked dissection tables in front of awkwardly posed, grossly exposed human corpses.[54]

Natural decomposition made a cadaver suitable for dissection only for the first couple of days following death – thereafter the stench became unbearable, a stench that would cling to the dissecting room, students' clothes, and their hands. Hence, dissection was a foul and mucky occupation. Not only was physical strength required, but most of all the capacity to withstand not only the stench of decomposing corpses, but also the inherent revulsion to work on such cadavers.

Apart from enduring the omnipresent permeating reek of decaying flesh, anatomy students during the eighteenth century were 'encouraged to feel the textures of various body parts and even to taste body fluids'.[55] In an era when scientific testing and examination was not yet an option, and microscopes were unreliable, anatomists relied heavily on their inherent senses. Prominent Scottish anatomist, surgeon John Hunter (1728-1793) – brother to William Hunter (1718-1783), renowned anatomist, physician and leading obstetric consultant in London – apparently routinely used his sense of taste during dissections, encouraging his students to do likewise. Wryly John Hunter pronounced that 'gastric juice was salty and brackish to the taste, while mucus from the urethra was strongly akin to the taste of sea-salt and semen appeared to have a maukish quality, producing a warmth similar to spices',[56] especially when held in the mouth for some time!

An important aspect of antomical dissection and medicine in general, is clinical detachment. William Harvey, one of the world's greatest anatomists and England's first true scientist,[57] reached his revolutionary findings by dissection and experiment. Taking clinical detachment almost to the extreme, Harvey is known to have dissected his own father and sister post-mortem 'which suggests the considerable extent to which he had become able to divorce himself from traditional attitudes to the human corpse'.[58]

Although the use of human corpses for dissection was customary on the Continent since the fourteenth century, circumstances and resulting occurrences were somewhat different in England. Here, dissection was prohibited until the sixteenth century, when a series of royal pronouncements granted physicians and surgeons limited rights to dissect corpses…

V

SURGEONS AND THE GALLOWS –
A SPECTACLE OF SUFFERING

The title of this chapter suggests a bizarre, horrific, almost unbelievable association between educated men of medicine and those pitifully executed at the gallows. This subject matter is confronting, tragic and immensely sad from a modern perspective. However, the bloody and appalling connection between surgeons and the gallows, although not generally known, forms an important and once prominent part of medical history.

In Scotland and England, the link between medicine and the gallows was first forged by sixteenth century legislation, which relates to the number of bodies supplied to anatomists and medical schools for dissection. In Scotland anatomists received royal patronage through James IV (1473-1513) in 1506, whereby the king formally granted the 'Edinburgh Guild of Surgeons and Barbers' the bodies of select executed felons for dissection. In England however, the process took a while longer and it was not until 1540 that the companies of 'Barbers and Surgeons' were united by Royal Charter and that King Henry VIII bestowed to them the annual right to the bodies of four hanged criminals. More than a century later Charles II added a further two corpses to the original grant. The dependence of surgeons and anatomists on the gallows, as the only legally accepted method of obtaining subjects for dissection, continued in England until 1832 – when the Anatomy Act was passed.

The Royal Charter by King Henry VIII granting the companies of 'Barbers and Surgeons' the annual right to the bodies of four hanged criminals marks the foundation of a relationship between the medical profession, the ruling elite, and exemplary punishment. Henceforth, dissection and the resulting public exposure and physical destruction of the corpse came to be associated in the eyes of the English people as a terrible punishment. Dissection was seen as an aggravation and an added penalty to the frightful sentence of execution. It was popularly perceived that surgeons acted as secondary executioners to the law.[1] Justifyably it can therefore be said that '…by the beginning of the eighteenth century, at the gallows standing at the conjunction of the Tyburn and Edgware roads, the history of the London poor and the history of English science intersect'.[2]

The Bloody Code – a sad history

Between 1770 and 1830 the legal system known as the 'Bloody Code' was implemented in England. The name speaks for itself, attesting to the enormous numbers of crimes for which the death penalty could be imposed. In 1815 the number of 'crimes' carrying the death penalty in England amounted to 225.[3] Whereas hundreds were executed annually[4] for relatively trivial crimes in eighteenth century England, this changed in 1837 with the abolition of the death penalty for theft – capital punishment was henceforth reserved mainly for murder.

Although the Company of Barber-Surgeons' right to six bodies annually from Tyburn was firmly endorsed by royal authority, the Georgian populace however by no means accepted it.[5] On execution days the working class poor would desperately struggle to preserve the respect for those put to death by the hangman at the Tyburn Gallows. South of London the scaffold at Tyburn, known as 'the deadly nevergreen', the tree that bore fruit all year long, was a grizzly reminder to all that life outside the law could indeed be, as English philosopher Thomas Hobbes (1588-1679) had described: '…solitary, poor, nasty, brutish and short'.[6] Tragically, Tyburn was a place of execution between 1169 and 1783 and it is estimated that between forty and sixty thousand executions took place there during that period – a terrible legacy indeed.

The groan of the gallows

To the early anatomists of Scotland and England '...the groan of the gallows was sweet music, and hundreds of condemned men and women who walked to the scaffold at Tyburn in London or elsewhere were horrified in their last moments as to what would happen to their remains after they had been cut down'.[7] Given the association of execution and dissection, the lowered perception of the anatomists' profession in the public mind is not surprising. Surgeons were well aware of what went on at the gallows and '...to gain their quarry they (often corruptly) obtained the apparent support of the panoply of law from executioners and others involved in public executions'.[8] Scenes of conflict were exacerbated by surgeons from various medical schools competing and vying for cadavers. Often the corpses of those executed were simply snatched for the purposes of dissection.

The total lack of respect and decorum – especially from medical surgeons – denoted to those put to death at the gallows, is highlighted over and over in various written accounts. According to *Barber Surgeon's Company Records* in *Annals of the Barber-Surgeons of London*[9] it is evident that major battles erupted continually around the gallows, usually when the felon was scarcely dead. These fights and clashes could be vicious, violent and bloody. Relatives and friends would be dragging and pulling the scarcely cold body forcibly from the surgeons who were desperate to procure corpses for dissection.

As much as what Leonardo da Vinci had used cadavers stolen from the gallows to produce his anatomical sketches, in Renaissance Italy, '...so eighteenth century London anatomists turned for their research requirements to Tyburn Tree'.[10] Although eighteenth century English history books generally mention the brutal, violent and unruly spectacles of public hangings at Tyburn, the direct involvement of anatomists in these brawls are not cited. Accounts of violence at these public execcutions are usually juxtaposed by the era's many achievements in the fine arts of music, literature and architecture.

Descriptions of life in eighteenth century England generally paint an idillic picture, emphasising '...the civility of life in well-landscaped gardens, the good sense of Hanovarian compromise, and the quiet accumulation quantified in account books of London and Bristol merchants [...]. Eighteenth century English history, slowly, inevitably, meanders on a broad river spreading peace and bounty'.[11] In truth however, death on the gallows was a messy, dismal and horrific experience: '...the choking, pissing, and screaming'[12] ignored and 'primly' secreted by polite society. In addition, the public brawls and fierce disorders on hanging days caused major disruptions, in which especially surgeons and their porters seem to have been the main targets.

In response to the apparent breakdown in law and order on the part of the authorities, the 'Murder Act' was passed by British parliament in 1752. This ensured that surgeons could henceforth only receive the bodies of felons who had been officially sentenced to dissection after execution. It also decreed that any attempt at rescuing such a corpse from the surgeon's custody would be punishable by transportation to one of His Majesty's colonies. Therefore, with the passing of the 'Murder Act' it was to be expected that the tumultuous rioting on hanging days would became a thing of the past. After all, anatomists were ensured those victims who had specifically been sentenced to dissection after their death on the gallows. But this was not to be.

A fate worse than death

Crowds at public executions blatantly disregarded legalities surrounding the corpses of executed criminals – unless the victim was a particularly unpopular criminal. One can almost imagine a literal tug of war enacted at public executions. And the reason for the violence is clear: anatomical dissection was seen as a fate much worse than death due to the fact that '...in no case whatsoever the body of any murderer shall be suffered to be buried'.[13] This robbed infamous victims of a grave and subsequently, according to popular belief, of all hope to attain an afterlife. Dissections remained fiercely unpopular and the additional disgrace of the surgeon's scalpel to the hangman's noose 'rendered the injustice of the law all the more loathsome'.[14]

To most English surgeons, the crowds who opposed them at the gallows constituted the scum of the people, a mob, loose and disorderly.

But, direct evidence survives as to who these 'disorderly persons', this 'scum of the people' were. They were none other than the felon's family, friends and fellow workers. Many convicted felons stated that they preferred being hung in chains and exposed, after death, rather than to be 'anatomised'[15] by the surgeons. Although the thought of serving as carrion to the birds must have caused as much anguish as being cut up after death. Either way a burial and, according to popular belief, any chance of salvation, was denied the victim.[16]

To protect their bodies from the dissection table, the condemned would go to great lengths, earnestly appealing to family, friends and acquaintances to secure their corpse immediately after death. Nothing was worse than to be publicly exposed on the dissection table, then cut and mangled, and later simply discarded and fed to the fishes in the Thames – as reported in the *Political Anecdotist* of 1831.[17] Many tragic stories of troubled prisoners' fears are documented in the *Newgate Calendar*, compiled by the Old Bailey's attorneys-at-law. All cases attest to prisoners' begging relatives and friends to rescue their executed corpses from the anatomist's scalpel at all costs. Apart from hatred towards dissection, the popular notion that the dead could 'come again' or be 'troublesome' after death – a last revenge of the dead upon the living so to speak – ensured that the living showed every last act of kindness possible to convicted felons before execution.

There are countless written records, tragic examples, of close family protecting the corpses of their executed loved-ones. For instance, shoemaker Matthew Lee, hanged in 1728 for stealing a silver watch, was guarded by his sister and brother after death and given a decent burial. 'Oliver White's father came down from Carlisle to protect his son's body from the surgeons and to watch over his grave at night'.[18] Samuel Curtis's father walked thirty miles to London to witness his son's execution and to take possession of his son's body beneath the gallows. His son had been hanged for stealing a mare.

Many sacrifices were made by caring relatives and friends to wrestle their loved ones from the arms of anatomists. Writing in 1741 novelist Samuel Richardson describes attending a mass execution at Tyburn[19] – it was common to hang several felons at the same time. At this occasion he witnessed the outbreak of rioting: 'As soon as the poor creatures were half-dead, I was much surprised [...] to see the populace fall to hauling and pulling the carcasses with so much earnestness, as to occasion several warm encounters and broken heads. These were friends of the persons executed [...] and some persons sent by private surgeons to obtain bodies for dissection. The contests between these were fierce and bloody, and frightful to look at'.[20] Although these gallows brawls against the surgeons never escalated in destroying metropolitan order, and were not considered dangerous enough to provoke government action, they were however always a potential flashpoint for full-scale rioting.

In other European countries there was no need for anatomists to vie for bodies at the gallows, as they were well supplied with cadavers (See chapter on Resurrectionists and anatomists). Unrest would generally only occur if the executioner bungled his duties, thereby causing the victim undue pain. Although there was undoubtedly a feeling of discomfort about dissection in general, the comparatively slow and orderly growth in demands made by other European anatomists, as opposed to the rapid expansion of anatomy schools in England, helped preserve the balance between the various different interests.[21] Another factor contributing to the relative lack of violence at executions in countries like France, the Netherlands and Germany was the fact that executioners generally remained in complete control. They either put the executed in coffins or prepared them for transport to the gallows field or personally handed them over to anatomists.[22]

The question arises, as to why there was such overwhelming fear on the part of the condemned, for family and friends to secure their corpse immediately after death? This has to be understood in the contemporary mindset of the time. The notion of keeping the physical body intact was strengthened in Christian Europe by a literal acceptance of Christian doctrine of the resurrection of the dead. At all costs the body was to be kept whole to await resurrection. To be buried with any body part missing was thought to incur a risk for the deceased of spending the whole of eternity without it. Therefore, many people even went to the extent of preserving all lost teeth so that these could be buried with the rest of the body.[23]

Not to be buried *at all* meant foregoing *any* chance of an afterlife. Therefore, dissection of the corpse was also seen as posthumous punishment of the criminal's soul – a soul which could never find rest. For this very reason, European anatomists had great difficulty, already during the Middle Ages, in obtaining corpses to pursue their anatomical studies. Hence, it was not unusual for condemned prisoners, who were not already under sentence of disection, to be offered money to leave their corpses to the anatomists. This course of action was however fraught with uncertainty as such bodies were frequently literally 'wrestled' out of the hands of surgeons and anatomists by crowds milling around the gallows.

Tragically many a prisoner sealed deals with surgeons before their deaths, selling their bodies in order to at least be able to purchase 'decent' clothes for their execution – something regarded with the utmost importance. Alternately, they would use the money to pay expenses in prison while awaiting their inevitable fate. Again this goes to show that business dealings in corpses was a shoddy, murky and tragic business – but one, which eighteenth century anatomy-study could not have done without in England.

Anatomists – instruments of death

Anatomists were also greatly unpopular because according to widespread beliefs *they* were often the instruments of death for the condemned. At times '…it was reasonable to regard the surgeon, not the hangman as the agent causing death',[24] because it was not uncommon for the noose to have done its work inadequately. There were numerous genuine cases of incomplete hangings where victims were brought to life again later by relatives and friends. Several seventeenth and eighteenth century accounts of hanged felons 'resurrecting' as it were after execution, are documented in *Proceedings from the Old Bailey, London Criminal Court.*[25]

Up until 1872, hangings using little or no drop were the general rule. It made no difference, whether prisoners were suspended from the back of a cart or a ladder or later by some form of trap door device, they usually got only a few inches of actual drop. It was therefore not uncommon for relatives and friends of prisoners to fiercely pull on their legs in order to shorten their suffering.[26] In other words, hanged felons died of asphyxia and not from a broken neck. Often however, asphyxia resulted in temporary unconsciousness, giving the impression that the victim was indeed dead.

At other times, there is evidence that the hangman was in collusion with victims and their families. In such cases, he could be coerced to exercise discretion as to how he placed the noose and the knot, so that fatal strangulation would in fact not take place.[27] It was therefore desirable to wrestle victims from the surgeons at all costs, as the function of anatomists was of course not to revive but to dissect the physical body. There were too many cases of 'miracle' revivals after hangings, which is why victims of the noose were terrified of a bungled, clumsy execution and the chance of being cut up alive on the anatomy table.

Numerous accounts have been recorded during the seventeenth and eighteenth centuries, of people waking up on the dissection table. For example, in 1651 Anne Greene was hanged in Oxford, for the murder of her bastard child. She dangled at the end of the rope for thirty minutes, while her friends pulled on her legs, to hasten her suffering and ultimate demise. Then her body was cut down from the gallows and brought to anatomists Thomas Willis and William Patty for dissection. To the astonishment of the anatomists, Anne woke up just seconds before the knife was thrust into her sternum. The doctors obtained a pardon for Anne, who later married and bore three children in wedlock.[28]

In November 1740 William Duell came back to life on the anatomist table, as he was being washed and prepared for dissection. It was noticed that he was breathing and had a faint pulse. Although still in pain he could soon sit up, eat, drink and converse. Sent back to Newgate Prison, he was later reprieved and sentenced to transportation.[29] Similarly, seventeen-year-old thief William Duell, after he was left hanging at the gallows for thirty minutes, revived on the anatomists' table in front of all assembeld surgeons. He was later sentenced to transportation.[30]

While many came back to life on the anatomy table and went on to live for many years, not all were so lucky. An article by Jessie Dobson titled *Cardiac Action after Death by Hanging*, published in the *Lancet* (December 29, 1951), reveals that out of thirty-six bodies dissected after hangings, between 1812 and 1830, the heart was still beating in ten. In spite of the fact that these felons were obviously still alive, the dissections went ahead anyway.[31]

Habitual commotions and violence at the gallows continued, with angry multitudes denying surgeons their quarry. Eventually, in 1783, this led to the transfer of all London executions from Tyburn to Newgate. Public hangings were forthwith carried out just outside the walls of the Newgate Prison – in close proximity to Surgeon's Hall. This facilitated the procurement of bodies for dissection and resulted in a tighter control over the condemned by authorities. If someone was sentenced to death and subsequent dissection there was now absolute certainty, that the condemned person would indeed undergo the sentence. However, surgeons continued to be loathed until the Anatomy Act of 1832 finally severed the connection between dissection, crime and punishment.

However, long before the passing of the Anatomy Act and in addition to the violent scenes at the gallows, England experienced a two hundred year period of terror and grief of a different kind, unique to this small island country...

RESURRECTIONISTS AND ANATOMISTS – A 'GRAVE' ALLIANCE

By the turn of the eighteenth century it was evident that English medical education had fallen far behind its continental rivals – aspiring young doctors rather studied abroad in Italy or Paris. Therefore, in order to compensate for England's lack of progress in the medical field, parliament dissolved the two hundred year-old 'Barber-Surgeon Guild' in 1745. This meant that surgeons broke away from barbers to form the 'Company of Surgeons', thereby opening the way for private medical schools to be established.[1] But, unlike in France, Germany and other European countries, licenses were not required in England to establish medical schools and soon they were cropping up in increasing numbers. As a result, the demand for bodies to be used in the various schools for anatomy classes, outstripped the supply of executed felons from the London and Middlesex areas.

Eighteenth century medical schools in England

Medical schools were highly competitive and sought to keep their students from joining rival schools at all costs, as students were a lucrative business. They paid general fees, as well as separate payments for each anatomy and dissection class. Therefore, to keep students in their respective schools it was imperative to have an adequate supply of corpses available. After all, '…anatomy was medicine's essential science and if it were not learned on the dead, then knowledge would need to be obtained by mangling the living'.[2] According to William Hunter – brother to anatomist John Hunter – founder of one of the largest anatomy schools in London, it was essential for a corpse to be 'heaved' through the back door of his establishment, for every new student that walked through the front entrance.[3]

In order to present a complete course in anatomy, 'fresh subjects' had to be provided in large numbers.[4] With an increasing number of students drawn to the study of medicine, not only private schools, but also the larger London hospitals such as St. Thomas and St. Bartholomew, began offering anatomy classes. The obvious result was soon apparent – a dire shortage in cadavers for dissection, creating a demand for something the common populace was simply not willing to surrender. Wendy Moore succinctly makes the point in her account of John Hunter in *The Knife Man*: '…the steady flow of petty felons condemned to the gallows could not keep pace with the growing demands of anatomists, other more devious methods had evolved'.[5]

As discussed in the previous chapter, anatomists initially resorted to the gallows. Such cadavers were in fact favoured. They were 'fresh', healthy specimens, usually in the prime of their lives, free of fatal diseases which had led to death. But this source of cadavers proved insufficient, especially after the passing of the Murder Act in 1752, when only those bodies specifically ordered for dissection – and their numbers were limited to only several a year – could be used. For example, as late as 1831 the number of corpses acquired from the gallows by medical schools for dissection in London still only amounted to eleven – a ridiculously low supply when considering that there were at least nine hundred students studying anatomy in the city at that time.[6]

After the passing of the Murder Act this created a situation where anatomy schools were practically forced to obtain corpses from other sources. In addition, the gallows could not provide the corpses of pregnant women, babies or young children, which were likewise necessary for dissection. Hence, the demand for bodies gave rise to the secret disinterment of corpses from graveyards – a clandestine activity, which became prevalent in England from the early eighteenth to the early nineteenth centuries. Ironically, due to their ability of raising vast numbers of dead from their graves, the perpetrators became known as 'resurrectionists' or body snatchers, who sold the exumed freshly buried corpses to medical schools for dissection and anatomy classes.[7] This created a situation in England, where '...from Land's End to John o'Groats, people lived and died in terror of the body-snatchers'.[8] The old saying, to be 'worth more dead than alive' was certainly true in those times.

Anatomy schools on the Continent

But, what was the situation in other European countries with regard to body snatching? As was the case in England, growing student numbers in medical schools around Europe led to a high demand in bodies for dissection. However, on the Continent an adequate supply of corpses to anatomists ensured that body-snatchers were indeed unknown there. On the Continent, the use of executed criminals was *never* the only source of anatomists' supplies, thereby eliminating from the outset any ill repute associated with dissection. For example, in France legislation decreed that the bodies of all persons who had died in hospital, should be made available for anatomical purposes – if they had not been claimed by relatives twenty-four hours after death. In addition, any would-be resurrectionists in that country would have been deterred by France's penal code, which imposed mandatory imprisonment as well as a fine for the violations of graves and burial sites.

Similar regulations applied in Italy. The bodies of those who had died unclaimed in hospitals were made available to anatomists and '...the relatively slow and orderly growth in the demands made by Italian anatomists, as compared to the sudden mushrooming and rapid expansion of foreign colleges',[9] maintained a healthy balance in the organisation of public anatomy sessions.

In Germany, anatomists were especially well supplied. They received the corpses of all who died in prisons, unless family or friends cared to pay a specific sum to release the body. They were also given all those who had been executed, as well as all those who could not afford to pay for a burial, and all poor people who had been supported in life by the public purse. In addition, the corpses of all prostitutes were used for anatomical purposes. The popular perception in this case was that these women had after all used their bodies in life to corrupt unsuspecting males, and therefore got their 'just deserts' so to speak, in death. In Austria, Portugal and the Netherlands bodies for dissection were made available from similar sources as in Germany.

In the United States, no regular supply of bodies to anatomy schools was legislated – in fact, the practice of dissection was illegal until the 1830's. After that date, medical schools openly purchased bodies from resurrectionists - authorities turned a blind eye. The poor, white or black, as well as southern slaves were the most vulnerable for exploitation. It was not uncommon for slave owners to sell the bodies of their slaves to medical schools.

'Sack-em-up gentlemen'

In the early days of medicine in England, the first body snatchers were the anatomists themselves. Not only teachers and surgeons at medical schools engaged in this nefarious activity, but also their students, who frequently paid for their tuition in corpses for anatomical use. The fact that students had probably been participating in this practice for some time is evidenced in a 1721 clause of the 'Edinburgh College of Surgeons'. The clause specifically barred students from robbing graves. In spite of these directives though, students continued 'resurrecting' bodies, although their methods were incompetent and easily detected.

In a report given by a young medical student in 1751, he describes an evening of drinking in the anatomy room and the subsequent decision later that night by all present to dig up the body of a woman executed for theft the day before. After midnight the students set out with spades and other paraphernalia. However, arriving at the appointed graveyard they had difficulty finding the correct grave. After locating what they believed to be the right grave, they inadvertently dug up a coffin which when opened proved to contain '…an old woman very foul' [10] – in other words, she was already decomposed. They had dug up the wrong grave and the bungling students hastily departed without even an attempt at covering up their underhand activities.

Although student 'sack-em-up gentlemen' were a valiant lot to jeopardise so much for science, the risks and dangers were too great, and with the ever-increasing demand, these 'gentlemen' body snatchers were unable to keep up. They were instead replaced by a group of low class rowdies, shifty criminals and deceitful gravediggers, generally referred to as 'rascals'.

At first only a handful of such men devoted themselves to stealing corpses for the purpose of dissection. But soon others, generally from the lower classes, joined in the trade, as financial inducements became more and more lucrative. Anatomy classes ran in winter, the cold temperatures delaying putrefaction of the corpses. Therefore, resurrectionists would work throughout the winter on dark, moonless nights, to the discreet glow of covered lanterns.

Professional body snatchers

The methods employed in body snatching are discussed at length in *The Diary of a Resurrectionist 1811-1812*: 'In the case of a neat, or not quite new grave, the ingenuity of the resurrectionist came into play. Several feet – fifteen or twenty – away from the head or foot of the grave, he would remove a square of turf, about eighteen or twenty inches in diameter. This he would carefully put by, and then commence to mine. […] Taking a five-foot grave, the coffin lid would be about four feet from the surface. A rough slanting tunnel, some five yards long, would, therefore, have to be constructed, so as to impinge exactly on the coffin head. This being at last struck (no very simple task), the coffin was lugged up by hooks to the surface, or, preferably, the end of the coffin was wrenched off with hooks while still in the shelter of the tunnel, and the scalp or feet of the corpse secured through the open end, and the body pulled out, leaving the coffin almost intact and unmoved. The body, once obtained, the narrow shaft was easily filled up and the sod of turf accurately replaced. The friends of the deceased, seeing that the earth over his grave was not disturbed, would flatter themselves that the body had escaped the Resurrectionist; but they seldom noticed the neatly-placed square of turf, some feet away'.[11]

On the other hand, the *modus operandi* did not always involve tunnelling, which was, after all, time-consuming and especially difficult in winter. Throughout England the poor were often buried in deep pit graves, up to twenty foot deep, where coffins were stacked on top of each other – easy pickings for body snatchers.

A canvas was first spread to catch all loose soil and then a hole dug at the end where head and shoulders lay. Once parts of the coffin had been exposed, a crowbar was used to pry the lid open, snapping it off against the weight of earth covering the rest of the coffin. To deaden the cracking noise of tearing wood, the thieves used sacking. Then the corpse was efficiently pulled out of the coffin, unceremoniously stripped naked, roughly doubled in half and thrust into a sack. Now the soil was neatly put back on the grave together with any markers or booby-traps, which may have been put there by concerned relatives, eager to prevent exactly what had just befallen their loved-one. This was carried out *not* to spare loved-ones grief and pain, but simply because the villains could then return again and again to the same graveyard.

The law of supply and demand

A single team of body snatchers could easily secure as many as ten bodies in a night's work or as many as three hundred in one year.[12] In 1828 police in London stated that over 200 resurrectionist gangs were operative. Considering that *The Diary of a Resurrectionist 1811-1812* records over four hundred bodies taken by the Crouch gang alone and that Bishop and Williams '…resurrected over five hundred bodies, it is estimated that between 1780 and 1832 the total numbers of bodies procured unethically by anatomists in Britain and Ireland would amount to around 200,000 at least'.[13]

In London a gang of resurrectionists confessed to stealing and selling hundreds of corpses to anatomists and surgeons at King's College, St. Bartholomew's Hospital, St. Thomas Hospital and others. Of course their motives were purely mercenary. During the early eighteen hundreds, a skilled worker in London, would earn a few shillings for a week of backbreaking labour and a merchant seaman received less than £2 a month.[14] However, a 'fresh' corpse – in a time when refrigiration was unknown – would collect a fee of between £6 to £9 for a single night's work. These were unbelievable takings for the average person. In addition, special requirements by anatomists ensured increased prices for specific 'items'. The corpses of pregnant women for instance were highly sought after and the corpses of children, known as 'smalls' '... were priced by the inch, while an unusual or rare medical condition could always command a premium'.[15]

Naturally, as the demand for corpses rose so did payments. The economic law of supply and demand catered to expanding resurrectionist ventures. Initially, only a few men engaged in body snatching because the demand was small. Accordingly, the price a cadaver fetched was 'pegged' at two pounds or less. But, once the number of students and teachers multiplied out of all proportion, this created a market scarcity. Not only did the cost of an individual cadaver skyrocket to as much as fourteen pounds,[16] but extortion was often also employed. As a result of the large amounts of money up for 'grabs' more 'rascals' were attracted to the trade.

There was also another lucrative niche in the market: various resurrectionists dealt solely in Jewish bodies, stemming from the tradition of early burial – within twenty-four hours of death – which leant these corpses the desired 'freshness', ideal for anatomical purposes. William Hunter told his class that every hour a corpse was kept '...it is losing something of its fitness for anatomical demonstrations. [...] the process of natural decomposition would quickly cause the blood to seep out of the tissues and vessels, rendering the various parts one indistinguishable soupy mass, while all the while putrefaction advanced, turning the flesh flabby and indistinct, not to mention noxious to the extreme'.[17] Hence, freshness of corpses was repeatedly stressed by anatomists, who were no doubt willing to pay slightly more for such specimens. Unfortunately, after handling human remains all day with their bare hands – their finger-nails still clogged with putrid flesh after a quick rinse – those students combining anatomy instructions with their ward rounds, would go on to 'pass deadly bacteria' to their hapless patients.[18]

Wicked money-making ploys

The wicked money-making schemes of resurrectionists knew no bounds. It would have been impossible for resurrectionists to provide the sheer numbers of bodies they did, had they not made shady deals, with the custodians of different cemetaries. Often these 'keepers' of burial grounds were handsomely bribed and complicit with nefarious goings-on. Also, as James Bailey states in *The Diary of a Resurrectionist* 'the ranks of resurrection-men were largely recruited from the keepers of burial-grounds'.[19] When not themselves functioning as resurrectionists, grave-diggers frequently supplied information as to who had been newly buried. In addition, it did no harm for resurrectionists to vigilantly listen out for 'passing-bells'[20] and to frequent ale-houses to learn who had died.

Often, the bodies of suicides or those who had met with accidental death, while awaiting the coroner's inquest, were stolen and sold to anatomy lecturers. Resurrection-men would then surreptitiously call on police, to inform them where the missing body was hidden, so the body could be restored to the coroner. After the inquest 'grieving relatives', who were in fact accomplices of the resurrectionists, would lay claim to the body for burial. In reality they would however resell the corpse to another medical school, thereby doubling their profit.

A further ploy, for which a female accomplice was generally engaged, was to lay claim to those who had died friendless in workhouses. Clad in mourning and overcome with grief, the female and her male accomplice would claim the body of their dearly departed relation, to provide him or her with a decent burial. Instead however, they sold the corpse straight to the nearest school. Of course this involved fee-splitting, which lowered the profit for individuals. Often corpses were obtained from complicit, unscrupulous undertakers, who kept the bodies of the poor until burial. Coffins, devoid of their legitimate content were then weighted down and sham funerals conducted for the grieving, unsuspecting families.

As body-snatching became more and more of a lucrative business for resurrectionists, it was inevitable that the money-making tables were turned by innovative individuals. Hence, there were those who willingly offered their bodies for anatomical purposes in return for an immediate 'downpayment'. Of course this was nothing but a swindle, as anatomists had no hold on those whose bodies they had 'bought' and they could certainly not force families to give up such a person's corpse after death. A written example of such a proposal to Sir Astley Cooper (1768-1841), renowned English surgeon, and professor of anatomy at St. Thomas hospital, is still on view in the Stone Collection at the Royal College of Surgeons of England: 'Sir, – I have been informed you are in the habit of purchasing bodys and allowing the person a sum weekly; knowing a poor woman that is desirous of doing so, I have taken the liberty of calling to know the truth'.[21]

In at least one documented case, body-snatchers actually performed an invaluable service to someone mistakenly buried alive. John Macintire, while in a state of trance, but consciously aware of all goings-on around him, had been put in a coffin and buried. Serendipitously, he was taken on the night of his 'burial' by resurrectionists and immediately sold to the surgeons for dissection. He was however suddenly and painfully brought out of his state of conscious immobility by the surgeons scalpel on the dissecting table – no doubt to the utter surprise and shock of teacher and students alike.[22]

Export trade in bodies

Bodies for dissection were also shipped from one destination to another, as prices varied from city to city. As bodies were abundant and cheap in impoverished Ireland, it was good business to ship them across to Scotland and England to sell there. Although such 'exports' depleted supplies in Ireland's own medical schools, Dublin had numerous badly protected burial grounds, which facilitated the trade. And so it was, that hundreds of consignments, artfully disguised as coming from dry salters, pork curers, fishmongers and fruit dealers, passed undetected from Dublin to the mainland. But, many bodies failed to make their destination to the surgeons' dissection tables. Due to faulty packing and lack of refrigeration such cargo was often uncovered, and then simply buried at sea. If an inquest did take place the findings usually read: 'Found dead in a box'.[23]

In October 1826 thirty-three human bodies were discovered in casks about to be shipped from Liverpool to Edinburgh. Accidental discovery was due to the foul odours emanating from several casks on Liverpool docks, while awaiting shipment to Edinburgh. As the casks were marked 'Bitter Salts', their sickening smell soon aroused suspicion. Although the bodies had been pickled in brine and packed in salt, they were partly decomposed. Although the police officially uncovered this particular corpse-exporting scheme, the perpetrators only received light jail sentences. Of course, the loss of a large consignment meant great financial loss to the consignees – on one occasion Dr. Knox (1791-1862), an instructor at Edinburgh's largest private anatomy school, was reputedly £800 out of pocket for bodies lost at sea.[24]

A strange interdependence

Once body snatchers had completed a successful night's work, it was convenient to shelter the bodies as close to the cemeteries as possible. For this express purpose many anatomy schools made 'out-houses' available to those resurrectionists who supplied them regularly. This raises questions about the affiliation and rapport between surgeon-anatomists and resurrectionists. Modern sensibilities find the relationship between educated, honourable men dedicated to scientific discovery and the criminal, wicked ruffians dealing in this ghastly trade, disconcerting to say the least. The relationship between surgeon-anatomists and their suppliers was one of strange interdependence. Although it seems to have been a necessary alliance, it contained an attitude of utter contempt and social disgust from the side of the anatomists towards the body snatchers.

Although anatomists were complicit in these actions, it was always the resurrectionists who took the brunt of popular sentiment against exhumation and the sale of the buried dead. In his diary Charles Darwin describes a riot witnessed in Cambridge in 1830. Two bodysnatchers had been arrested by police and '…whilst being taken to prison had been torn from the constable by a crowd of the roughest men, who dragged them by their legs along the muddy and stony road. They were covered from head to foot with mud, and their faces were bleeding either from having been kicked or from the stones; they looked like corpses, but the crowd was so dense that I got only a few momentary glimpses of the wretched creatures...'.[25] Resurrectionists were the ones hated and resented by the general populace for the exumation and sale of the buried dead, while surgeons and anatomists wielded powerful connections behind the scenes.

The relationship between physicians and high-ranking officials is epitomised by the following account. In 1801 a gang of resurrectionists supplying Sir Astley Cooper with anatomy subjects, implemented a plan whereby corpses packed in large baskets were left in his courtyard every night, awaiting transportation to the hospital. One evening they were interrupted by a police officer. When questioned by the officer, the famous surgeon claimed to have *no* responsibility for anything left in his courtyard. The subdued officer left, but stated his intent of reporting the matter to the Lord Mayor of London the following morning. Sir Astley Cooper however, forestalled the officer by arranging a breakfast meeting with the Mayor, during which he recounted the incident. The Mayor assured Cooper that police would not bother him again,[26] thereby strengthening the prevailing opinion amongst members of the medical profession that they were legally justified in such actions. It was even rumoured that Home Secretary Sir Robert Peel went out of his way to avoid prosecuting surgeons and resurrectionists.

Similarly, orders were frequently passed down to police officers to turn a blind eye to the thefts of bodies from public burial grounds and not to be overzealous in seeking out those responsible for, or the whereabouts of, stolen bodies. Officers who disobeyed could loose their positions.[27]

Sometimes, anatomist-surgeons were known to openly consort with resurrectionists. Anatomist John Hunter, was recognised as a great 'favourite' with the body snatchers, 'hobnobbing' with them as it were.[28] One particularly indiscreet entry in one of his casebooks confirms this. In September 1758 he writes '...we got a stout man for the muscles from St. George's ground'.[29] John Hunter's obscure 'we' suggests that he may well have been part of the group of men obtaining the corpse. He was well known to have 'body snatched' on many occasions,[30] when procuring corpses for his brother's anatomy school. As his treatise *The Anatomy of the Human Gravid Uterus* indicates, William Hunter dedicated much of his life to investigating the pregnant womb. However, not one to get his hands dirty, it was his anatomist brother John, whose intricate network of contacts amongst resurrectionists afforded him the opportunity of obtaining such 'specimens' – female bodies in various stages of pregnancy. How many other anatomist-surgeons were thus overtly involved in body snatching is obscure.

Until the passing of the Anatomy Act in 1832 in England, there *was* no alternative to body snatching. Anatomy was an integral part of medical students' training. Body snatching was high in demand and anatomists paid well. However, where possible surgeons stayed in the background and avoided any direct dealings with resurrectionists. The schools' porters and students placed a modicum of distance between body snatchers and the surgeons they supplied. Porters generally negotiated price and took deliverance of sacks and bags containing the 'goods', or picked them up at a designated spot. However, many records attest to direct contact between resurrectionists and anatomists. Often money not only changed hands on receipt of a corpse, but unabashed, resurrectionists regularly waited for anatomy lessons to be concluded in order to claim what was known as 'finishing money' from teachers at the schools. In documentation relating to renowned surgeon Sir Astley Cooper we read: 'May 10th, 1827, paid Hollis Vaughan and Llewellyn finishing money, £6 6s od. June 18th 1829, paid Murphy, Wildes & Naples finishing money £6 6s od.'[31]

But costs to medical schools did not end here. When a group of resurrectionists regularly supplied specific schools, anatomists often felt obliged to pay them a weekly allowance if they got caught and were forced to serve a minor sentence – which was however rare. Technically the theft of dead human bodies did not constitute a crime, because a corpse did not represent 'property'. While poachers, who often acted out of necessity and desperation to feed their families, were sentenced to death and those aiding and abetting them to transportation, robbing a grave of its body resulted in *no* form of punishment.[32] Unless clothes, coffin or valuables on the corpse itself had been stolen, the act of robbing a grave did not constitute a felony. Resurrectionists were well aware of this and were always careful to remove only the corpse devoid of all clothing or any other 'accompaniments'.

Dead-houses and mortsafes

Apprehension for the newly buried was widespread. Hence, the ever-increasing need to protect deceased loved ones soon led to an industry of specialised coffins, iron grids and additional cemetery buildings. Stone-houses, 'dead-houses' or mort houses were erected in graveyards. Here coffins could be stored for a few weeks until their content was of no use for dissection. Naturally, this service did not come free and demanded a fee from those wishing to ensure the safety of their newly-deceased loved-ones. Frequently these 'dead-houses' served several villages at once. Alternately, graveyards housed watch towers where guards could look after fresh graves at night. Unfortunately these individuals were often persuaded by lucrative bribes to look the other way. Wealthier families had mortsafes – huge pieces of stone or iron grids – placed on fresh graves. Some of these can still be seen in English, Scottish and Irish graveyards to this day. Another option for the well-to-do was to purchase special iron coffins.

Some relatives would literally sleep next to the grave of a loved-one for several nights after burial to deter any prospective body-snatchers. Some families employed 'watchers' in burial grounds to protect new graves from being robbed. Others would subtly place an unobtrusive object in a certain position on the grave of a loved-one, able to discern after a night or two whether the object had in fact been moved. But resurrection-men were wise to such ploys and able to spot them immediately. After robbing such a grave of its content, they simply carefully replaced the hidden clues in their exact spot.

Unable to afford comparable modes of protection for their loved-ones, the poorer classes were painfully aware of their vulnerability when it came to the nocturnal avtivities of body snatchers. After all it was they who helped in the construction of iron coffins, delivering them to the houses of the wealthy; it was they who built mortsafes, elaborate vaults or dug deeper graves. Feelings of resentment against those responsible for the outrage of marketing the dead, those who had betrayed their own class, ran deep in the social fabric of England at the time. Repeated assaults on resurrectionists and violent public riots, expressed a deep, ingrained frustration and helplessness with the order of things.

Essential funerary ritual

To understand the immense pain and grief caused by body snatching, popular death culture of the time needs to be illuminated. It was a culture coloured by the prevailing religious belief of a strong tie between body and soul after death. 'This belief underpinned the central role of the corpse in popular funerary ritual, and gained added power from confusion and ambiguity concerning both the definition of death and the spiritual status of the corpse. The result was an uncertain balance between solicitude towards the corpse and fear of it'.[33]

The popular notion that the dead could 'come again' or be 'troublesome' after death was regarded as the last revenge of the dead upon the living. Hence, 'proper' burial by adherence to funerary ritual was essential. Especially amongst the poorer classes superstitious fear dictated that everything possible be done to ensure the safe passage of the soul of the deceased into the afterlife, particularly because the deceased were considered far more powerful in that state than they ever were during their lifetime. As a result, complex and universally extensive customs evolved in all cultures around the dying and deceased. Scrupulous attentions to the proper rites of burial were by and large thought to ensure the peaceful departure of the deceased and the assurance that the dead did not return to the realm of the living.[34]

Burial practices were carried out carefully according to the belief that the deceased would ascend to heaven on Judgement Day. Especially the notion of keeping the physical body intact was strengthened in Europe by a literal acceptance of Christian doctrine of the resurrection of the dead. A widespread notion persisted that the destruction of the body could result in the loss of identity after death. Added to that the lingering dread that on the Day of Judgment the dissected corpse would be seen wandering around searching for its lost parts.

As Christians believed in the literal rising of the dead, the souls of dissected bodies could not go to heaven. Affecting and dictating how most people lived their lives, was the firm conviction that all those who had died and were buried, awaited Resurrection Day in their grave. In other words, graveyards were seen as solemn waiting grounds, from whence everyone would eventually be called to Judgement and eternity.

And the Church constantly reinforced this belief, preaching that humankind should lead pious Christian lives, in order that everyone would eventually be saved and 'go to heaven'. One can therefore barely imagine the terrible anguish and pain, caused to thousands of grief-stricken people by money-hungry body-snatchers, who were robbing loved-ones from their ultimate resting place.

The ultimate depravity

Sadly and perhaps predictably, the considerable amounts of money to be made from body snatching eventually led to murder. In 1752 Helen Torrence and Jean Waldie shocked the English people by murdering a child and selling the body to an anatomist.[35] Edinburgh resident John Wilson killed unsuspecting travellers, by offering them arsenic mixed with snuff and then selling the bodies to the medical school.[36] Two of the most famous and well-documented trials however, are those of Burke and Hare, as well as Bishop and Williams.

William Burke (1792-1829) and William Hare (c.1792-c.1858) launched into their crime spree quite by accident, when one of the tenants, in the boarding house they ran in Edinburgh, died. The deceased, an old man, owed rent and Burke and Hare decided to bring him to Dr. Robert Knox, a well known instructor at Edinburgh's largest private anatomy school. To their surprise and delight they were paid seven pounds for the corpse. Overjoyed at how easy it was to make so much money, they were spurned on by greed, committing sixteen murders over the next couple of months in 1828. For each corpse brought to Dr. Knox, they received between £7 and £14 – a small fortune for men of their standing.

Although they are often described as body snatchers, Burke and Hare's corpses had actually never been buried – some of the victims had never even left the boarding house, which the two men ran. Once Burke and Hare had singled someone out, the subject was asphyxiated – the men used their own form of strangulation, which later became known as 'burking'. Once the subject was dead and the right opportunity presented itself, the cadaver was sold to anatomist Dr. Robert Knox.

The first question which comes to mind is that surely the good doctor, who was a reputable anatomist after all, must have known or at least suspected that the corpses supplied to him had met with a murderous end. It could be argued that there must have been some evidence of foul play, glaringly obvious for a medically trained individual to discern. But, he asked no questions and unsympathetically turned a blind eye. At the time of Burke's confessions a sixpenny pamphlet titled *Echo of Surgeon's Square*, appeared on the streets, purporting to expose certain hitherto unknown facts pertaining to the murders, as well as much information about the running of the anatomy establishment.

Apart from general information, two disclosures made, added to the suspicions surrounding the person of Dr. Knox himself. Firstly, it was stated that several of the bodies supplied by Burke and Hare showed blood around the mouth, nose and ears, and secondly, that the body of one Jamie Daft – a well known street character in Edinburgh – had had both feet as well as his head severed prior to delivery at Knox's school. Today it is known that the source of these writings came from a doorman at Knox's school, probably eager to exonerate himself of any blame. Awaiting execution Burke told his jailers that the doctor asked no questions and that when a body was delivered they were always told to bring more.[37]

The murders eventually came to light in 1828 when one of the tenants in Burke and Hare's boarding house, found a corpse 'awaiting' delivery. The culprits were soon arrested. Hare turned state witness and testified against his associate in exchange for amnesty. Burke was tried, convicted, hanged and his body publicly dissected and displayed. His complete skeleton, as well as his death mask, taken a day after he was hanged – the bite of the rope around his neck clearly visible in the plaster cast – are still on display at the University of Edinburgh's Anatomical Museum. While Burke's actual dissection was witnessed by a number of select ticket-holders, the general public eagerly viewed his sliced up corpse on the next day. In a macabre spectacle at the 'grand public exhibition' more than thirty thousand people passed through the anatomical theatre in Edinburgh to stare at the partially dissected body on the black marble slab – the murderer's dissection fittingly justified in the eyes of the public.

Dr. Knox, who did not deem it fit to voice an apology, went unpunished. Failure of the authorities to investigate Knox at the time, led to disbelief, bitterness and anger. This was an era in England, when poor people were routinely hanged, imprisoned or transported for even the smallest of misdemeanours – the Knox case simply highlighted again that there seemed to be separate laws for the rich and for the poor. Public opinion favoured an obvious cover-up. Widely held resentment and outrage against Knox in Edinburgh soon turned to rioting and rowdy demonstrations.[38] Change was inevitably on the cards. But a similar murder case was yet to occur again, before Parliament was forced to act against the desecration of robbing corpses from graves and acquiring corpses through murder.

In 1831 John Bishop (died 1831) and Thomas Williams (died 1831) killed three people in London in order to sell their bodies for dissection. As was customary, they had pulled out all teeth from the cadavers, but the fact that the corpse of one of the victims, a young boy, had been 'knocked around' in transit, while the perpetrators offered it to various anatomy schools, caused a huge public outcry. For the first time, ill treatment and desecration of a corpse by body snatchers, as well as by members of the medical establishment, was publicly reported for all to read. Bishop and Williams were convicted for murder, hanged and their bodies given up for dissection. The case was reported in all newspapers and pamphlets of the day.

A lack of decorum

Written references to the thousands of cadavers dissected over time are oblique, as though the subject matter was far too offensive to discuss. In most cases, even in medical literature, allusions as to how and where bodies for dissection were obtained and how they were discarded are either totally absent or blurred. The language used was one of unemotional and detached indifference. Never was mention made of the humanity of the subjects, on which students would after all spend hours carefully cutting and slicing away.

Many indignities were perpetuated on bodies brought for dissection.

The body of a young woman, voluptuous Edinburgh prostitute Mary Paterson, whom Burke and Hare had smothered and brought to Dr. Knox in Edinburgh for dissection, was displayed naked at the school for all to see. 'Because of her beauty, the corpse was kept in whisky for three months before she was dissected'.[39] Since her 'attributes' were particularly shapely, several artists came to paint her. In fact, Dr. Knox personally brought an artist to paint her and several sketches of Mary Paterson are still in existence. 'The dissecting room was a place in which gross indecencies were performed and not only by medical men'.[40] There are even reports of subjects being raped on the dissecting slab in front of students.[41] Sexual indecency was not the only degradation propagated on the bodies of the dead. Many reports told of naked bodies crammed into crooked, twisted, perverse positions in sacks or small confined spaces, lacking all dignity and respect.

In addition, as there is no evidence that they were in fact buried, the widespread belief prevailed that the remnants of dissected victims were treated as offal, fed to the dogs, or made into manure. In 1829 *Medicus Magazine* wrote that 'human remains from dissection were cast away as mere filth or given as food to animals.' Similarly the *Political Anecdotist* of 1831[42] stated: 'The Anatomica Department of King's College will be situated nearest the Thames, for the greater facility, it is supposed, of feeding the fish.' Also, the widespread notion persisted that soap and candles were made from human fat harvested from the dissection table.

However, there were those in the medical profession who while recognising that dissection was a necessary learning tool, nevertheless had a profound distaste for the practice. George Guthrie (1785-1856), professor of Anatomy and Surgery at the Royal College of Surgeons in London, in his 1832 pamphlet on the *Anatomy Bill*, denounced the hypocrisy of doctors 'who recommended dissection for the poor, yet who went to considerable pains to ensure that their own bodies did not even undergo post-mortem examinations.[43] Progressive intellectuals such as Jeremy Bentham[44] (1748 –1832), founder of University College London, were the first to donate their remains, thus helping to overcome the stigma attached to dissection.

Jeremy Bentham left instructions that after his death, his body be turned over to anatomists for dissection, expressing the hope that his body might be of use to science after it had ceased being of service to his own person. In addition though, he made stipulations, which were somewhat out of the ordinary to say the least: after dissection his skeleton was to be kept intact; his head and hands preserved. Furthermore, he should be dressed in his customary attire, and be placed in his old familiar chair in his habitual pose. Bentham's specific conditions regrading his corpse arose from his odd personal notion that the dead should not be hidden deep in the ground, but surrounded by relatives and friends.

Following his death in 1832 at the age of eighty-four, his trusted friends conscientiously carried out Bentham's requests. After his body had been dissected, a replica wax head was placed on his skeleton; he was then dressed in his own clothes and placed in his old armchair, which was enclosed in a glass and mahogany case – he is still on permanent display in the Anatomical Museum of University College Hospital in London. Attempts to preserve his real head were unsuccessful. However, the mummified head is also on view in the Anatomical Museum – although parched and withered, it is lying at the skeletal feet of the seated Jeremy Bentham.

Approaching legislative changes

We have to ask ourselves in earnest, why the ruling classes in England did not legislate sooner for a solution to the supply and demand problem of corpses for anatomists. Making the robbing of graves a criminal offense would have been sufficient and highly effective in putting an end to much misery and fear. But, authorities turned a blind eye. After all, body snatchers rarely interfered with the graves of those in authoritative positions or the well-to-do. Also, the army and navy were desperately short of skilled surgeons, and the need for them to master their craft was appreciated.

Similarly, established Churches displayed a flagrant lack of interest in the activities of body snatchers. Had ecclesiastic institutions reacted to public outcry, which grew in intensity over the decades, or had Church leaders expressed strong concern and promoted law adjustments to the legal supply of unclaimed bodies for anatomical purposes, change would have been effected over a century earlier.

Although many have attributed the passage of the Anatomy Act to the numerous murders committed, in order to supply anatomists, it should be kept in mind that the heinous Burke and Hare murders already occurred in 1828, while the Anatomy Act was not implemented until four years later in 1832. Again this may be attributed to the fact that the murdered or 'burked' victims stemmed from the lower classes of society and not from the ruling elite. As body-snatching activities increased, the wealthy simply protected their own more efficiently, thus choosing not to address a widespread social problem. It was only when Sir Astley Cooper arrogantly revealed his ability to obtain the body of *any* person regardless of their station in life, that the attentions of the ruling classes were alerted. He haughtily proclaimed that '…there is no person, let his situation in life be what it may, who, if I were disposed to dissect, I could not obtain'.[45] Indeed, it seems certain that '…the bodies of wealthy, intellectual, eccentric, insane, aristocratic or otherwise medically interesting people from the middle and upper classes were obtained by various means'.[46]

A perusal of the strange Hunterian Collection at the Royal College of Surgeons in London, adequately proves this point.[47] Renowned anatomist and founder of the Hunterian Collection, John Hunter, fostered his personal relationship with resurrectionists, and was known to offer '…the highest prices to ensure a regular supply of dissection material for himself and his students. In particular he was notorious for paying above the odds for any kind of anatomical curiosity, whether rare human deformities or the result of a pioneering, but ultimately fatal operation'.[48] Hunter actively sought out the unusual and extraordinary for his collection. For instance he bought the 'remains' of the Irish Giant while the huge man was still alive. But, when the man felt his death to be imminent, he regretted having 'sold' his soon to be dead body, and tried to escape from his London quarters. However, Hunter's servants shadowed him until his death and subsequently brought the body home 'in triumph'.[49] Today the huge skeleton is still on exhibit in Hunter's Collection.

With the passage of time, alternatives to grave robbery were earnestly sought as anatomists increasingly tried to distance themselves from the odium of exhumation and the exorbitant prices demanded for cadavers. Artificial corpses, models, animals and props were tried as substitutes for the 'real thing'. In addition, various means were tried to preserve human flesh in order to delay purtrefication, so existing cadavers would last longer. But, these methods and alternatives proved frustratingly inadequate. Anatomy schools in the early nineteenth century continued to rely on bodies supplied by underhand practices until the Anatomy Act was finally passed in 1832, making unclaimed bodies from poor houses available to anatomists. The gruesome age of body snatching was finally over in England.

The following chapters deal with repulsive examples of medications that dominated medical directives right up to the eighteenth century. For centuries, orthodox medical practitioners made use of various forms of excrement, human and animal, as well as human flesh, blood, bone and fat in prescriptive medications.

VII

SEWER PHARMACOLOGY – FILTHY MEDICINE

In the developed world faeces, whether animal or human are considered dirty and disgusting, their proper place being in a sewer or septic tank. However, societies in rural areas, which are closely connected to the land, see this type of waste as a prized resource. Millions of people use excrement as a fertiliser and as one of the world's foremost cooking fuels when dried. In addition, excrement is made into bricks or used in road building.[1] It may however come as a surprise that not only animal dung, but also human faeces, urine and other bodily excretions were once extensively used internally and externally to cure numerous ailments, and that this practice is still adhered to in various cultures.

Medical historians generally refer to the practice of using excrement in medications as 'sewer pharmacology'. Surprisingly, this healing option was not only used by the ancients, but also popularly and most abundantly utilised by physicians during medieval and later times. What is even more surprising is the fact that this treatment is finding a partial resurgence in modern medicine.

Ancient 'filthy' medicine

In past medicinal practices, repulsive, disgusting and mystifying examples of 'medications' often dominated directives. Urine, excrement, saliva and various other bodily secretions appear in the pharmacopoeias of many cultures. In India and Middle Eastern countries, urine and excreta from animals and humans have been used for centuries as a medicinal cure, and to maintain good health. Advocates of urine therapy generally refer to the Biblical recommendation: 'Drink waters out of thine own cistern'[2] to strengthen their argument. Similar 'self-remedy' appears in all ancient religious and medical texts. Ancient Indian holy texts, like the *Atharva Veda*, *Charaka Samhita*, and *Sushruta Samhita* advocate the drinking of cow urine to treat various ailments, while the ancient Chinese used urine medicinal therapies more than two thousand years ago.[3]

Similarly, in ancient Egypt, the 'cure' sometimes seems to have been far worse than the disease itself – excrement of human and animal derivation was widely used in medications. On the surface, the dominant ancient Egyptian approach to healing lay in magic. But this should not distract from the vast amount of information in ancient Egyptian records on internal medicine, surgery, as well as a pharmacopoeia based on millennia of experience. Sewer pharmacology had its rightful place in Egypt and according to the principles of sympathetic magic[4] contemptible mixtures of excrement were thought to successfully drive out disease-causing demons. In time, it seems that many of these remedies were indeed found to have a positive healing effect, which is perhaps why their use was continued.

The *Ebers Papyrus* (circa 1550 BCE), alone, contains fifty-five specific prescriptions in which faecal matter and urine are primary ingredients. Many of the preparations are as putrid and repulsive as they are confounding. Interestingly, instructions in the *Ebers Papyrus* are surprisingly specific in expressly recommending the excretions from specific animals to treat a singular disease or condition.

Various prescriptions call for one or two of the following to be mixed with other components: fly, pelican and gazelle droppings, lizard and crocodile excrement, human faecal matter and urine – to be used internally, as well as externally. For example, male semen, utilised as a flavouring agent in a mixture of various other substances, was prescribed to relieve abdominal obstruction; human excrement, to be mixed with yeast and honey, was recommended as a dressing for wounds; human urine was to be used specifically to treat acute burns, as this invocation suggests: "Your son Horus has burnt himself in the desert." "Is there any water here?" "There is no water here." "Water is in my mouth, a Nile is between my thighs, I have come to extinguish the fire." "Flow out, burn."[5, 6] As ancient Egyptian physicians *did* record many recoveries on such specific treatments, it seems that in spite of their repulsive nature, these practices and medications proved effective in many cases.

Excrement and urine were also widely used by ancient Greek physicians in treating various ailments and medical conditions. In his book *The Water of Life,* John Armstrong relates '…The wiser of the ancient Greeks used nothing but urine for the treatment of wounds'.[7] The widespread use of excrementous material during the times of Hippocrates may be deduced from the writings of his contemporaries. For instance, playwright Aristophanes (c. 446-386 BCE), whose powers of ridicule were feared by influential contemporaries, stigmatised all medical practitioners as 'excrement eaters'.[8] Greek physician Xenocrates of Aphrodisias, who lived to mid-first century CE[9] is said to have made constant use of human and animal excrement in his medical practice and also recommended human sweat, earwax and menstrual fluid to be used externally and internally.[10]

Although Galen did not agree with Xenocrates's 'filthy medications' he did advocate the '…ordure of a boy, dried, mixed with Attic honey. The urine of a virgin boy or girl is an invaluable application for affections of the eyes, stings of bees, wasps and other insects'.[11] Greek physician and pharmacologist Dioscorides (c. 40-90 CE), author of the well known *De Materia Medica,* devotes a whole chapter in listing dozens of different ordures and their medical values: stork dung as a remedy for epilepsy; mouse dung to expel calculi; dog dung used against angina; hen dung for dysentery; crocodile dung to be used as a cosmetic; fresh human excrement to be applied to wounds; the patient's own urine for a variety of conditions, especially against poisons of all kinds, and the urine of an undefiled boy commended for various purposes, especially when mixed with honey – the list is endless.[12]

Roman historian and prolific writer Pliny the Elder (23-79 CE) is a veritable mine of information on the subject of 'sewer pharmacology', listing: camel, goat, dog, bull, mouse, dove, swallow, pigeon, wolf, calf and hyena dung, as well as human excrement, urine and other bodily fluids, to alleviate and cure all manner of physical ailments. He notes for instance that the seminal fluid of athletes is a 'sovereign remedy for the sting of scorpions' and recommends that fresh excrement voided at the moment of birth by an infant, made into a pessary, is invaluable for curing sterility in women.[13] The list of hundreds of possible combinations of dung, urine, blood and other ingredients', to be applied externally or to be ingested, is never-ending, indicating how established these remedies were at the time.

Pliny relates the various theories regarding human urine and its medical utilisation prevalent amongst contemporary physicians, stating unequivocally: 'Our authorities attribute to urine great power.'[14] Warm urine, cow dung, and goat dung were to be applied to scrofulous sores. The urine of boys below the age of puberty had many special uses '…added to fenugreek it is prescribed for swellings of the hypochondria, […] to sinews it is applied with juice of henbane, for freckles, in vinegar and honey. […]. It is used warm, in red wine, for the stings of scorpions, spitting of blood, and for tracheal affections. For a cough, goat-suet or butter is added'.[15] Furthermore, it was thought that men's urine relieved gout, and old urine added to the ash of burnt oyster-shells was used to treat rashes on the bodies of babies and for all running ulcers. Pitted sores, burns, affections of the anus, chaps, and scorpion stings, were all treated by applications of urine.

The most celebrated midwives have declared that no other lotion is better treatment for irritation of the skin, and with soda added for sores on the head, dandruff, and spreading ulcers, especially on the genitals'.[16] The urine of eunuchs was regarded as highly beneficial to promote 'fruitfulness' in women, while the urine of children was a 'sovereign remedy' in treating snakebites. Pliny writes '…each person's own urine, if it be proper for me to say so, does him the most good,' thereby advocating the ancient practice of urine therapy.[17]

Medieval and early modern sewer pharmacology

Strange as it may seem from a modern perspective, the utilisation of 'sewer pharmacology' continued for centuries beyond ancient Greek and Roman times, and was still in vogue during the mid-eighteenth century. The widespread use of such confronting medical directives may perhaps be easier to understand when considered from a framework of contemporary living conditions. For centuries people in European towns and cities lived in 'stinking' environs, surrounded by squalor and filth. Cities and towns smelled strongly of sewage, human faeces, urine and rotting matter.

What would offend modern sensibilities as intolerable was once accepted as a matter of course: 'The streets stank of manure, the courtyards of urine, the stairwells stank of mouldering wood and rat droppings, the kitchens of spoiled cabbage and mutton fat; the unaired parlours stank of stale dust, the bedrooms of greasy sheets, damp featherbeds, and the pungently sweet aroma of chamber pots. The stench of sulphur rose from the chimneys, the stench of caustic lyes from the tanneries, and from the slaughterhouses came the stench of congealed blood. People stank of sweat and unwashed clothes; from their mouths came the stench of rotting teeth, from their bellies that of onions, and from their bodies, if they were no longer very young, came the stench of rancid cheese and sour milk and tumorous disease. The rivers stank, the marketplaces stank, the churches stank, it stank beneath the bridges and in the palaces. The peasant stank as did the priest, the apprentice as did his master's wife, the whole of the aristocracy stank, even the king himself stank…'.[18]

Hence it is almost not surprising, that sixteenth and seventeenth European pharmacopoeias abound with recipes containing the most revolting, disgusting ingredients. In London the official Latin *Pharmacopoeia Londinensis*, produced in 1618 by the Royal College of Physicians, lists hundreds of recipes to be used by physicians – and physicians *did* prescribe these remedies. Not only are countless exotic constituents such as worms, dried snakes, fox's lungs, oil of ants and many others listed, but also ingredients obtained from human cadavers; human semen, human fat, human earwax and spittle, human perspiration, and fasting-saliva,[19] human and animal urine, and excrement or 'turds'.

One of the chapters in the *Pharmacopoeia Londinensis* catalogues: '...Parts of living Creatures and Excrement' apothecaries should keep in their shops at all times.[20] Among these are: '...Dogs Turd, Vipers flesh, the brain of Hares and Sparrows, Crabs claws, the runners of a Lamb, Kid, Hare, Calf and Horse [...] a Cocks comb the tooth of a Bore, an Elephant and a Sea Horse [...] stone in an Ox gall, stones in the bladder of a man, the Jaw of a Pike [...] the pizel (penis) of a Stag, of a Bull, Fasting Spittle, blood of a Pidgeon, of a Cat, of a Goat, of a Hare, of a Heifer...'.[21]

In addition: '...the Turds of a Goose, of a Dog, of a Goat, of Pidgeons, of a Stone Horse, of a Hen, of Swallows, of Men, of Women, of Mice, of a Peacock, of a Hog, of a Heifer...'.[22] Also: 'all Turds in general especially Pidgeons and Goats dung',[23] '...the piss of a Boar, of a she Goat, of a man or woman that is a maid...'[24] '...Bullocks dung made in May, Swallows, Earth worms, Magpies, spawn of Frogs'.[25] The list continues with cleansing medicines such as '...Honey, Sugar, Salt, Urine, especially your own Urine, white Wine, these generally cleanse all wounds and Ulcers...'.[26]

The *Medicus Microcosmus*, a work by physician Daniel Beckherius (1594-1655), published in London in 1660, extols at length the many virtues of excrementitious preparations. The book promotes countless recipes, mixtures and lotions made with one's own urine and the urine of others. The book also advocates the drinking of stale urine, washing with urine, urine baths, as well as the distillation of urine and salt of urine for remedial uses.

Daniel Beckherius recommends urine especially from healthy young individuals, as well as plasters made from human urine and a variety of other ingredients. He cites a case where dried human excrement, powdered and drunk in wine for three days cured a man of yellow jaundice. For angina he prescribed the white dung of dogs powdered, mixed with human ordure, swallow droppings and liquorice. Goat urine drunk regularly for a time, was prescribed to expel *calculi* of the bladder, while hawk dung and cow urine alternately were applied to sore eyes.[27] Dozens of similar recipes mixed with equally popular ingredients such as potable gold or mercury, are contained in Daniel Beckherius's *Medicus Microcosmus*.

In his popular work *Complete English Dispensatory* (1721), English apothecary and medical writer John Quincy (died 1722) advocates innumerable different urine therapies. In a chapter titled 'Distillation of Urine', John Quincy recommends salts obtained from 'the urine of a sound young man' in the treatment of rheumatism and arthritis.[28] Human or animal urine was to be evaporated or distilled, fermented or drunk fresh. Quincy advocates the minerals alum and kali mixed with urine to provoke vomiting;[29] cow's 'piss' was to be drunk as a purge.[30]

Furthermore, the ingested dung of various animals is commended as the prevalent medicine against dropsy, pleurisy, jaundice, scurvy as well as bladder and kidney stones. Excrement and droppings made into plasters were utilised in the localised treatment of swellings and pain. It should be pointed out to the sceptics that Quincy's *Complete English Dispensatory*[31] was so widely used by physicians that the twelfth edition of the book was published in 1749 – twenty-eight years after initial publication.

On the Continent, repulsive medical directives did not differ from those prescribed in England. The following quotation by Martin Luther (1483-1546) attests to the once popular use of medicines consisting of human excrement and other bodily secretions: 'Truly, it surprises me that God has put such superior medication into filth'.[32] Similarly, flamboyant Swiss-born Renaissance physician Paracelsus writes: 'Man's dung or excrement, hath very great virtues, because it contains in it all the noble essences'. Of man's urine he declares: 'The salt of man's urine hath an excellent quality to cleanse, it is made thus'.[34] Although he was an advocate of the medicinal properties of human excrement and urine, Paracelsus nevertheless reviled the physicians of his day who '…made very many medicines of most filthy things, as of the filth of ears, sweat of the body, of women's menstrues, spittle, flies, mice…'.[35]

The filthiest book in world literature

Unquestionably one of the 'filthiest' books in world literature is the *Heilsame Dreck-Apotheke* or *Therapeutic Dirt Pharmacy*',[36] written in

1696. Its author, German born Franz Christian Paullini (1643-1711), was an eminent physician, well travelled and highly regarded in European countries. Paullini's book is full of nauseating, revolting prescriptions, when taking modern sensibilities into consideration. But, the book was hugely popular at the time. Just how popular is proven by the printing of the fourth enlarged and revised edition published in 1734. This revised edition of the *Heilsame Dreck-Apotheke* consisted of double the volume of its original. Two further editions were published a couple of years later. Paullini's book was translated into English and the practices and recipes it contained widely discussed, used, and disseminated. The '...numerous references in the book to individual doctors, demonstrate that the *Dreck-Apotheke* was indeed a widely practiced form of medicine in popular culture'.[37]

According to its title *Heilsame Dreck-Apotheke* or *Therapeutic Dirt Pharmacy*, the purpose of the book was to successfully cure almost all ailments, even the most serious diseases, from head to toe, internally and externally, with human as well as animal excrement and urine. However, the *Dreck-Apotheke* is not exclusively devoted to faeces and urine but to a variety of bodily secretions such as menstrual blood, mucous, pus, perspiration and earwax. Giving hundreds of examples from his own medical practice, as well as from medical texts, Paullini promotes the exceptional virtues of human stool and urine and all the other 'delightful' secretions mentioned. Apart from human 'by-products', Paullini also recommends the excrement and urine from domestic and other animals, such as squirrels, cuckoos, peacocks, owls, wolves, bears, lizards and spiders – many of these recipes supplemented with non-repulsive substances such as wine, herbs, honey and vinegar.

Similarly, renowned German physician Michaelus Ettmüller (1644-1683) considered medicines made from human excrement and urine highly effective. But, whereas Ettmüller expounded at length on the *reasons* behind the use of ordure in general, Paullini collected and listed cases in which human and animal excreta were employed.

Aureomycin – the 'golden fungus'

Remarkably, several discoveries made during the twentieth century suggest that physicians of the past were not far off the mark in their medicinal directives. Ancient Egyptian doctors may well have been on the right track thousands of years ago, when they fought various types of infection by using excrement, urine, as well as 'mud from the Nile'. In 1948 the discovery of the antibiotic aureomycin was hailed as one of *the* most significant medical breakthroughs. This finding significantly changed modern evaluation of ancient medicine, leading to a new perspective on Egypt's medical achievements.

The antibiotic aureomycin was introduced to the world by Benjamin Duggar (1872–1956) professor of Plant Physiology at the University of Missouri and Washington University. He became widely known for his work with moulds and *fungi* and later turned to research new antibacterial drugs. Although penicillin and streptomycin were being widely used to treat bacterial infections, a number of diseases and strains of bacteria were resistant to these treatments. Duggar focused his research on specific groups of moulds found in soil and mud particularly in the vicinity of cemeteries. After testing thousands of samples, he was successful in finding a mould active against the *staphylococci* and *streptococci bacilli*. Duggar named the substance he had discovered 'aureomycin', from the Latin word *aureus* meaning 'gold', and the Greek word *mykes* meaning 'fungus'.

Overnight, the 'golden fungus', aureomycin, became the new wonder drug. Dr. Duggar's discovery brought to light that waste products resulting from the metabolic processes of particular moulds in soil and mud have an annihilating effect on specific bacteria. Similar waste products are found in mud and soils where once living material has decayed – especially in earth from around cemeteries. Furthermore, the same principle holds true for bacteria living in a human or animal body. Bacteria release their excretory products into the host's excrement. In other words, the excrement of various animals and humans contains different antibiotic substances.[38]

Bacillus subtilis – dung to the rescue

Similarly, the detection of the *bacillus subtilis* makes fascinating reading. *Bacillus subtilis* is a bacterial micro-organism commonly found in the environment rather than in humans. The Nazi German medical corps discovered the *bacillus* in 1941, toward the end of their African campaign. Although German military victory was at its height, hundreds upon hundreds of soldiers in this campaign suddenly began dying every week – not by battle conflict, but from uncontrollable dysentery. Naturally, the Germans were aware that this problem was caused by pathogens in the local food and water supply. Yet strangely, none of the local Bedouins seemed to get ill.

Shortly, a contingent of scientists, chemists, biochemists, bacteriologists and other experts were sent from Germany to help solve the problem. It was soon discovered that the Bedouins *did* contract dysentery, but that they followed a peculiar practice at the onset of symptoms: they would immediately ingest warm camel dung, following the animal around until the dung could be collected fresh and still tepid. This curious procedure successfully purged their dysentery almost overnight. Apparently the custom had been followed for generations – in fact for as long as anyone could remember. Upon scientific examination it was discovered that camel and horse dung teem with a powerful bacterial micro-organism, which later became known as *bacillus subtilis*. This bacterial micro-organism is so potent that it eliminates all harmful micro-organisms in the human body, including pathogenic bacteria like the virulent strain causing dysentery in the German troops.

Soon hundreds of gallons of active *bacillus subtilis* cultures were produced for the German troops to ingest, resulting in the total eradication of dysentery. Cultures of *bacillus subtilis* were sold worldwide as a medicinal product for many years to come until the advent of synthetic antibiotics in the late 1950's. Nonetheless, *bacillus subtilis* remains one of the most potent and beneficial of all health-promoting and immune-stimulating bacteria.[39]

Similarly urine has been used in various cultures around the world for centuries, as a medicinal cure and to maintain good health. Interestingly, various modern studies with regard to this bodily fluid have been found to support the claims of past medical practitioners.[40] It seems that not only were physicians of the past on the right track with their disgusting medications, but the practice is finding a modern resurgence: twenty-first century doctors treat bowel infections through fecal transplant procedures. These involve taking stool samples from healthy people, mixing them with saline solution and transferring the mixtures into the colons of those infected with the superbug *Clostridium difficile*, a nasty bacterium, which is speedily developing resistance to antibiotics. In clinical trials conducted, such fecal transplants successfully cured ninety-one per cent of patients of their bowel infections.[41]

Given some of the unusual modern findings and discoveries relating to the so-called 'sewer pharmacology' of ancient, medieval and later times, this may give profound new meaning to the old saying: 'Where there is muck, there is luck!'

VII

Corpse medicine –
medical cannibalism

In modern times our immediate reaction to this topic is one not only of revulsion, but also the resolute conviction that such remedies were surely restricted only to the illiterate masses. Corpse medicine or 'medical cannibalism' is a topic not widely discussed or even recognised in modern medical circles. Those vaguely aware of this subject matter, relegate corpse medicine to the realm of superstitious practices by common people. Nothing could however be further from the truth.

Widely used by ancient cultures and popular from medieval times until the late eighteenth century, corpse medicine was once an important part of mainstream medicine, accepted and in most cases advocated by educated physicians at the time. Ironically, corpse medicine was most persistently used in Europe after the fifteenth century '…in an era when reports of New World cannibals were circulating amidst the outraged Christians of Rome, Madrid, London and Wittenberg'.[1] For the sceptics it may be added that references in medical textbooks, to what is today known as 'corpse' medicine by historians, are far too numerous and detailed to doubt that these medications were not simply written about – they were in fact earnestly prescribed and actively recommended by medical establishments for centuries. Acknowledgement and acceptance of such medical practices is clearly evident from the total lack of repulsion and distaste affirmed in the numerous written accounts.

Rich and poor alike enthusiastically partook in 'medical cannibalism', which was not '…limited to the fringe groups of society, but practiced in the most respectable circles'.[2] This point is aptly illustrated by numerous prescriptions from the highly popular *Complete English Dispensatory*, first published in 1721. The recognition this book received from physicians is attested to by the fact that its twelfth edition appeared in 1749, twenty-eight years after its initial publication.

The *Complete English Dispensatory* recommends countless human body parts to be used medicinally. For bruises its author, apothecary and medical writer John Quincy, recommends the 'fat of a man',[3] as well as fat from the bodies of dogs, vipers and bears; he advocates distilled human skull,[4] as well as powdered human skull mixed with powder of mistletoe, snake-root, elk's-hoof, red coral and various oriental stones for the treatment of epilepsy.[5]

Furthermore, he prescribes the powdered 'bones of a man', mixed with turpentine, sugar and senna in the treatment of arthritis.[6] Similarly, a powder for epilepsy made up of peony-root, native cinnabar, and powdered man's skull.[7] Another of Quincy's recipes to cure epilepsy and vertigo contains powdered human skull, to be taken twice-daily.[8] Countless such examples are contained in European pharmacopoeias from centuries past.

For hundreds of years medical prescriptions, or 'recipes', providing instructions on how to process human bodies, were as familiar as the use of plants, herbs and roots. On 30 January 2009 the German magazine *Der Spiegel* published an article titled *Europe's Medicinal Cannibalism* declaring: 'Research shows that up until the end of the 18th century, medicine routinely included stomach-churning ingredients like human flesh and blood.'

Orthodox physicians extensively used human flesh, blood, fat and bone as curative, medicinal agents. In fact, '…dead bodies, those of convicts as well as those of children, were the object of procedures within popular medicine, and of official pharmaceutical prescriptions. What was sought after above all was the fat, but also blood, teeth, hair, burnt skull, the umbilicus, and other parts and substances of the body that possessed specific healing properties'.[9] Human flesh was commonly pickled, dried and powdered or cut into thin strips to be chewed and ingested. Similarly, human blood was a popular medicinal. Other forms of 'corpse medicine' were equally popular: Egyptian mummy for instance, was in such high demand for prescriptions, as to warrant a sizeable counterfeiting market, with fraudulent substitutes still for sale well into the eighteenth century.

Skulls, powdered, grated or distilled, were used as effective 'physick' – an obsolete term for medicine. Whole human skulls, often partially covered with moss – considered especially effective in curing nosebleeds – were for sale in apothecary shops. Similarly human fat, in the form of ointment, was a popular remedy to alleviate rheumatism and arthritis. Other parts of human cadavers were likewise used. For example, *Corium humanum*, or human skin, tanned and cut into strips was in demand by licensed midwives and pregnant woman in general, to ease the pangs of childbirth – the skin strips worn like a belt during labor. In addition, strips of human skin, worn around the joints were thought to alleviate arthritic pains.[10]

It is therefore not surprising that William Shakespeare in his tragedy *Macbeth*, has the third witch adding human body parts to the cauldron, in addition to those derived from animals and plants. Apart from 'Witches' mummy – made from mummified human flesh, she throws in 'Liver of blaspheming Jew', as well as 'Nose of Turk and Tartar's lips' and 'Finger of birth-strangled babe' – a babe, which had been delivered by its whore-mother in a ditch and then killed.[11] It is difficult to believe, but human body parts were still routinely prescribed for various ailments during the late eighteenth century.

Human cadaver parts and blood were available in every pharmacy, and recipes of the times routinely included so-called 'corpse medicine'. The *Pharmacopoeia Londinensis* produced in 1618 by the London College of Physicians included numerous human body parts, such as mummy, skull, bone, fat and blood – to which new ones were added on a yearly basis.[12] Fundamentally, it was not until the 1721 edition of the *Pharmacopoeia Londinensis* that any significant changes were made: botanical names of herbal remedies were added to the official ones and distilled liquids were prescribed in a uniform strength. But, although many of the previous remedies were omitted, the use of excrement and various body-parts such as mummy,[13] human fat,[14] human blood,[15] human skull[16] and moss obtained from human skulls[17] were still maintained and recommended in the *Pharmacopoeia Londinensis* 1747 edition.

In 1662 Johann Joachim Becher (1635-1682), personal physician to the Elector of Mainz, Germany, recommended that apothecaries should keep at least twenty-three different kinds of human materials in store '...indeed, apothecary inventories and pharmacopoeias confirm that a ready supply of human raw materials was on hand'.[18] As undisputable proof of medical exploitation of the human cadaver, the official pharmacopoeia of the imperial city of Nüremberg, Germany, dated 1652, lists: '...whole human skull (*Cranii Humani Integri*), and prepared human skull, human grains (*Granii Humani*), mummy or "marinated flesh" (*balsamiertes Menschenfleisch*) human fat (*Pinguedo Hominis*), salt from human grains (*Salii Granii Humanis*), and spirit of human bone (*Spiritus Ossium Humanorum*)'.[19]

Similarly, *Lemery's Medical Dictionary*, a standard authority in Europe during the eighteenth century lists virtually all parts of the human body, as well as many of its products, for medicinal use.[20] A medicinal recipe written by German professor of medicine at the University of Marburg, Oswald Crollius (c. 1563-1609) [21] prescribes the flesh of a 'reddish' young man, who had died a violent death and had then been exposed to the moon's rays for a day and a night. After such exposure the body was to be cut into small pieces, sprinkled with herbs and soaked in a mixture of wine and turpentine. The pieces were to dry in an arid and shady place, after which they would be without any stench.[22] The emphasis in this recipe is on the young man having died a violent death – a common factor in medicinal recipes of the time.

The healing power of the human body

But where does the belief in the healing powers of the human body originate and how did physicians explain these perceived healing powers? In addition, why were especially executed individuals sought after for their curative 'powers'? Nobody can answer these questions with any degree of certainty, but various explanations exist. During the sixteenth and seventeenth centuries, doctors and jurists agreed that a body after death retained a certain degree of 'sensitivity'.[23,24] According to learned physicians at the time, the healing power of a newly deceased corpse stemmed from the life force, which remained in the body after the moment of aberrant death. In other words, it was postulated that all organisms have a predetermined life span. If a body died in an unnatural way, the remainder of that person's life force could be 'harvested', as it were – hence, the preference for the executed.

Paracelsus expressed this belief most concisely, arguing that '…the healing life force was strongest in the body of a young and healthy person who had died a sudden, violent death. He condemned the medicinal use of cadavers of persons who had died of natural causes, comparing their flesh to skinner's carrion'.[25] Belgian physician Jean Baptiste van Helmont (1577-1644) in his work *A Ternary of Paradoxes* similarly provided the succinct answer that it is: '…the originary, implantate and confermentate spirit safely remaining and in an obscure vitality surviving in bodies extinct by violence'.[26]

While the more fortunate and educated acknowledged the explanations of physicians, regarding the curative powers of the human cadaver, a reason based on magic probably appealed more to the common masses. At a time when little was known about the origins of illness and disease, it was popularly believed, that evil entities were the root cause of all maladies. It was also firmly held that perpetrators, executed on the gibbet or block, were themselves wicked or evil. Hence, according to the principle that 'like affects like', evil could dispel evil. In other words, using the various body parts of those executed could successfully cure illnesses, thought to originate through malevolent forces. Such examples of 'sympathetic magic' abounded in the social setting of times past and were commonly accepted.

Up until 1868, when hangings in England ceased to be public, many offenders, sentenced to be gibbeted after execution, were left suspended indefinitely, coated with tar to delay the process of decay – to passers-by this conveyed the very clear message that crime definitely did not pay.[27] While in this suspended state many deliberate indignities took place, inflicted on the exposed corpses of convicted criminals. Often their teeth would be pulled out and kept as charms against toothache, according to the principle that 'like affects like'. Frequently various body parts of gibbeted corpses were simply cut off, without any scruples, especially hands and thumbs, but also private parts and pubic hair, to be used for varying nefarious needs.

The mere contact with the corpse of someone who had been executed was once considered to be curative. Amongst the common people, the hand of someone who had died a violent death was considered to have the power of dispelling most diseases, especially skin diseases, birthmarks and growths or swellings of various kinds. Apothecary and medical writer John Quincy laconically confirms this widely held belief in his popular work *Complete English Dispensatory* first published in 1721: 'A dead man's hand [...] is supposed, from some superstitious conceits amongst common people to be of great efficacy in dispersing scrophulous tumours. The part forsooth is to be rubbed with the dead hand for some time. And report furnishes us with many instances of cures done hereby; some of which may not improbably be true [...] as the imagination of the patient contributes much to such efficacies'.[28]

It was still customary in England during the late nineteenth century for sufferers of various ailments such as goitre, bleeding tumours and other conditions, to crowd around a gallows in the hope of receiving the 'dead stroke' on execution days, paying the presiding hangman handsomely for his services. This meant that the ailing person had to be touched by the hand of the executed felon, which was guided by the hangman. With crowds pushing and shoving this could not have been easy to accomplish.

Public hangings in England and the Continent, were festive occasions in those days, attended especially in the large cities, by thousands of jeering, taunting and applauding men, women and children – for instance, some 30,000 spectators attended an execution in the German city of Mainz in November 1803.[29] Cheering spectators were crowded around the wooden platform of the gallows or had paid a sum of money to perch on lamplighter's ladders, hired out on hanging days, to afford a better view of proceedings. Paradoxically, during such demonstrations of justice, pickpockets were especially active amongst the heckling crowds, thereby clearly suggesting that the example of punishment in no way intimidated delinquents.

Crowds often took matters into their own hands, if executioners did not comply in speedily supplying the blood and gore they craved for various medicinal purposes According to a typical seventeenth century account from Charing Cross – today's Trafalgar Square in London – the hanged prisoner was cut down by the crowds while still alive '… his privy members cut off before his eyes, his bowels burned, his head severed from his body, and his body divided'.[30]

Human blood – the elixir of life

Rich and poor alike once partook in the consumption of human blood, known as *elixir vitae*, the 'elixir of life'. For thousands of years, the drinking of human blood was thought to imbue with strength and vigour, to rejuvenate the old and decrepit and was used as a sought-after cure against epilepsy. During the Middle Ages and centuries beyond, human blood was ingested fresh from someone's body or in powdered, dried or distilled form and often mixed with spices and herbs to make it more palatable and perhaps easier to digest. Apart from the execution block, human blood could be obtained from barber-surgeons and blood-letters – in an era of routine bloodletting. Dried and then powdered, it was sold by apothecaries, although it was also recommended 'fresh' for certain medical conditions.

During the fifteenth century the well-known Italian Renaissance scholar, Marsilio Ficino (1433-1499) – himself the son of a physician – advocated that human blood should not only be used as a specific medicinal. He suggested that the elderly might restore their vigour and strength by sucking directly from the vein in the arm of a healthy youth: 'Why should not our old people, namely those who have no [other] recourse, likewise suck the blood of a youth? A youth, I say who is willing, healthy, happy and temperate, whose blood is of the best but perhaps too abundant. They will suck, therefore, like leeches, an ounce or two from a scarcely opened vein of the left arm; they will immediately take an equal amount of sugar and wine; they will do this when hungry and thirsty and when the moon is waxing. If they have difficulty digesting raw blood, let it first be cooked together with sugar;

or let it be mixed with sugar and moderately distilled over hot water and then drunk'.[31]

But the practice of rejuvenation after drinking the vital fluid was not always successful. In 1492, when Pope Innocent VIII (1432-1492) was on his deathbed, his physicians reputedly bled three young boys and had the pope drink their blood.[32] Unfortunately, the boys as well as the pope died – but probably for different reasons.

Since antiquity, human blood was also used as a sought-after cure against epilepsy. In his *Natural History*, historian Pliny the Elder confirms this belief with some revulsion when he decribes gladiatorial combat in Roman arenas: 'While the crowd looks on, epileptics drink the blood of gladiators, a thing horrible to see, yet they think it most efficacious to suck it as it foams warm from the man himself'.[33] It was common for sufferers, to drink from the veins of slain gladiators 'as though from living cups'.[34] Gladiators' blood continued to be the sought-after medicianl for epilepsy until the final ban on gladiatorial combat around 400 CE, after which the execution block became the logical replacement.

During medieval times, and for centuries to come, the practice of drinking fresh blood to cure epilepsy was still in widespread use in Europe. In the mid-eighteen hundreds, German philologist Jacob Grimm (1785-1863), famous collector of German folklore, confirmed the accepted, widely acknowledged cure for epilepsy: 'It is good for epilepsy to drink the blood of a beheaded man'.[35] For epileptics, this form of treatment was so popular that executioners routinely had their assistants catch the blood in cups as it spurted from the neck stumps of dying offenders. 'Epileptics waited at the scaffold as a beheading took place and drank the poor sinner's blood immediately while it was still fresh and warm'.[36] Well into the nineteenth century, public executions by sword or guillotine offered macabre spectacles, featuring dozens of people, their faces smeared with blood like vampires, after drinking the fresh blood gushing from the neck-stumps of the newly executed.

In their book on executions in the German state of Hessen,[37] Christiane Wagner and Jutta Failing recount numerous such ghoulish examples. In September 1812, after notorious robber Conrad Werner's decapitation by sword, the executioner handed out cups of fresh blood from the pulsing neck stump, to epileptics. Apparently, at the time, this occurred by official permission from the reigning monarch.[38] During the mass execution by guillotine of twenty robber gang members in the German city of Mainz, in 1803, epileptics were frantically pressing through the throng of people milling around the scaffold, holding up their glasses for the executioner to fill with fresh blood.[39]

In his autobiography, the Danish writer of fairytales, Hans Christian Andersen (1805-1875), reported witnessing a public execution in 1823. He saw the father of an epileptic child collect a cup of the dead man's blood and administer it to his child as a potential cure.[40] The same scenario was witnessed in 1859 in the German city of Göttingen, after the execution of a woman accused of murdering her victims with poison. Two years later, people were recorded as stumbling onto the execution platform in Hanau, Germany, to drink the still warm blood after the beheading of a thief. [41]

For centuries, human blood remained the medicine of choice in Europe, where the axe or the sword fell regularly on the necks of criminals, innocent unfortunates, as well as royals. As previously mentioned, anything associated with death was considered to have healing ability – but especially so, if combined with sanctity. The exalted status of monarchs and rulers was held to impart distinctive excellence on them. Hence, they were credited with healing powers, which their subjects thought them capable of passing on even after death, by their touch[42] or their blood.

This is why immediately after the beheading of Charles I in 1649, people were swabbing the king's blood with handkerchiefs, wiping every small fragment from the execution block. Not only the bloodstained sand and sawdust, but even strands of his hair and threads from his clothes, were sold for their perceived healing properties.[43] The painting by John Weesop, titled *An Eyewitness Representation of the Execution of King Charles I* clearly shows the crowds eagerly mopping up the blood of Charles I.

Although there are numerous accounts relating such scenes surrounding execution platforms, monarchs and royals on the scaffold were generally protected from the crowds' mad rushes to glean blood and other body parts. However, similar scenes to those surrounding the execution of Charles I also took place when Louis XVI (1754-1793) lost his head during the French Revolution – eager spectators dipping handkerchiefs, linen and even dice into his freshly spilled blood.[44] Many miraculous cures were reputedly accomplished with these blood soaked cloths and objects.[45]

Similarly, at the public execution of a murderer in the provincial town of Hanau near Frankfurt in 1861, a crowd of women had to be prevented by police from dipping rags into the freshly spilled blood.[46] After a public execution in Berlin in 1864, the executioners' helpers dipped strips of cloth in the running blood still gushing from the neck stumps of two criminals. These dripping little bits of material could not sell fast enough – even at exorbitant prices – among the throng of people milling around the execution platform.[47]

In order to put these bloody scenes into perspective, let us not forget that they took place in eras, which boasted literary and musical greats such as Goethe, Kant, Schiller, as well as Mozart, Hayden, Beethoven and Chopin. As Richard Sugg so eloquently puts it: 'While the polished violins of the great concerti, string quartets and monumental symphonies flashed in stately harmony in the salons and palaces and concert halls of Hanover and Salzburg and Vienna [...] the sick raised steaming cups to their lips and bloodied handkerchiefs were handed down from the spattered scaffold'.[48]

Other sources of relatively cheap human blood could be obtained from battlefields, barber-surgeons and blood-letters – in an era of routine bloodletting. Dried in an oven and then powdered, this blood was sold by apothecaries.

Human skull – in great demand

A human body part much in demand for hundreds of years, as a popular medical ingredient in orthodox medicine, was the human skull. Whether powdered, grated or distilled, it was prescribed against epilepsy, convulsions and various diseases of the head. As far back as 77 CE, Roman historian and naturalist Pliny the Elder recommended powdered fragments of the human skull, to be administered as a cure for epilepsy. Alternatively, if removed altogether, the skull should be used as a drinking cup for epileptics, to affect a cure.[49] Again, it was preferable that the bone particles or pieces belonged to someone who had suffered a violent death, in order to achieve a successful outcome for the patient – a belief that persisted for hundreds of years. For that reason, the bones of executed persons were obtained, usually at high prices. They were pulverized and mixed with various oils, especially for the treatment of gout and arthritis. In 1686, the English court-apothecary requested the head of a child-killer after her execution in order to make a special salve for his royal patients.[50]

As with all other body parts, human skull was used by orthodox medicine as a curative agent. Listed in the *Pharmacopoeia Londinensis* as part of the 'catalogue', which apothecaries should keep in their shops, we find '…the skull of a man killed by a violent death'.[51] Furthermore, the official list of medications in the *Pharmacopoeia Londinensis* recommends '…that small Triangular bone in the Skull of a man, called *Os triquerum*, so absolutely cures the Falling sickness, that it will never come again;'[52] as well as '…stone taken out of a Mans bladder, Vipers flesh […] Virgins wax, […], the moss on a mans Skull'.[53] Also advocated is '…the Skull of a man that was never buried being beaten to Powder and given inwardly, the quantity of a dram at a time […] helps Palsies and Falling sickness'.[54]

Whereas physicians advocated the use of powdered human skull for the 'falling sickness' or epilepsy, the general populace once thought it sufficient to simply drink from a human skull to effect a cure. It was still firmly held by some locals in the Scottish Highlands, in the early nineteen hundreds that well water drunk from the skull of an ancestor was a certain cure for epilepsy.[55]

Some bizarre treatments regarding the human skull were advocated by renowned German-Swiss physician Paracelsus, probably as a result of his many appropriations from folk magic.[56] He would come across such 'remedies' on his lengthy travels, remedies, which were firmly embraced by the common people across Europe. To treat wounds, Paracelsus recommended mixing red wine and earthworms with powdered fragments from the skull of a man recently killed or hanged. However, strange as it may seem, this 'ointment' was not applied to the wound itself, but to the weapon which had caused the wound in the first place. But, more on that subject in Chapter 11 titled Medical magic – healing by touch and sympathy.

'Usnea' skull moss recommended by physicians

Often human skulls, which had been exposed to the elements for a length of time, would have moss growing on them. Known as *usnea*, this moss was highly prized for its healing properties. London druggists sold such skulls covered with green moss for eight to eleven shillings each, depending on their size and the amount of *usnea* they contained.[57] The moss, from these skulls, was dried and powdered and used as a cure for ailments as varied as the plague and toothache. It was also used as snuff to cure headaches and as a wound dressing in battle, which was probably useful – in modern times there is general awareness of the powerful antiseptic properties of moss.[58]

None other than philosopher and statesman Sir Francis Bacon (1561-1626), considered the father of modern science, in his work *Sylva Sylvarum*, advocates that '…the moss which groweth upon the skull of a dead man unburied, will staunch blood potently'.[59] In *A Ternary of Paradoxes,* Belgian physician Jean Baptiste van Helmont recommends grated human skull, deliberating on the reasons for its effectiveness '… the usnea, or moss, is to be selected onely from the skulls of such, as have been hanged. […] in strangulation the Vital spirits violently retreat into the skull and there constantly shroud themselves for some time, until the moss shall, under the open canopy of the Air, grow up and periwig the Cranium.' He further elaborates that '…by multiplied experience we are confirmed, that usnea gathered from the skulls of such who have been broken on the wheel is in virtue no whit inferior to that of men strangled with a halter'.[60]

Usnea could be readily obtained from charnel houses. In many European countries burial spaces were limited. Hence, to make room in consecrated grounds for the recently dead, existing graves were unearthed after a time and skeletal bones moved and stored in charnel houses. These were vaulted buildings usually situated in the vicinity of churches and adjoining graveyards, where stacked skeletal remains lay in damp dark surroundings for years on end – ideal for the growth of moss.

Although charnel houses delivered adequate supplies of *usnea*, the main supply of this moss – still attached to the skulls – in all probability came from battlefields. This is especially true in view of the many wars fought on the Continent and in England. With the beginning of the English Reformation in 1536, when Henry VIII broke with Papal authority, came a determined effort on behalf of the English to conquer and colonise Ireland. The conflict and animosity between Catholics and Protestants was to last for hundreds of years.

Civil war in Ireland during the seventeenth century, as well as the wars which pitted Irish Catholics against British forces and Protestant settlers, killed hundreds of thousands. The large numbers of men who lost their lives in a single battle could not all be interred – it would have been a physical impossibility. Therefore, as time passed, hundreds of Catholic and Protestant skulls covered in moss could be found lying around in remote areas. Ironically, as one moss-covered skull does not differ much from another, it seems more than likely that a multitude of these skulls were shipped back to Protestant England to be powdered into medicine and eagerly swallowed by their nearest and dearest.

Hence, due to the many wars fought on the British Isles for several hundred years, powdered, grated or distilled human skull was not in short supply during the sixteenth, seventeenth and eighteenth centuries. An article in the *Irish Examiner Newspaper*, dated 25 May 2011 titled *Skulls the best medicine for Irish exports in the past*, discusses the export of skulls from Ireland: 'Long before the British Empire shipped living slaves to the West Indies, the Irish victims of English occupation became mercantile commodities after their deaths.'

In an attempt to anglicise Ireland under English rule and make the 'Emerald Isle' into a peaceful and reliable possession, the system of 'Plantations' was established, wherever the policy of surrender applied to the Irish had failed. This meant that confiscated lands were colonised by English settlers following the suppression of rebellions. As a prelude to the 'Plantations', Sir Humphrey Gilbert (1539-1583) slaughtered thousands when he arrived in Ireland in 1566. During the three weeks of his campaign, all enemies were treated without mercy and Gilbert's attitude towards the Irish was one of relentless oppression. He did not distinguish between soldiers and civilians, but would happily cut off the heads of soldiers, woman and children alike.

To further cow all rebel supporters he devised a particularly gruesome spectacle: he had the heads of all those unfortunates who were captured, severed, and stacked in long rows, like a wall, leading to his tent – a powerfully effective warning to any chieftain who did not bow to English rule. The skulls piled up outside his quarters soon decomposed in the damp conditions and became overgrown with moss – and so began the very lucrative export of 'cannibal medicine' from Ireland. It was *so* profitable in fact, that it was not long, before the English introduced an import tax of one shilling for each skull. The article *Skulls the best medicine for Irish exports in the past* comments: 'As late as 1778, the commodity [of skulls] was still liable for duty and was also listed amongst goods which were imported into England, before being exported elsewhere'.[61] Obviously the English had few scruples about cannibalising their subject neighbours.

The human skull remained a popular medical ingredient for around two hundred years, with the moss growing on some of them especially hailed to stop severe nosebleeds – a treatment tried and enthusiastically advocated by none other than Anglo-Irish philosopher, chemist, physicist and inventor Robert Boyle (1627-1691). He is largely regarded as one of the founders of modern chemistry, although his research clearly had its roots in the alchemical tradition. Boyle was badly afflicted with nosebleeds and decided to try the 'moss of a dead man's skull, which had been sent from Ireland' and found to his surprise that he could halt the bleeding by simply holding the moss in his hand instead of inserting the powder into his nostrils as was the conventional method.

Powdered and distilled human skull

Powdered skull, 'of a dead man burned' was also used to cure epilepsy, and came highly recommended by surgeon George Barrough in 1583.[62] Similarly, powdered human skull mixed with nutmeg and other 'powerful' ingredients, all to be ingested, was recommended by the surgeon Thomas Brugis (c.1620-c.1651). In his work *The Marrow of Physick* (1651) he wrote: 'A Mans Skull that hath been dead but one yeare, bury it in the Ashes behinde the fire, and let it burne untill it be very white, and easie to be broken with your finger; then take off all the uppermost part of the Head to the top of the Crowne, and beat it as small as is possible; then grate a Nutmeg, and put to it, and the blood of a Dog dryed, and powdered; mingle them all together, and give the sick to drinke, first and last, both when he is sick, and also when he is well, the quantity of halfe a Dram at a time in white Wine'.[63]

The recipe for distilled powder of the skull was closely associated with well-known English physician Jonathan Goddard (1617–1675), army surgeon to the forces of Oliver Cromwell, active member of the Royal Society and physician to Charles I of England (1600-1649). Jonathan Goddard reputedly sold the instructions for the formula of distilled powder of human skull to Charles II of England for the sum of £6,000[64] – an extraordinary amount of money in those times.

Charles II delighted in science and medicine, becoming the founding force behind the Royal Society, 'although not its financial benefactor, and made science fashionable'.[65] Hence the regent was not averse to dabbling with tinctures and other mixtures, which is confirmed by Raymond Crawfurd in his book *The Last Days of Charles II.*[66] Apparently the king applied the distillate, widely known as 'the king's drops', regularly. But, they were not effective in saving his life. Many years later, early on Monday 2 February 1685 King Charles II, feeling unwell went to his 'closet to get some of the famous King's Drops [...] made up in the King's own "laboratory" after a formula devised by Dr. Jonathan Goddard, in high repute on the Continent, and commended by no less an authority than Sydenham'.[67] Racked with convulsions on his deathbed, his doctors administered all manner of cures and potions, including the guaranteed cure of forty drops of 'spirit of human skull'. But, even this proved unsuccessful in saving the king's life and he died five days later.

'Oil' of human bones – a prized medication

Pioneer archeologist John Aubery (1626-1697) who excavated the prehistoric burial mounds near Avebury in Wiltshire, England,[68] recorded an interesting case relating to medical cannibalism. Dozens of bodies were laid to rest in the burial mounds near Avebury, all in distinct social groups. But it soon became apparent to John Aubery that the bones had not only been jumbled up, but that there was a significant discrepancy between the numbers of skulls and long bones buried there. Some bones had obviously been taken and in his work *Monumenta Britannica*, John Aubery tells us by whom: in Aubrey's time, the barrow was being systematically looted by the local doctor for the purposes of making medicine from the bones.

At the time the acquisition of these ancient bones was not seen as improper at all. In fact, the culprit, a Dr. Toope, wrote to Aubrey in 1685 and told him that he had attained many 'bushels' of bones from the barrow, with the help of workmen, '...of which I made a noble physick that relieved many of my distressed neighbors.' Exactly what his 'physick' consisted of, apart from human bones, he does not mention. Little did the good doctor realise the archaeological damage he had wrought by digging up countless mounds – often to no avail as he did not delve deep enough – hence leaving a destructive legacy which survived long after his death. It is indeed not far-fetched to imagine that '...in rural areas, far from the busiest scaffolds of London and Edinburgh, other more or less qualified practitioners may well have shown a similar intuitive'.[69]

Substantiating this theory, historian Richard Sugg names various sources, amongst them physician Edward Bolnest, who in 1672 stipulated the use of '...bones of a man which hath not been buried fully a year'[70] to make the medicinal 'oil of bones'. In addition, the unabashed Bolnest instructed the bones should be '...well washed and dried'.[71] As this quote clearly suggests, the good doctor and his associates had to have deliberately robbed a marked grave of its musty remains, to be certain that the corpse was less than a year old. Also, his blatant instructions to carefully clean the bones, suggest that there was nothing untoward about his actions. It is well documented that the most horrible extremes of commercial and organised grave robbing occurred in the late eighteenth and nineteenth centuries, which strongly suggests that the practice was just as popular, although not as widely written about, in earlier centuries.

Human fat – in ointments and medications

Apart from the human skull, bones and blood, another human resource was highly prized in the past. From the sixteenth through to the beginning of the nineteenth century, human fat was mentioned in European pharmacopeias as an important component of ointments and other medications. Human fat was also advocated in all medical books of that time.[72] The German doctor Johann Agricola (1496–1570) specifically described the recovery of human fat and its applications. In his book *Parnassus Medicinalis Illustratus*, physician Johann Becher advocates human fat especially for lame joints, but it was also advocated for use internally for lung ailments and general pain,[73] as well as for treating bone pain, toothache, gout and rheumatoid arthritis. The use of human fat is also mentioned in the British Royal Society's official pharmacopoeia, the *Pharmacopoeia Londinensis*, which lists various medications made from human fat, advising that '...the Fat of a man is exceeding good to anoint such limbs as fall away in the flesh'.[74]

Abhorrent as it may seem, infants' fat was advocated in cosmetics, deemed suitable '...for those desiring a youthful appearance'. Interestingly, human fat[75] was still used for the surgical treatment of scars and wounds in 1909.

At first glance, cannibalistic medical practices of the past seem far removed from our own culture. However, the utilisation of body parts for medicinal purposes still persists in modern times, although in different forms. Despite the fact that blood transfusions or organ transplantations may seem dramatically different than drinking the blood or eating the flesh of another human being, these medical practices do share one fundamental common belief: the human body as an instrument of healing.[76]

Another aspect of cannibalistic or 'corpse medicine' is discussed in the next chapter, namely powdered mummy...

IX

'YUMMY' MUMMY

For hundreds of years powdered mummy was actually just 'what the doctor ordered' although this subject matter has received very little historical attention. For centuries 'medicinal cannibalism' was part of mainstream western medicine and 'mummy' remained a popular standard-issue drug by medical practitioners until well into the eighteenth century. As renowned Egyptologist Sir Earnest Wallis Budge (1857-1934) confirms in his classic book *The Mummy: A Handbook of Egyptian Funerary Archaeology*: 'Egyptian mummy formed one of the ordinary drugs in apothecaries' shops'.[1]

An article titled *Anthropophagy in Post-Renaissance Europe: The Tradition of Medicinal Cannibalism,* states: 'One of the most common human substances used by apothecaries during the early modern period was mummy, a medicinal preparation of the remains of an embalmed, dried, or otherwise "prepared" body that had ideally met with sudden, preferably violent, death'.[2]

Although mummification may be found on almost every continent, in the minds of most people, the process itself is inextricably linked with the culture of ancient Egypt.[3] In fact, for many, the word 'mummy' is synonymous with Egypt itself. Whereas the wealthy were artificially mummified and placed in specially built tombs, the majority of Egyptians were simply buried in hollows in the sand, somewhere far away from the cultivated areas near the banks of the Nile. In the scorching desert they were mummified by natural means, as corrosive body fluids drained away into the hot dry sand, which desiccated and preserved skin, hair and nails. In modern times the term 'mummy' is used to describe all human remains, which retain their soft tissue, either by natural means or artificial preservation.

'Menstruation of the dead'

The English word 'mummy' is derived from the Latin *mumia*, which comes from the Persian word *mūm*, meaning 'bitumen'. The term 'mummy' originally referred to the bituminous substances, seeping from Egyptian mummies – medieval sources generally referred to such leakage as 'menstruation of the dead'.[4] Over time the meaning of the term 'mummy' changed and by the fifteenth century it included the whole mummified body, permeated with these fluids. It is this – in powdered or alternate form – that early modern physicians prescribed in their medications.

But, why was 'mummy' such a sought after commodity? For the very reason that it was believed to contain bitumen, which was considered to have healing properties since ancient times. Because the skin of mummies appears blackened, it was once believed that bitumen was extensively used in ancient Egyptian embalming procedures. However, Egyptian mummies were incorrectly assumed by Europeans to be embalmed with bitumen – in reality most mummies, at least those dating to before 500 BCE, were coated with various resins, which lent the dark tone to a mummy's skin. It was only when the ancient Egyptians started running short of resins, some time around 500 BCE, that they began coating mummy wrappings and filling body cavities with bitumen, which they sourced from the Dead Sea.[5]

The firm belief in the healing properties of bitumen goes back thousands of years. In Ayurvedic medicine, the oldest and most holistic medical system dating back to about 3000 BCE, bitumen or *shilajit* [6] was used extensively as an analgesic, an anti-inflammatory, an antibacterial and a diuretic agent. Indian physicians also used it externally and internally as a wound cleaner; an expectorant, to stimulate bowel movements; in the expulsion of kidney and bladder stones; as a respiratory stimulant; to cure cystitis, diabetes, epilepsy, haemorrhoids, skin diseases, menstrual disorders and digestive disorders – in fact almost any medical condition they were aware of.

Similarly, the Romans were enthusiastic about the medicinal qualities of bitumen for preventing and curing a number of ailments including boils, toothache and ringworm. Taken in wine it was thought to soothe chronic coughs and to relieve shortness of breath and mixed with vinegar it reputedly relieved rheumatism and lumbago. The first century Greek physician Dioscorides, as well as second century physician Galen, whose medical discourses were slavishly followed by physicians for more than one 1500 years,[7] recommended bitumen for its therapeutic qualities.

Desiccated mummy flesh and bones

Consequently, the presence of bitumen, which was incorrectly assumed to be contained in all mummies – irrespective of age – was partly responsible for this popular form of 'corpse medicine'. Desiccated mummy flesh and bones were used in medical treatment since antiquity, advocated by renowned physicians such as Avicenna [8] who advised treating medical problems from broken bones to paralysis with tinctures and powders laced with powdered mummy.[9]

Similarly, centuries later, renowned German-Swiss physician Paracelsus advocated 'balsam of mummy' as well as 'treacle of mummy' to his patients for certain medical conditions. In fact, Paracelsus declared no remedy more fitting to cure the human body, than the human body itself, when reduced to a medication.[10] Mummy was also applied locally for various ailments and highly recommended in Europe for the treatment of coughs, throat ailments, wounds, contusions, fractures, liver, stomach and intestinal disorders, palpitations, poisoning, paralysis, migraine, rashes and ulcers.

Therefore, bizarre as it may sound, mummy powder or paste became a sought after edible commodity in Europe between the twelfth and eighteenth centuries, widely prescribed by physicians. The Royal College of Physicians' official *Pharmacopoeia Londinensis*, lists various entries of 'mummy' to be added to recipes.[11] In his popular work *Complete English*

Dispensatory (1721) John Quincy recommends '...sealed earth, dragon's blood, mummy, rhubarb', mixed into a powder against bruises,[12] and mummy mixed with lead, calamine oil, silver, wax, resin and other exotic ingredients against ruptures.[13]

Any possible taboos regarding the ingestion of 'mummy' were mitigated by two factors: firstly, the great unfathomable expanse of time lying between these ancient bodies and those consuming them; and secondly, the fact that the bodies evidenced nothing of the odour and texture of normal dead flesh. Mummies, which had been buried in hot sand for centuries and had dried out, were shipped across the Mediterranean to apothecaries in incredibly large quantities in medieval times, right up to the eighteenth century. Literally hundreds of thousands of mummies were destroyed – shedding a whole new meaning on Shakespeare's quote in *Hamlet* '...a King might go a progress through the guts of a beggar'.[14]

Mummy brown – the ultimate pigment

But mummies also had other uses. Human as well as feline mummies were powdered and added to artists paints – a practice popular since the sixteenth century. In France, after the Revolution in 1792, even the mummified hearts of numerous French kings and their family members were sold to painters by revolutionary authorities – the hearts[15] of French kings, and their family members, which had been kept in various cathedrals in Paris. As a pigment in paints, mummy powder produced a colour popularly known as 'mummy brown'[16] – one of the favourite colours of the Pre-Raphaelites.

Not only was mummy used in paints. Powdered mummy mixed with morsels of minced bird meat was also considered first-rate fish bait, while mummified cats, found in their thousands in Egypt, were shipped to Europe to be used as fertilisers in 'distinguished' gardens. Mummies exported to the US on the other hand ended up in the papermaking industry. In his book *The Scientific Study of Mummies* Arthur Auf der Heide writes that in 1855 '...mummy wrappings could be bought in Egypt and shipped to New York for about three cents per pound, approximately half the price of local rags'.[17] Furthermore, during the American Civil War, several shiploads of Egyptian mummies were imported to American paper mills, stripped of their wrappings and together with the papyri in the wrappings thrown into the paper beaters. '...the resulting coarse brown paper found its way into the regional and other stores'.[18] Probably the most well known use of mummies appeared in Mark Twain's novel *Innocents Abroad*. He recounts how mummies were used by the British as fuel to power Egyptian locomotives: 'I shall not speak of the railway, for it is like any other railway – I shall only say that the fuel they use for the locomotive is composed of mummies three thousand years old, purchased by the ton or by the graveyard for that purpose'.[19]

Medicinal mummy – powder, paste, balsam and treacle

To make the various medications prescribed by physicians, mummies were first unwrapped, all remaining hair burnt and the bodies crushed. Ashes from the burnt hair were subsequently added to the mummy powder. Instructions for preparations containing various mummy products are well documented in fifteenth and sixteenth century pharmacopoeias. Mummies could be boiled and the resulting oily liquid used as a medicinal agent. Or, most popularly, the mummy was powdered and used as such internally or externally. Apparently it did not taste too bad. The 1747 edition of the *London Pharmacopoeia* describes the taste of mummy as 'somewhat acrid and bitterish'.[20]

As an alternative to pure mummy powder, physician prescribed tincture of mummy, elixir of mummy, mummy treacle or balsam of mummy. These mixtures often involved complicated and time-consuming processes. For instance, in order to make 'balsam of mummy', mummy tincture was mixed with specific quantities of powdered coral, musk, *terra sigillata* and what English apothecaries called 'Venice treacle'. Venice treacle known as 'theriac' in the ancient world, was one of the most expensive medications available.[21] It contained sixty-four different ingredients, amongst them opium, viper flesh, cinnamon, numerous herbs, certain fungi and exotic varieties of dried mushrooms, as well as *gum arabic*, the hardened sap from acacia trees originating in Arabia and Asia. The fact that 'Venice treacle' had to mature for six months to a year or longer, made it exorbitantly expensive.

Apart from Venice treacle, another ingredient of 'Balsam of Mummy' was *Terra sigillata*. This was medicinal soil obtained from the Greek island of Lemnos, high in mineral content and prized as a medicinal component for hundreds of years by surgeons and physicians. According to popular belief, the resulting 'balsam of mummy' possessed such intense qualities '…that it pierceth all parts, restores wasted limbs, heckticks, and cures all ulcers and corruptions'.[22]

Pure mummy, without additives was given as a powder to treat vertigo, palsy and epilepsy, as well as externally applied to wounds. Elizabethan physician William Bullein (c.1525–1576) advocated the use of mummy in his work *Bulleins Bulwark of Defence against all Sickness, Soreness, and Wounds that do Daily Assault Mankind*.[23] He suggested that mummy be especially added to the ingredients of 'Theriaca Galeni',[24] to successfully treat migraines, jaundice, falling sickness and other complaints.

Shakespeare mentions 'mummy' in *Othello, The Merry Wives of Windsor* and *Macbeth*. In Macbeth the third witch places various ingredients into the cauldron. Amongst them: 'Scale of dragon, tooth of wolf, witches' mummy, maw and gulf'.[25] Mummy powder was still widely sold by European druggists in the eighteenth century although the list of ailments it was believed to cure had by then been narrowed down to gastric pains and bruises – for which the 'miracle powder' was to be taken internally or applied externally respectively. Although he was generally a staunch opponent of corpse medicine, sixteenth-century French royal surgeon, Ambroise Paré, noted that mummy was '…the very first and last medicine of almost all our practitioners' against bruising.[26]

Because 'powdered mummy' was in great demand, a lucrative trade had developed by the late Middle Ages in mummified remains coming from the Middle East. This continued well into Victorian times when mummies were first seriously studied and examined, and wealthy travellers sometimes brought them back as souvenirs from Egypt.[27] It seems that for centuries no one in Europe felt any misgivings in desecrating pre-Christian bodies. Although criticism came from many quarters, the trend continued unabated, leading to varied fraudulent practices. Hence, when Egyptian mummies became hard to acquire, a new market for the dearly departed very swiftly opened up, with anything even remotely resembling old, brown, crumbly dust being passed off as the 'real' thing. In addition, the substance did not come cheap, thus encouraging many apothecaries to substitute genuine mummy with low-cost imitations.

The constant, large demand led to an ever-ready supply: mummies were now 'manufactured', as traffickers simply dealt in the flesh of contemporary Egyptians who had died: executed criminals, the poor, the aged and those who had died of disease – all marketed as 'genuine' mummies. The corpses were pickled, resinated and powdered, to meet the great European demand. Egyptologist Sir Earnest Wallis Budge confirmed this: 'In the year 1564 a physician called Guy de la Fontaine made an attempt to see the stock of mummies of the chief merchant of mummies at Alexandria, and he discovered that they were made from the bodies of slaves and others who had died from the most loathsome diseases'.[28]

Sir Earnest Wallis Budge further details the nefarious practice of traders, who in certain cities were '…chiefly Jews […]. After a time the supply of mummies ran short and the Jews were obliged to manufacture them. They procured bodies of all the criminals that were executed in goals and who had died in hospitals, Christians and others. They filled the bodies with bitumen and stuffed the limbs with the same substance; this done they bound them tightly and exposed them to the heat of the sun. By this means they made them look like old mummies'.[29]

However, claims also abounded that mummy products consumed during the late sixteenth century, when the counterfeiting trade in mummies had begun, came from France. It was alleged that mummy was regularly prepared in that country from '…bodies stolen at night from the gibbets, the brains and entrails removed, and the bodies dried in a furnace, and then dipped in pitch'.[30] But, wherever they may have originated, by the end of the seventeenth century inferior wares, sold as the genuine article had become so widespread that buyers were being officially warned to '…choose what is of a shining black, not full of bones and dirt, and of a good smell'.[31]

Corpse medicine did have its opponents and critics, with some physicians describing these remedies as 'unnatural'. Referring to counterfeit mummy, French royal surgeon, Ambroise Paré, protested in 1585 that '…we are […] compelled both foolishly and cruelly to devour the mangled and putrid particles of the carcasses of the basest people of Egypt, or such as are hanged'.[32] A few years earlier, in his essay *Of Cannibals* French thinker Michel de Montaigne (1533-1592) had attacked the duplicity of those Europeans who condemned New World natives as cannibals, while indifferently partaking in 'corpse medicine'.[33] Some time before his death in 1566 German physician and botanist Leonhard Fuchs (1501-1566) had attacked the '…gory matter of cadavers […] sold for medicine', wondering '…who, unless he approves of cannibalism, would not loathe this remedy?'.[34]

However, in spite of various cries of opposition, there was no question of banishing the practice – it was simply too popularly pervasive and embedded. Even Ambroise Paré only objected to mummy products partly due to the fact that mummy did nothing to help his patients. He implied, that he would have been prepared to use it, had he found it effective. On another occasion, he noted that one of his patients complained when he was not prescribed mummy after a fall from his horse.

By the late eighteenth century, orthodox practitioners stopped consulting the *Complete English Dispensatory*, which prescribed 'three drams of [crushed] human skull' for epilepsy, or 'two ounces of mummy in a plaster against ruptures'.[35] During this time general hostility to corpse medicine amongst the medical establishment became widespread – although still practiced in popular culture for some decades – and 'such feculence', was eventually banished from the pharmacopoeias. No doubt this was also necessitated by an arbitrary tax imposed on the illegal mummy trade by the Egyptians, once it had been exposed to local authorities there.[36]

Unfortunately, lost behind the various shocking uses for mummies, is the fact that these captivating, astonishing 'artefacts' were once living people – their preservation in as lifelike a way as possible considered a way of providing a permanent home for the soul and ultimately defying death itself.

Whilst 'corpse medicine' was popularly widespread and has frequently been described as a medieval therapy, it survived well into the late eighteenth century and even lingered on persistently into Victorian times. In the procurement of human body parts, such as blood, fat and other substances to be turned into medications, executioners once played a vital part. In fact, they once occupied a very strange and paradoxical role in marginal and alternate medicine which merits discussion…

THE EXECUTIONER'S HEALING TOUCH

An amazing, yet little known reality – almost inconceivable in its contradiction – is the fact that executioners in various European countries once functioned as renowned healers. Although public execution defined their prime social function in their local districts, executioners made an additional tidy profit by making their own medications and successfully treating patients.

The executioner's 'dishonourable' status

In the framework of their officially recognised healing skills, it is appropriate to discuss executioners' official social standing, as well as their duties under the law, in centuries past. During the Middle Ages executioners, together with skinners, linen-weavers, customs officials, gravediggers, prostitutes, shepherds and actors, were among those regarded as 'dishonourable', in other words socially unacceptable. Similarly, the families of these groups of 'dishonourables' were looked upon as publicly objectionable. As such, members of the aforementioned trades suffered various forms of social, economic and legal discrimination.

The low status of executioners in the past was particularly widespread, although not wholly universal. For instance, executioners in the Ottoman Empire enjoyed a relatively high social standing.[1] Although contempt for executioners was present in most western European countries, the notion of 'infamy' or 'dishonour' was most prominent in German-speaking countries, and affected not only the executioner himself but also his whole family. The idea of infamy was like a contagious disease, spreading to all who came into contact with the executioner, his family or even objects associated with him. Consequently his sons could not follow 'honest' trades, as all guilds refused entry to the offspring of infamous and despised men.

Due to meticulous record keeping, most data regarding western European executioners has been collected in Germany – the oldest documentation concerning this office dates back to 1276 in the *Stadtbuch* or town records of the city of Augsburg.[2] Here the executioner was clearly grouped or categorised amongst the *unehrliche* or 'infamous' persons. Accordingly, he was responsible for carrying out various 'mean' tasks apart from his usual office. It should be added that nobody in Europe voluntarily committed to the duties of being an executioner. These men always came from the lowest classes and the occupation inevitable passed from father to son, which is how whole dynasties of executioners came into being in various countries.

Imperial laws in Germany occasionally attempted at limiting the number of infamous occupations. For instance, a '...diet held in Frankfurt in 1577 ordered that linen-weavers, barbers, shepherds, millers, publicans, whistlers, trumpeters and bath-keepers and their children should not be barred from the guilds, provided that they lived an irreproachable life'.[3]

Generally, in European countries, people avoided all dealings with executioners. Social isolation went so far as to shun any physical contact with these men and their families. In local pubs they even had their own table, at which no one else *ever* sat, as well as their own mug to drink from. In 1500 a decree in the German town of Strassburg made the executioner's disreputable status quite clear, requiring that he stand separately at the back of the church. Even worse, the Bamberg criminal code of 1507 indicated that he might be denied salvation altogether and many a parish priests refused the executioner Holy Communion.

Executioners were usually given a house in which to live, and generally this was situated outside the confines of the city or near the pillory. In

France, executioners were forced to wear a red or yellow coat in order to differentiate them from 'decent' citizens. However, their sinister role also ensured certain privileges. In Paris, the executioner had the right to take for himself all he could hold in his hands from every load of grain, brought into the marketplace. In order to preserve the grain from his reprehensible contact he usually used a wooden spoon instead of his bare hands. In addition, the executioner received all personal property of the condemned – meaning all they had on their person during the execution – as well as the rents from shops and stalls surrounding the pillory, where the retail fish trade was usually carried out. As in other European countries, the takings from these various duties amounted to a considerable source of revenue for executioners, establishing them as generally wealthy individuals.[4]

Notoriety or infamy extended from the executioner to his equipment, through to the scaffold. Christiane Wagner and Jutta Failing, in their book on executions and executioners in the German state of Hessen, *Vielmals auf den Kopf gehackt – Galgen und Scharfrichter in Hessen*, recount numerous such examples. Workmen were usually almost impossible to recruit for the re-building and renovations of older scaffolds, as well as the construction of new ones, and many of the tasks had to be performed by 'dishonourable' persons. However, trades people would by necessity have to be involved in these constructions. The problem of their defilement was usually solved by forcing *every* tradesman to hammer at least one nail into the proposed gallows.[5] Hence, the 'burden of guilt' was evenly spread between all partaking in the construction of the 'killing platform'!

The 'contagion' of infamy was even thought to be transmitted through objects such as money, which is why money was never taken directly from the executioner's hands. Similarly, there are accounts of hangmen being refused burial as no 'honourable' person was prepared to carry their body to the grave. Ultimately, the infamy associated with the executioner also extended to the convicted. In past centuries, evidence of crimes committed, rested not on circumstantial proof but solely on the confession of those accused. Hence, torture was extensively used to elicit affirmation of guilt. If however a subject did not confess, even under the most horrendous physical torment devised by the executioner, this person would be released back into society. Tragically, because of 'close' personal contact with the executioner during the horrendous tortures, the victim was now also deemed 'dishonourable' and usually ostracised from society[6] – a cruel blow indeed.

In spite of the executioner's 'dishonourable' status, people were apparently not afraid to make contact with him, on specific occasions. As indicated in chapter 8 on Corpse Medicine, the blood, skin, fat and flesh of the convict, even the finger of a condemned man or the hangman's rope, were thought to have curative powers – and these were supplied for their desired curative effects by the executioner himself. Consequently, attitudes towards the executioner were ambivalent to say the least

A proclivity for medicine

This ambivalent attitude towards executioners is also evident in the fact that executioners, in spite of their social isolation, were paradoxically consulted for medical reasons in various European cultures. It seems incongruous and absurd to think that the executioner's role as someone who was apprenticed to kill was offset by his function as a healer in the community. Bizarrely, the very person whose official function was to torture, maim and take life, spent much of his spare time practicing medicine. On the other hand, the common ground shared by executioners and the medical profession in the early-modern period should not be surprising – both professions were after all expert at practising their skills on a common object: the fragile human body.

As hereditary healers for many generations, executioners occupied a sanctioned *niche* in the medical infrastructure of medieval and early modern towns. In *Defiled Trades and Social Outcasts: Honour and Ritual Pollution in Early Modern Germany*, Kathy Stuart describes how executioners' gift of healing enabled them to come into contact with people of the highest social echelons. In their curative capacity executioners entered the homes of patricians and aristocrats.[7] This took place in spite of the fact that people had a wide variety of authorized medical practitioners to choose from. Many executioners even published their cures and methods of healing. For instance, over many generations, the executioner family Seitz, from Kaufbeuren in Bavaria, Germany, collected in excess of 500 medicinal recipes.[8]

But, what led to executioners' proclivity for medicine? Expert in torture, disfigurement, and killing by profession, they were closely familiar with the human body, and thus well versed in anatomical knowledge. Every executioner had to be able to judge the physical condition of a prisoner in deciding which tortures to apply. Victims were often made to suffer intolerably for days. Therefore, executioners were compelled to know exactly how to refresh the tortured person in order to continue their gruesome task, but still have the poor victim 'fit' enough to be executed. For this reason, the responsibility given them in the criminal justice system provided executioners with immense opportunity to study the human body.

Skill, know-how, and medical knowledge would be passed down from fathers, grandfathers and great-grandfathers. When Bishop Ernst from the German town of Hildesheim was embalmed in July 1471, it was the local executioner's task to remove the bishop's entrails, thereby attesting to his recognised and undisputed anatomical knowledge.[9] Several years later, in Febuary 1477, the annals of Hildesheim record that the executioners' office was under orders to treat all women postpartum.[10]

The healing skills of executioners are widely documented in medieval chronicles and in writings by legal experts and theologians. Numerous cases of executioners practicing medicine are documented in Dutch, as well as French, Danish, and Norwegian records between the late sixteenth and late eighteenth centuries. Many executioners who had distinguished themselves in their community through proven healing skills, were officially declared 'honourable' citizens and went on to become surgeons and even highly respected physicians.[11]

Executioners were thought to be able to cure various illnesses: '… notably they reset broken or dislocated limbs [...]. People in need of this service visited him willingly [...]. Of course surgeons' guilds protested against this infringement on their monopoly'.[12] One of numerous examples comes from the Netherlands in 1676, when the provincial executioner presented a petition to the *burgermasters* (town council) of the city Haarlem. After consulting with the surgeons' guild the *burgermasters* made public their decision to grant permission to the provincial executioner, Tobias Ran, to practice as limb-setter without anyone being allowed to hinder him in this exercise.[13]

The executioner's healing and medical skills

On the whole, the majority of available literature about executioners and hangmen comes from Germany by way of thorough record keeping over the centuries. Although there are hundreds of references in German city chronicles and annals about the healing skills of executioners in that country, only select examples are cited here.

A well-known case was the executioner in the German town of Eger. Throughout his lifetime, Karl Huß (1761-1838) attempted to escape the social exclusion imposed by his office. Hazel Rosenstrauch, in her book *Karl Huß, der empfindsame Henker – Eine böhmische Miniatur*, describes his remarkable life and great achievements, which defied all odds at the time. Karl Huß was a victim of circumstance, as well as a perpetrator. Apart from his 'bloody' occupation, he was renowned for his healing skills and wrote several books, amongst them a chronicle of the town of Eger, as well as leaving behind a sizeable museum collection.

Although he was eventually honoured when he was an old man, receiving recognition for his diligence, passionate moral rectitude, and deep religiosity, Huß bore the burdens of his 'dishonourable' origins throughout his life. Not able to attend public school due to this 'dishonerable' status, Huß received private tuition in his youth. He successfully carried out his first execution at the age of fifteen and took up the post of town executioner for Eger at the age of twenty – a position which he held for forty-seven years. He and his wife lived in social seclusion, their little house typically segregated from other houses and situated against the town wall. Commendably, Huß used his social isolation to his advantage for study and self-education, and started building up a numismatic collection from numerous old coins he would receive for his extensive medical services. Known for his medical skills, people flocked to him from near and far.[14]

German archival records cite numerous references to executioners performing duties, which were ordinarily carried out by surgeons and barber-surgeons. Furthermore, to the annoyance of the medical establishment, executioners did not limit their treatments to external injuries and broken bones, but impinged on the field of internal medicine, the monopoly of physicians. In 1661, a petition was given to the city council of Augsburg in Germany, by outraged physicians who voiced their infuriation at the insolence of the local executioner. Annoyingly, he was writing prescriptions, advising patients, mixing and distributing medicines as well as examining urine.[15] In addition, throughout the seventeenth and eighteenth centuries German executioners were permitted to perform autopsies on the bodies of criminals.[16]

German archival sources quote many examples of 'executioner medicine', including patients' recommendations from the highest social spheres. For instance, '...in 1711 King Frederick I of Prussia (1657-1713) appointed the Berlin executioner, Martin Coblenz, as his personal physician, and in 1744 his grandson Frederick the Great, disregarding the protests of barber-surgeons, issued a decree reaffirming executioners' traditional rights to practice as long as they passed a medical examination – a somewhat surprising move for an enlightened despot in what is commonly held to be an age of medical professionalisation'.[17] Executioner Johann Bast (died 1703) from the German city of Giessen, was so successful in his healing skills, that Emperor Leopold granted him the licence to practice medicine.[18]

A yearbook from the northern German city of Stade[19] refers to Johann Christian Zippel, who was the town's executioner from 1766 until 1782. It appears that he treated numerous patients from all social classes every year, giving them powders, tinctures and creams for their various ailments. Similarly, a petition for legitimation in 1624, for the Nüremberg executioner Franz Schmidt (1555-1634), included amongst his patients imperial councillors, cathedral cannons, aristocrats, patricians and city council members.[20] German, Dutch and French records suggest that while the poor may have kept their distance, the wealthier classes were not reticent to consult an executioner for medical purposes.

When Duke Julius of Brunswick-Lüneburg (1528 –1589), founder of the Universität of Helmstedt, in the erstwile Dutchy of Brunswick-

Wolfenbüttel, was sent to the Netherlands to further his university studies, he heard of the extraordinary medical skills of 'Meister Peter' in the city of Antorff (the Antwerp of modern times). As Julius had suffered from a crippling, debilitating condition in his leg since childhood, the young man soon sought out this renowned healer. According to city annals,[21] Meister Peter attached Julius to various instruments and pulleys for several pain-filled hours a day for many weeks, resulting in a straightening and re-alignment of the limb. Although Duke Julius continued to limp for the rest of his life, his gait and general function of the leg were thereafter greatly improved. There is no question as to who 'Meister Peter' could have been – a German euphemism for an executioner is either 'Meister Hans' or 'Meister Peter'.

Many executioner families distinguished themselves over many generations through their excellent medical acumen. One such family in Germany was the Fuchs family, which spawned like no other, several generations of doctors: excutioner Samuel Christoph Fuchs in 1727, received the emperors priviledge because of his medical acumen and was permitted to study medicine. He passed both *Doctorandus Medicus* exams and duly received his medical degree. In addition, both his brothers – who had also functioned as executioners – graduated as physicians.

Similarly, in the German town of Thedinghausen, executioner Meister Philipp Hartmann distinguished himself with his medical aptitude to the extent that the emperor decreed that Hartmann was able to officially practice as *Medicus*.[22] Another noteworthy example, where generations of executioners functioned as healers, was the Uder family. Georg Uder, executioner of the German city of Magdeburg in 1795, was known for his medical skills and proficient use of medicaments. Before him, his father, uncle and grandfather, all executioners in Osterode, a district in Lower Saxony, Germany, were renowned far and wide in neighbouring towns, to cure all patients who could not be helped by orthodox physicians. Georg Uder's son, who functioned as executioner in Königslutter, similarly made a name for himself as being 'cleverer' than all the medical doctors, resulting in people coming to him from near and wide for therapeutic aid.[23]

In France, not only the executioner, but also to a limited degree his servants were officially permitted to perform duties normally reserved for surgeons – when they were not engaged in their primary function as executioners. In Denmark, executioners were similarly involved in the healing arts. For example, '...as early as 1579 the hangman of Copenhagen, Anders Freimut, received permission to set fractures and treat old wounds'.[24] In time, over the centuries this diversion of Danish executioners was to become traditional, and in the seventeenth century, King Christian V (1646-1699) legitimately conferred a salary on Copenhagen's hangman, thereby rewarding his continued medical services.[25] Another example comes from the Norwegian city of Bergen, where the official executioner obtained a royal writ in 1732, allowing him to practice minor surgery.

Skinners, like shepherds and smiths, who constantly examined sick, dying or dead animals, aquired intricate knowledge about the physiology, as well as the various illnesses and conditions affecting domestic animals. Because many executioners also functioned as skinners, and were usually the first to consider the causes of the various ailments and illnesses afflicting domestic animals, this is why so many executioners not only attended to the medical needs of humans but also those of animals. In 1618, the executioner of Wolfenbüttel, Meister Dietrich, besides fulfilling his duties as executioner, was appointed by Count Friedrich Ulrich as vetenery surgeon for his extensive stables. Similarly, in 1820, Karlsruhe executioner Franz Wilhelm Widmann officially served as the Grand-Duke's vetinary surgeon.[26]

Although the official medical ordinance of 1782 in Bavaria forbade skinners to medically treat the general populace, they were however frequently sought out for advice on medical matters. Christian Probst cites numerous such examples in *Fahrende Heiler und Heilmittel Händler – Medizin von Marktplatz und Landstraße*. Many skinners gave up their dishonerable trade after years of successful part-time medical practices, and upon being declared honourable by the reigning monarch, went on to study as surgeons.[27] Skinner Anton Falk, after declaring that he had never 'personally' carried out the dishonourable trade, but had merely overseen it, was permitted to study and later practice surgery and midwifery in the German city of Reichenberg in the late eighteenth century.[28]

Harvesting human 'ingredients' for medications

In addition to practicing various forms of medicine, executioners derived many of the basic ingredients for their remedies from the bodies of executed criminals. From the fifteenth to the nineteenth century, human blood, human body parts, and human fat, were used in mainstream medicine to cure a variety of ailments (see Chapter 8 on Corpse Medicine). It is a tragic fact that the bodies of the executed were usually totally disseminated and the various body parts would be on their way to apothecaries, only hours after an execution.[29] In 1578 the official executioner in the German city of Nürnberg applied for state permission to open the bodies of executed felons and to remove whatever 'ingredients' he deemed fit for medicinal use.[30] Especially human skin and human fat, mixed with herbs and roots were much in demand as medicaments.[31]

'Poor sinner's fat'

Reputedly, many executioners recovered fat known in Germany as 'Armsünderfett' – 'poor sinner's fat' – from the bodies of their victims and sold it, thereby making a tidy sum on the side, together with all the other body parts in demand at the time.[32] Neither did trained physicians consider human fat inefficacious. Executioners sold human fat to apothecaries by the pound until the mid-eighteenth century – surely an indication of its popularity in medical circles. In 1747 the Munich city executioner Johann Georg Trenkler petitioned to be allowed to continue harvesting fat from those he executed. However, the petition was turned down by the city council, due to the fact that physicians were now regularly performing dissections and would therefore adequately provide apothecaries with the human fat they needed to make up the various salves and ointments – again an indication of how widespread the use of human fat was.[33]

Similarly, executioners sold human fat as a potent painkiller in early modern Italy: '…human fat, […], was generally extracted from the bodies of convicts by the executioner – sometimes as the last act of the execution – purified, and then sold as a pain-killer'.[34] It seems incongruous to say the least, that something extracted under the most excruciating pain during the last seconds of the poor victim's life, was harvested specifically for intended pain relief – cruel times indeed.

Until 1737 the collection of human blood and fat was facilitated in Germany by the executioner's undisputed right to '...dissect' the bodies of those he had put to death.[35] In *A Hangman's Diary: Being the Authentic Journal of Master Franz Schmidt, Public Executioner of Nuremberg 1573– 1617*, Franz Schmidt refers to cadavers of felons, which he regularly 'dissected' after their executions.[36] However, the executioner's right to dismember the bodies of those he had put to death was soon to be taken away, when by the mid-eighteen hundreds medical practitioners began impinging on this traditionally held privilege of executioners.

Executioners were henceforth ordered to deliver the dead bodies of criminals to local doctors for dissection.[37] Consequently this dealt a serious blow to the lucrative side-line business of many executioners, who were dependent on cadavers to glean the various human body parts needed to make their own medications, as well as to abundantly supply various apothecaries. Dissections, dismemberment and the consequent concoctions of medications by executioners ended in the early eighteen hundreds in European countries.

The following chapter deals with 'medical magic' – specifically, 'healing by touch' or transfer', and 'healing by sympathy', concepts once widely accepted and approved by physicians and other medical practitioners…

MEDICAL MAGIC –
HEALING BY TOUCH AND SYMPATHY

Until the early eighteenth century, 'medical magic' was acknowledged and accepted by the uneducated and scholars alike. It was firmly believed, that disease 'could be transferred, transplanted or transformed'.[1] In the minds of the general populace as well as the educated, therapeutic magic also functioned together with religion and superstitious practices. For instance, Richard Napier (1559-1634), parson and physician, learned academic, and graduate from Oxford University, not only prayed for the recovery of his patients, but also supplied them with various charms and amulets to protect them against 'evil spirits, faeries and witcheries'.[2] In the European best seller *Religio Medici,* The Religion of a Doctor, published in 1643, newly qualified physician Sir Thomas Browne (1605-1682) expounded on Christian faith, hermetic philosophy, alchemy and astrology. In accordance with the vast majority of seventeenth century European society, Browne confirmed his belief in the existence of angels, witches and witchcraft.

In a similar vain, Samuel Pepys, London dignitary,[3] and president of the Royal Society of London, finding himself in exceptionally good health at one particular time – Pepys suffered from chronic ill health throughout his life – was at a loss to explain such good fortune. In his diary he wondered, whether this luck was due to the hare's foot he always carried, or due to 'taking every morning a pill of Turpentine'.[4]

The following chapter deals with two forms of 'magical therapeutics': the once popular concepts of healing by transfer, as well as healing by sympathy, both of which were eagerly endorsed and propagated by physicians and other medical practitioners, as well as the general populace.

Healing by touch

Healing by touch – in other words, transferring perceived healing qualities – was once a firmly held conviction, persisting for many centuries. In the past the touch of the reigning monarch, the king's hand, was thought imbued with healing powers. The implicit belief in the supernatural healing powers of sovereigns is a relic of the ancient doctrine of divinity of kingship.[5] The reigning monarchs of England and France were the only Christian rulers who claimed the divine gift of healing by touch.

Deemed to be the chosen representatives of God, the exalted status of kings and queens was held to impart distinctive excellence on them. Hence, they were credited with healing powers, which their subjects thought them capable of passing on, by their touch. While English and French monarchs healed by touch, alternate miraculous healing powers were attributed to the kings and queens of other European sovereign houses. Members of the royal House of Habsburg reputedly cured stutterers by giving a kiss on the mouth, while Hungarian royals were specifically known to restore jaundiced individuals back to health and Castilian monarchs were known to successfully exorcise demons.[6]

The touch of English and French monarchs was believed to heal especially scrofula, a tubercular disease of the lymph glands, which on this account came to be called 'The King's or Queens Evil'. In pre-industrial Europe, scrofula was characterised by slowly festering abscesses and a significant number of deaths from the Evil were recorded throughout England in the sixteenth and seventeenth centuries.[7] In France the first monarch to be credited with the power to heal scrofula was Philip I (1059-1108) and in England, according to legend, the first king to apply the healing touch was Edward the Confessor (c.1003-1066).[8]

Generally, English kings performed the royal touch less frequently than their French counterparts. It should perhaps be mentioned at the outset that the elaborate healing rituals, regularly performed by reigning sovereigns, as well as the resulting 'cures', were invariably recorded and supported – by conviction or perhaps under duress – by physicians at the time.

The Royal Touch for healing purposes was usually performed between Michaelmas and Easter, when the cold European weather was thought to make contracting the disease from infected sufferers less likely. Generally, monarchs laid their hands on the heads, or stroked the sores of those affected, and wished them better health. During the reign of the English King Edward III (1312-1377), the Archbishop of Canterbury, John de Stradford, gave testimony to the authenticity of the practice: 'Whoever thou art O Christian, who denyest these miracles, come and be an eyewitness to their truth'.[9]

Throughout the many centuries when the Royal Touch was performed, the concepts of 'touching' and 'healing' were always considered synonymous and attributed to all Christian kings. After Henry IV's (1366-1413) accession to the throne, the Lord Chief Justice Sir John Fortescue wrote that 'the kings of England at the time of unction receive such divine power, that by the touch of their hands, they can cleanse and cure those who are otherwise considered incurable of certain diseases, commonly called the king's evil'.[10]

Decades later, Henry VII (1457-1509) of England was the first monarch to establish a service of ceremony, later printed in the *Book of Common Prayers*, to accompany the healings. However, he only touched a small number of sufferers annually and there were times when the 'touch' was suspended altogether. This monarch also introduced a tradition which was adhered to henceforth during these ceremonies: he presented sufferers with an 'angel', a gold coin, also known as a 'touch-piece'.

Royal touch-pieces

Touch-pieces were coins believed to bring good luck and to cure diseases, but, they had to be 'touched' in order to convey or transfer their power, which was then thought permanently imbued in the object. Such touch-pieces reputedly cured many disesases and often remained as treasured possessions in families for many generations. Such touch-pieces or 'angels' were worn by recipients until the end of their lives and failure to do so was thought to bring on the return of the original ailment. With symbolic significance, gold 'angel' coins featured St.Michael slaying a dragon on the reverse side – St.Michael was held as guardian of the sick and associated with casting out devils, which were often held responsible for causing diseases in the first place. Angel coins minted for the King's Evil ceremonies were pierced – the size of the hole an indication of the amount of gold the jeweller took as payment for his efforts – and worn around the recipient's neck.

During the reign of Henry VIII the practice of the Kings Touch died down somewhat and the rite was performed sporadically. For instance, between early January 1530 and late December 1532 the king only touched fifty-nine sufferers – a miniscule number compared to other English monarchs.

Despite chronic ill-health suffered since puberty, the first queen of England, Mary Tudor or 'Bloody Mary' (1516-1558) – as she soon became known – eldest daughter to King Henry VIII, began performing 'the touching' for the King's Evil in 1536. She took this duty very serious and usually fasted beforehand. During her reign the royal 'miracle-working' took place on Good Friday or Easter Sunday, Pentecost and the Feast of Michaelmas – it was believed that the healing process was more effective if performed on holy days.

Strict procedural protocol was usually followed: a church official would bring the sufferer to the seated queen; and several passages would be read from the Gospels; Mary would then lay hands on the afflicted, caressing the raw wounds several times and finally brushing them with a gold 'angel', threaded on a ribbon.

It was however believed that apart from curing scrofula, the queen's touch could also prevent illness. Therefore, in addition to touching scrofula sufferers, the queen would bless large containers of rings, at these healing or 'touching' services. These 'ring' containers were habitually placed close to the high altar, where the queen sat. The queen expressly provided hundreds of rings for this purpose. But, rings were also presented by their owners and marked with their names for recovery after the service. Mary would devoutly pray and first pass her hands several times over the ring containers, and then would individually finger the gold and silver bands, touching and carefully separating them with her fingers. Her subjects cherished these so-called cramp-rings – as they were known – regarding them as powerful charms, which contained 'the power intrinsic to the touch of an anointed monarch. Mary's sanctified rings were uncommonly coveted, not only in England but in foreign courts as well, especially in Scotland'.[11] This fact is not surprising, as cramp-rings were considered a cure for 'diabolical sicknesses',[12] such as cramp and epilepsy.

The ritual performed by various monarchs

Although the practice of the King's Touch had died down somewhat under her father King Henry VIII, it was eagerly taken up by Elizabeth I (1533-1603), probably to confirm and demonstrate that despite excommunication from the Roman Catholic Church by the Pope, the rule of monarchs in England was nevertheless divinely sanctioned. Elizabeth's representation of herself as healer 'reinforced her position as a Christian monarch, suggesting that her virtue made her a fitting vessel for God's power'.[13]

However, she had two issues to deal with in post-Reformation England: her healing power provoked the hostility of the Roman Catholic minority, which considered Elizabeth an heretic; and the healing rite also roused radical Protestants – who later formed the Puritan movement – in her realm, who saw the practice of the healing touch as a most abominable superstition. It is ironic that the queen, whose government rejected the Roman Church's doctrine of adoration and worship of images and relics, as well as the invocation of saints, 'herself became the living embodiment of the sacred virgin healer'[14] – an irony not lost on the Puritans, for whom the 'touching' ceremony signified Elizabeth's failure to truly purify the Church'.[15]

In answer to those who risked damaging the prestige of English royalty, archdeacon William Tooker, wrote the *Treatise on the healing charisma* (1597) dedicated to the monarch, in which he exalted the royal miracle. The treaty was a justification of power inherent in English sovereingns. Five years later, one of Elizabeth's surgeons, William Clowes (c.1643-1604), published his *Treatise on the Struma*,[16] citing hundreds of cases where actual healings had taken place subsequent to queen's touch.

Clowes described meeting one of his former patients, a man whom he had unsuccessfully attempted to cure of struma or scrofula. Astoundingly, the man, whom he did not recognise at first – as he looked so well and healthy – was now completely healed of his former ailment.[17] The man described that he had been presented to Elizabeth 'our Sacred and Renowned Prince' and 'through the gift and power of Almightie God' she had cured him 'within the space of five months'.[18] The patient also added that he had not applied any medication, but had simply kept his sores clean. In his *Treatise on the King's Evil*, the queens surgeon strongly argued for the 'monarch's touch for strumas, when physic and surgery did not prove effective'.[19] Although Clowes's flattering vernacular was no doubt in part linked to his attempts to gain favour with the monarch, he *did* intend for his various accounts of actual healing in his book to be taken quite literally,[20] because there were dozens of analogous stories circulating in England at the time.

Charles I (1600-1649) is said to have surpassed all his predecessors in the divine gift, curing not only by his touch but also without physical contact through his divine blessing. Like other monarchs before him, he instituted several changes to the ceremony: Charles refused to touch the diseased part of the body, choosing rather to lay hands anywhere else on the bodies of sufferers; he also had the angel minted in silver, rather than in gold. In addition, no less than eleven different Proclamations relating to the cure of the King's Evil were issued during his reign. In an attempt to somewhat restrain the growing public demand the Proclamations addressed various matters: whether those seeking cures should bring certification from their parishes, vicars and church-wardens; and on which specific days or in which particular season divine cures should take place.

Under Charles I's reign the healing service of the King's Touch was integrated into the *Book of Common Prayer* in 1633, so that anyone besides the sovereign, touching for the King's Evil was considered guilty of a crime. Among the king's curative achievements, later recorded by John Browne (1642-1702), surgeon to Charles II, and at St Thomas hospital, was that of publican John Cole. Cole's neck was covered in open festering sores and when the monarch, after his arrest by Scottish forces, was passing through Winchester as a prisoner, Cole endeavoured to obtain the King's Touch. But Charles's escorts would not allow anyone to approach the king and Charles could only oblige the man's persistent solicitation with the prayer 'God bless thee, and grant thy desire'[21] – it is recorded that Cole's disease soon began to recede.[22] Even after the monarch's capture, when he was a prisoner at Holmby House, crowds of sick people congregated to see him, although to no avail, as a declaration had been drawn up under the new Parliament condemning the 'touching' ceremonial as mere superstition.

However, although Parliament could divest the king of his crown and also take his life, it was incapable of impeding the belief in his gift of healing. Immediately after the beheading of the monarch in 1649, as soon as the axe had fallen, people were swabbing the king's blood with handkerchiefs and wiping every small fragment from the execution block. Not only the bloodstained sand and sawdust, but even strands of his hair and beard, as well as threads from his clothes, were kept or sold for their perceived healing properties. These items were perceived as permeated with the same forces that dwelt in his touch when he was alive.

The popular fervour of Charles the martyr was repeatedly utilised as Royalist propaganda in the years following Charles' execution. Numerous miraculous cures were reported as having taken place – recorded, and published in 1684 by surgeon John Browne – by means of pieces of cloth stained or soaked with the king's blood. All of these were an affront to the existence of the Republic and confirmation of the legitimacy of the Royalist cause. Charles I was distinctive as the *only* 'post-Reformation monarch to be accredited with healing miracles after his death'.[23] It is interesting to note that as late as 1838, several coins, handed down through generations, bearing the effigy of Charles I, were still used to treat the 'Evil' in *lieu* of the Royal Touch in England.[24]

It is not surprising, that his son Charles II used the King's Touch above all to reinforce the general belief in the divine right of kings –

especially in view of his father's execution. 'Given Charles' cynicism it is impossible to tell whether he believed in his divine power to heal, but he was enough of a realist to understand its propaganda value'.[25] Although he initially performed it in exile Charles judiciously invigorated the royal touching ceremony.

The 'potency' of the monarch's gift was publicised by clergy, writers and physicians and it was even believed that the king could cure diseases such as syphilis, rickets and scurvy. Richard Wiseman (1621-1676), honoured as the 'father of English surgery', and surgeon to Charles II witnessed and recorded the touching of hundreds of scrofula sufferers on the Continent – and later in England – and accounted for a multitude of cures resulting from the king's touch. He thereby greatly boosted Charles's appeal throughout Britain even before the king's arrival on home soil.

Under no monarch and in no reign did the practice of the Kings Evil prevail in England to the extent that it did under King Charles II – the only English king to apply the royal touch more than the French monarchs. King Charles II touched for the King's Evil on every Friday in the Banqueting House at Whitehall and his surgeon Richard Wiseman kept painstaking records of the numbers attending, in the 'King's Register of Healing'. The king is reputed to have 'touched' as many as 600 people at one sitting and it is recorded that 'from May 1660 to September 1664 he touched twenty-three thousand persons'.[26] The throng of the crowds was so large at a sitting in 1684 that six or seven people were trampled to death.[27]

Thousands more came to see him in ensuing years, 'perhaps as many as one hundred thousand, seemingly half the nation, during his twenty-five year reign'.[28] People from every part of England, as well as the Irish, Scots, Welsh, Germans, and French came to be healed. In surgeon Browne's list of cures, mention is even made of a woman crossing the oceans from Virginia in the New World to receive the Royal Touch – she was subsequently restored to health.[29] The king also granted private healings by special request, as his father Charles I had done before him.

Ironically, although King Charles II diligently performed his duty as a monarch, the *Bills of Mortality* – weekly lists of deaths and their causes in London, compiled by pioneering statistician John Graunt, which included bizarre entries such as having been 'frighted' to death, or dying of 'itch' – during this period recorded that more people died of scrofula during his reign than at any other time. This may perhaps be attributable to the fact that total reliance was placed on the 'healing touch' during Charles's reign, thereby neglecting any alternate measures of a cure.[30]

Further endorsements by royal physicians

However, both his surgeons, Wiseman as well as Browne, claimed an abundant measure of success for Charles's therapeutic interventions, although they also added that cures were not always consistent especially at the first touch.[31],[32] John Browne (1642-1702), surgeon to Charles II, and royally appointed surgeon to St. Thomas Hospital, was probably the most ardent advocate of the monarch's healing powers, declaring that 'I do humbly presume to assert that more souls have been healed by His Majesties Sacred Hand in one year than have ever been cured by all the Physicians and Chirurgions of his three kingdoms ever since his happy Restauration'.[33]

Browne dedicated his book *Chirurgical Treatise of Glandules and Strumaes, or King's Evil Swellings* to his sovereign, substantiating the unquestioning belief in the 'King's Touch' by the medical establishment. At the time the book, listing some ninety thousand cases of strumas, was endorsed by Thomas Coxe, president of the Royal College of Physicians, and various other physicians and surgeons. In order to confirm effectiveness of the royal touch, Browne discussed eighty-six cases[34] in detail, although he gave scant descriptions of the nature of the various diseases. The remainder of cases were mostly based on hearsay evidence of laypersons, which leads to the assumption that failure was perhaps a regular, though not predictable outcome of cases.

Not to be overlooked in connection with all reports of successful healing by touch, is the fact that scrofula on its own was hardly ever deadly. The disease was naturally prone to extensive periods of remission and even spontaneous cures. In addition, those seeking to be cured may have been suffering from something totally different. It is safe to assert, that scrofula, as it is known and established in modern medical terms, was not always correctly identified. The majority of the population would not have had the means of consulting a surgeon or physician, hence sufferers would simply self-diagnose their condition. Medical practitioners' themselves were unsure about definitively diagnosing 'struma' or the 'King's Evil'. Hence, a wide range of benign and readily curable ailments, as well as many gruesome ones beyond the range of medicine and surgery, were evaluated as 'struma', all explained according to contemporary humoral theory and understanding.

According to Browne's view, all glands in the human body were actively involved in 'foraging' evil humors from the blood. Excessive ingestion of acid humors could lead to glandular swellings – in other words strumas. As glands seemed to be located in hairy parts of the body, Browne concluded that the hairs were conduits by which humors were excreted as perspiration. He asserted that strumous swellings could occur in the pituitary and jugular glands, the tonsils, breast glands, salivary glands, glands in the groin and joints, as well as organs such as the liver, spleen, kidneys, pancreas and prostate[35] – as opposed to a modern medical diagnosis which defines 'scrofula' as a tubercular disease of the lymph glands only. Each of these strumous swellings was given a proper name according to its location on the body or its characteristics.

Browne's curative treatments were in accordance with contemporary ideas and methods: internal remedies for purging and cleansing, as well as external plasters, ointments and poultices, made from typically seventeenth century ingredients such as various forms of animal dungs, herbs, tinctures, calamine, oil, silver, wax, resins and other exotic ingredients. (See chapters 8 and 9). Additional treatment, in line with humoral theory, related to specific dietary recommendations – abstinence from all foods creating 'gross humors' such as onions, leeks, beans, cheese, beef, fish and salted meat to name but a few.

Medical men like Wiseman and Browne seem to have accepted the royal gift of healing as a tenet of their creed. 'Every surgeon who attended Charles the Second was a man of high repute for skill; and [...] has left us a solemn profession of faith in the king's miraculous power. [...] The cures were so numerous and sometimes so rapid that they could not be attributed to any natural cause [and] the failures were to be ascribed to want of faith on the part of the patients'.[36] The mindset of Charles's doctors indicates that few men in history, however distinguished, are able to free themselves from the prejudices imposed by their time – a time when the belief in 'magical medicine' was still extant, finding its echo as late as 1633 in physician Thomas Browne's aforementioned popular work *Religio Medici,* or 'The Religion of a Doctor'.[37]

Eventual scepticism by the medical establishment

Decades later, King William III (1650-1702) of England was publicly disdainful of the customary royal touch, referring to it as a 'silly superstition'. The king 'had too much sense to be duped, and too much honesty to bear a part in what he knew to be an imposture'.[38] One Easter, when told that a large crowd of sufferers besieged his palace, his command was to 'give the poor creatures some money, and send them away'[39] and on the one and only occasion he was harassed into laying his hand on a sufferer, he was heard to say 'God give you better health, and more sense'.[40]

As a consequence to William's derisive stance in regard to the Royal Touch, the medical establishment began voicing their reasoned scepticism quite openly. In the late sixteen hundreds, physician Richard Carr, addressing the Royal College of Physicians objectively declared that 'the King's Touch may still be beneficial, if ever it was; often it is apt to be ineffectual, but it can never be harmful'.[41]

One and a half centuries later renowned British historian, Baron Thomas Babington Macaulay (1800-1859), contemptuously denounced the gross gullibility of those 'medical men of high note [who] believed or affected to believe in the balsamic virtues of the royal hand' and went on to say 'we cannot wonder that, when men of science gravely repeated such nonsense, the vulgar should have believed it. Still less can we wonder that wretches tortured by a disease over which natural remedies had no power should have eagerly drunk in tales of preternatural cures: for nothing is so credulous as misery'.[42]

The last monarch in England credited with the 'healing touch' was

Queen Anne (1665-1714). In the year 1712 she is reputed to have touched 200 sufferers, among them the then infant Samuel Johnson, who was later to become one of England's great literary figures. King George I (1660-1727) condemned the ceremony as superstitious and the custom of touching for the King's Evil ended forthwith in Britain.[43]

As strange as the belief in healing by touch may seem from a modern perspective, so healing by sympathy, or at a distance, seems equally bizarre. But, there is no doubt that this practice of 'magical medicine' was very popular and widely used by physicians during the sixteenth and seventeenth centuries.

Healing by sympathy

The 'wound salve', 'weapon's salve', or 'powder of sympathy' are fitting examples of healing by sympathy or at a distance, whereby ailments, as well as remedies, could be transferred as it were, from one body to another. This form of magical medicine was especially promoted in the writings of Paracelsus[44] (1493-1541) during the sixteenth and seventeenth centuries. At the time, the hypotheses and therapies of Paracelsus represented the most complete and wide-ranging alternatives to the traditional Galenic system of therapeutics.

Paracelsus propagated the principle of preserving harmony between man and nature – between microcosm and macrocosm. He believed that '…man resembles heaven and earth because he was made from them – "hence we must have all their nature and all their parts, down to the last hair"'.[45] Furthermore, he postulated that microcosm and macrocosm were linked through man's astral body, thus effecting an influence from nature and the cosmos on man, and similarly from man to his surroundings. 'Therefore, even though the macrocosm is the greater, the microcosm remains similar both in power and in composition.[46]

Through the interconnectivity between man and the natural world, all constituents of the external world were thought united in man, hence forming a 'sympathy' between himself and external objects. That is why the Paracelsian Agrippa von Nettesheim (1486-1535)[47] declared that 'it is well known amongst physicians [...] that the right eye of a frog helps the soreness of a man's right eye, and the left eye thereof, helps the soreness of his left eye, if they be hanged about in a cloth of its natural colour'.[48] For the same 'sympathetic' reasons, physicians during the second half of the sixteenth century, still gave smallpox the 'red treatment',[49] wrapping patients in scarlet clothes and red sheets, while red bed-coverings were employed to bring the pustules to the body's surface.[50]

The therapeutic practice of healing 'at a distance'

Based on these principles of 'sympathy', Paracelsus propagated 'healing at a distance' or 'action at a distance'. The pseudo-Paracelsian book *Archidoxis Magica*, published in 1570, first introduced the curative weapon salve and lists the following ingredients and method of preparation: moss which had grown on a human skull – preferably someone who had been executed or killed violently – human fat, mummy powder, human blood, linseed oil, oil of roses and bole-armoniack,[51] to be mixed to a smooth ointment.

However, strange as it may seem, this 'ointment' was not applied to the wound itself, but to the weapon which had caused the wound in the first place. If the weapon could not be found, a stick poked into the wound and thereby coated with the victims blood, was deemed a suitable substitute. By treating the instrument responsible for the injury, the wound itself healed 'sympathetically' – or so it was thought. Since one had caused the other, weapon and wound were sympathetically connected. The therapeutic practice of healing by 'sympathy' – advocated by physicians and learned men at the time – was clearly a form of 'sympathetic magic', universally also practiced in magic rites and folk medicine.

Although this, to modern thinking seemingly ridiculous method of 'healing', was arguably of very little use to someone severely injured in battle, because the weapon may not have been accessible, it was definitely deemed of benefit to a clumsy butcher, carpenter or other handyman. In administering this treatment it was of great importance that the weapon still be 'bloody' – the sympathetic bond between blood on the weapon and blood in the wound allegedly strengthening the efficacy of the salve.

In his overbearing manner, Paracelsus had couched such folk healing remedies in 'philosophical' gloss and interpretation: he rationally explained that the salve united the vital spirits in the blood on the blade with the spirit in the victim's body, whereby healing would take place. 'If you allowed that invisible influences could act at a distance – try explaining magnetism in any other way – it all made perfect sense'.[52]. According to the pseudo-Paracelsian *Archidoxis Magica*, the wound itself was to be bound with linen and washed every morning with the patient's own urine and 'it shall be healed, be it never so great, without any Plaister or Pain'.[53]

Regarding the seemingly outlandish, gruesome ingredients for the salve, they had been chosen for their sympathetic correspondence to the course of healing. The use of human blood, fat and mummy, reflected the notion that these possessed essential forces to accomplish the therapeutic process. For centuries, blood was regarded as an elixir, imbued with strength and vigour. But, the rejuvenating qualities of tissue from those who had died at a young age were particularly valued. This is why recipes generally called for the use of body parts from those who had died an aberrant death, as the healing life force was thought to remain in such a corpse for some time. (See chapter 8 on Corpse Medicine)

Strange as it may seem, various compositions for sympathetic cures, all with specific instructions, were prescribed by different physicians. Generally mixtures contained human fat and blood, mummy, moss of dead man's skull, or bull's blood and fat, as well as other 'exotic' ingredients. Often these had to be exposed to the sun for up to 365 days. Astoundingly, serious discussion was maintained in the sympathetical school of thought '…whether it was necessary that the moss should grow in the skull of a thief who had hung on the gallows, and whether the ointment while compounding should be stirred with a murderer's knife?'[54]

In Paracelsian philosophy the idea that 'like attracts like' produced a number of adherents in sixteenth and seventeenth century Europe. Not only was the original wound salve formula modified several times, but it also found its way into the books of numerous physicians and various erudite followers of Paracelsus. One of his ardent advocates was Oswald Crollius, professor of medicine at the German University of Marburg, who recommended the wound salve in his *Basilica Chymica*. This text was very popular in Europe at the time and was translated into several languages.[55, 56]

The 'Powder of Sympathy'

Another strong advocate of the wound salve and a believer in natural magic was Rudolf Goclenius (1572-1621), professor of physics, medicine and mathematics at the University of Marburg in Germany. Although he dedicated much of his time on cures for the plague, he became famous for his 'Powder of Sympathy', based on the postulates of Paracelsus.

The concept of 'action at a distance' to heal wounds, was brought to England by Paracelsian physician, astrologer and mathematician Robert Fludd (1574-1637). Fludd argued that the existance of magnetic force was proof for the efficacy of the weapon salve. He explained that just as magnetic force could unite particles over a distance, so the vital essence contained in blood could be transferred from the wound to the weapon. Decades later, English physician and writer Christopher Irvine (1620-1693) strongly advocated astrological components involved in the healing process, and expounded his theories in *The Rare and Wonderful Art of Curing by Sympathy*,[57] in 1656.

In 1657, Sir Kenelm Digby (1603-1665),[58] was one of many early scientists propagating 'action at a distance'. Before an assembly of nobles and learned men at the medical faculty of the University of Montpellier in France,[59] Digby lectured on his 'Powder of Sympathy' – to cure wounds by anointing the weapon that caused the injury. Digby's remedy was a powder, as opposed to the traditional Paracelsian salve.

Sir Kenelm Digby's chief aim before the doctors at Montpellier was to denounce magic and other supernatural means in the recorded healing abilities of the Wound Salve and to rather put its perceived positive effects down to natural causes.[60] When considering that surgeons in those times seem to have been impeded rather than facilitated by their modes of treatment in healing wounds, it seems miraculous that positive healing was recorded at all – even in connection with the wound salve. However, reported cures by 'sympathetic' doctors are easily explained when considering their directives regarding the Wound Salve or the Powder of Sympathy. Although these medications were smeared on the weapon responsible for inflicting the wound, the wound was to be washed, the edges of the wound brought into apposition and held in place by bandages, then kept undisturbed, the body maintaining rest – in other words, this fascilitated the natural healing process.

As late as 1730, a 'Sympathetic Liniment' was still advocated by apothecary and medical writer John Quincy. In his *Complete English Dispensatory* he instructs how to prepare this mixture: 'Take oil of roses, fine bole, linseed oil, Man's grease, moss of human Skull, of one killed by violence, in powder, mummy and man's blood, make a liniment'[61] – the mixture seems almost identical to that recommended by Paracelsus two hundred years earlier. Furthermore, Quincy recommends using the 'liniment' on the weapon itself.[62]

The medical debate rages on

As the concept of 'action at a distance' was heatedly debated in England and on the Continent, an argument soon developed as to whether the perceived effects of the wound salve should be seen as 'natural' or demonic. A number of treatises written by doctors and scientists appeared in close succession, but soon the purely medical discussions became embroiled in religious, denominational controversy, pitting Catholicism against unorthodox Protestantism. Goclenius published his first treatise affirming the efficacy of the Paracelsian wound salve in 1608. Subsequently, between 1615 and 1625 seven attacks and counterattacks were exchanged between Goclenius and the Jesuit Johannes Roberti (1569-1651), who condemned the salve as 'devil's deceit'. Protagonists of the wound salve were repeatedly accused of consorting with demons. In many cases such charges had a lasting effect. Because of his advocacy of the magnetic cure of wounds, renowned Belgian physician Jean Baptiste van Helmont suffered ecclesiastic prosecution from the Spanish Inquisition from 1625 onwards.

Physicians were still debating the apparently absurd remedy of 'action at a distance' furiously in the 1630's, when Anglican pastor William Foster published *A Sponge to Wipe Away the Weapon-Salve* – only to be energetically refuted by Fludd. In his efficacy criticism Foster did not denounce the weapon salve as inefficacious but rather as the product of witchcraft.[63] He argued that the cure was not in accordance with Church teachings; that none of the ancient authorities spoke of medicine that could cure from a distance; and that a remedy, which did not work by means of corporeal contact, could not be natural – hence it must be demonic.

During the second half of the seventeenth century, due to a growing interest in the explainations for the causes of various phenomena in nature, discussion and debate on the effectiveness of sympathetic cures eventually died down and ceased.

The following chapters offer a glimpse into three of the many, dreadfully virulent epidemics and diseases that swept over the European continent in past centuries – each disease evidencing its own distinctive medical and social implications and consequences …

THE GREAT MORTALITY – THE BLACK DEATH

In medieval times the dreaded plague was known as the 'great mortality', or the 'great pestilence'. The great plague epidemic of 1347-1351 was first referred to as the 'Black Death' only around 1550 – the term probably due to the sinister nature of the disease: the black colouring of the victims' swollen glands, the discolouration of the skin and the black tumours or buboes that occurred on the second day of initial outbreak.

The history of this deadly disease, which swept over Europe, Southwest Asia and parts of North Africa in the mid-fourteenth century, with lightning speed, was not characterised by medical success. On the contrary, physicians mired in traditional views held for over a thousand years, were utterly helpless and dismally failed the general population in the face of this overwhelming epidemic. Why then, is a chapter on the Black Death included as part of this book? The answer lies in the consequences of the epidemic. They were far-reaching and lasting, and any book dealing even marginally with historic concepts of disease and medical practices cannot fail to discuss this horrific outbreak. But historians have been divided over the impact of this contagion.

A couple of decades ago the traditional view of the pivotal role played by the Black Death on the fabric of European society was challenged. Revisionist historians recast this catastrophe as a '...necessary and long-overdue corrective to an overpopulated Europe'.[1] In other words, the plague was not an unexpected, outbreak, but consequential to a population that had outgrown the agricultural ability to feed itself. Post-revisionist historians have since swung the pendulum back again, validating the Great Mortality's impact on the Western world as *the* major turning point in the transition from medieval to early modern Europe. The Black Death effected many changes in the medical establishment, as well as manifest political, economic, social and cultural transformations.

Initial outbreak and spread

The sheer enormity of human loss and devastation between 1347 and 1351 is inconceivable. According to estimates by modern historians, the plague killed between twenty-five and forty-five percent of Europe's population – over 25 million people in Europe, and another 25 million in Asia and Africa.[2] This leads to the question of when the first outbreak of plague was recorded. In ancient times, many diseases referred to as 'plague' were simply a general name for varying forms of murderous epidemics, which could not easily be differentiated in those days.

Although outbreaks of infectious diseases were important in their impact on European history, their combined role was dwarfed by the arrival of the plague in 542 CE.[3] Plague is probably one of the most virulent and deadly diseases and it comes not in isolated epidemics but in pandemics, which strike in cyclic fashion – until the eighteenth century the Black Death returned again and again in Europe.

By the end of the twelfth century, diseases like smallpox, measles, leprosy, malaria, tuberculosis, typhus, scarlet fever and a few others had reached a tentative equilibrium within the European populace. That is to say, that the disease pool had stabilised and even the greatest killer of them all, the plague, had temporarily disappeared. But then, the prerequisites for utter calamity came into being: to begin with, a change in climatic conditions in earlier centuries had begun to vary the Eurasian insect and rodent ecology.

In addition, important social and economic changes had taken place in Europe: closer trade connections had been forged with Asia and

Africa. Therefore, as the demand for luxury goods rose in Europe, more ships and caravans journeyed to these continents, thereby changing the epidemiological balance for the European continent. These factors would combine to forever alter the course of Western history during the fourteenth century.

Spreading along the trade routes from Asia into southern Russia – the region between the Black and Caspian seas – the Black Death probably reached the port of Alexandria in Egypt by late 1347. Chroniclers report that the number of deaths in Alexandria soon rose to about 1,000 a day. Other towns in the Nile Delta were equally devastated. In Cairo more than a third of the population perished. From Cairo the epidemic spread to the Middle East.

Once the contagion arrived in Europe it spread quickly along the major trade routes, reaching France and England in 1348. The scale of losses is brought into perspective when considering some of the numbers: according to Church records fifteen hundred people died in the French town of Avignon in three days and in 1350, two years after the plague first reached Europe, the population in London was half of what it had been before the plague. Florence probably lost at least 40,000 of its nearly 90,000 inhabitants; Paris, the largest city west of the Alps, lost more than 50,000 of its 180,000 inhabitants.[4]

Not only contact with infected individuals, but also rats and gerbils coming off ships, played a considerable part in the rapid spread of the plague. The disease is carried by a variety of rodents and can pass on to humans when fleas carrying infected rodent blood attach themselves to a human host. Rodents provide the mode of transport for fleas, which share their 'accommodation' between humans and rodents.[5]

Symptoms – repulsive, fearsome and lethal

All symptoms associated with the Black Death were repulsive, erupting in such a fearsomely visible manner as to leave victims with no doubt that the mark of death was upon them. Although some sufferers survived, most people died within three days of the onset of symptoms. The pestilence seemed especially well appointed to debase and humiliate its victims who became objects of detestation rather than of pity, and in the words of a French chronicler, everything '...which exuded from their bodies let off an unbearable stench: sweat, excrement, spittle, breath, so foetid as to be overpowering'.[6]

A vivid description of the plague and its terrors in 1348, comes to us from plague survivor Gabriele de' Mussis, an Italian notary from Piacenza: 'Those of both sexes who were in health and in no fear of death, were struck by four savage blows to the flesh. First, out of the blue a kind of chilly stiffness troubled their bodies. They felt a tingling sensation as if they were being pricked by the points of arrows. The next stage was a fearsome attack which took the form of an extremely hard solid boil... as it grew more solid, its burning heat caused the patient to fall into an acute and putrid fever, with severe headaches. As it intensified its extreme bitterness could have various effects. In some cases it gave rise to an intolerable stench. In others it brought spitting of blood, for others swelling near the place from which the corrupt humors had arisen...Some people lay as if in a drunken stupor and could not be roused. Behold the swellings the warning signs sent by our Lord. Some died on the very day the illness took possession of them, others on the next day, others – the majority – between the third and fifth day'.[7]

The Black Death differed from other epidemics in its extent, severity and ubiquity. Leprosy, for instance was also widely feared in the eleventh, twelfth and thirteenth centuries, but affected fewer individuals who could then be segregated from the general community in leper houses and leper colonies. The plague on the other hand spread rapidly and struck swiftly, harshly and with fatal results. Life was in total chaos. Entire families were wiped out in a matter of days; hundreds of villages and towns were destroyed. Once a family member had contracted the disease, the entire household was doomed to die. Many people ran away in vain attempts to save themselves.

Chroniclers of the time described how those left alive struggled to bury the corpses of the hundreds who died each day. In some towns and villages dead bodies simply piled up, with no one to bury them and no priests to say mass over them. Neither was the plague a respecter of rank and riches; it '...seizes young and old alike, sparing no one and reducing rich and poor to the same level', King Edward III wrote after his fourteen-year-old daughter succumbed to the disease in 1348.[8]

The wrath of God

As may be expected in the face of such mortality, people were shocked, stunned, bewildered and terrified. As with all other major diseases, explanations for the causes of such devastation were frantically sought very soon into the outbreak. Like leprosy, this epidemic seemed weighed down with Scriptural associations, as well as moral metaphors. Hence, the plague was interpreted as requiring public atonement. Explanations for the origins of this 'great pestilence' were taken from Biblical exegesis and the high mortality was explained away as divine judgement – this *was* God's punishment of a sinful humanity. Obviously, the general populace had strayed from the straight and narrow path of true belief. It should be noted that most, if not all medieval authorities at the time assumed that the pestilence was an act of chastisement for humanity's wickedness.

Medical specialists like Guy de Chauliac (c.1300-1368), a member of the faculty of medicine at the University in Paris and personal physician to the Pope, acknowledged that medicine could not help when such contagion was sent by the will of God. In the autumn of 1348, at the initial spread of the contagion to England, King Edward III had a letter known as *Terribilis* circulated to all southern dioceses, urging the power of prayer and masses against the invasion of plague to his realm. In Avignon, Pope Clement VI (1291-1352) commanded devout processions with the chanting of litanies. While the Pope himself took part in some of these processions, thousands walked with him, tearing their hair, smearing themselves with ashes, wailing and whipping themselves bloody, in order to halt the spread of God's wrath.[9] As a further suggestion the Church '… stated that it was foolish to flee from the Black Death because it was God, not men, who disseminated the disease'.[10]

The call to repentance was loud and clear and consequently the ever-present medieval apocalyptic outlook deeply intensified. The European populace were preoccupied with death, the final judgement, heaven and hell. Because people became so acutely aware of the inevitability of Judgement Day and the omnipotence of God, the clergy and Church were seen as a conduit to salvation – notably medicine and its potential to help in this situation could not supplant theological issues. Salvation seemed more important than ever before, as death was lurking everywhere and people were dying by the hundreds and thousands every day.

Demonstrations of piety

Visible demonstrations of piety increased; good works and devout charity blossomed. The Church advised that time in purgatory could be shortened by charitable donations and bequests to hospitals and the like. Those financially able to make donations were therefore 'killing two birds' with one proverbial stone, by helping plague victims and contributing towards personal salvation.

Another channel to grant time off from purgatory was the sale of indulgences in the 1350's – drawing from the 'treasury of merits', which constituted the good deeds accumulated by saints and church fathers. However, there were pardons to suit the size of every purse. If indulgences proved too expensive for some individuals, churchmen offered cheaper options. They brought these 'options' to their congregations in glass bottles, so they could be seen but not touched. Alternatively, for a halfpenny of payment, the glass bottles would be handed around to be kissed by the penitent: '…bones from the skeletons of saints, hairs from hallowed heads, fingers from sacred hands, and pieces of wood from the cross of Christ […] a fragment of the veil of Our Lady, or perhaps her shoe or the ring of St. John the Evangelist or even the very finger which John the Baptist had pointed at Christ'.[11]

Many believed that extreme measures were called for in this time of crisis, which is why groups of Flagellants appeared in great numbers.. Flagellants, although in existence long before the eruption of the plague, dramatically increased in numbers during the Black Death outbreak. The movement spread quickly across Europe and '…the public seemed unable to get enough of the Flagellants [...]. From mid-August to mid-October 1349, fifty-three hundred Flagellates reportedly passed through the town'[12] of Tournai in France.

Similarly other towns saw large processions every week. Processions varied in size from a handful of people to hundreds. Each Flagellant carried a 'scourge', a wooden stick with a couple of leather thongs attached to one end. Fastened to each thong was a sharp iron spike, which when hitting the Flagellant's back drew blood almost immediately. This self-punishment was to pay for their own, as well as humanity's sins, in an effort to reduce the incidence of pestilence.[13]

As is apparent from preceding paragraphs, medicine played very much a secondary role during this crisis. The Church's stranglehold on all realms of life and education also firmly applied to the field of medicine. In the face of this calamity, the Church hammered home its harsh irrefutable message of a sinful humanity, public atonement, divine judgement and punishment. The position of doctors was not facilitated by the '...stern determination of medieval churchmen to keep the physician in his place'.[14] Contemporary physicians were helpless in the face of such mortality and implicitly agreed with theologians that the epidemic had religious causes. Although physicians also advocated physical causes for the contagion, theology ensured that medicine played a lesser role.[15] The function of medicine and physicians during this great mortality shall be discussed at length in subsequent paragraphs.

Popularly perceived causes of the plague

Although divine judgement was a generally accepted cause of the plague, the general populace also zealously sought other reasons for the origin of this catastrophe. Scapegoats were soon found amongst various minority groups, especially among the European Jewish community. Regrettably, '...the Great Mortality occasioned one of the most vicious outbreaks of anti-Semitic violence in European history'.[16] In medieval Europe, little if anything was known about the local Jews, especially about their various traditions and their culture. As is often the case, such ignorance gave rise to gross mistrust and misconception. In addition, Jews were perceived as representing social non-conformity, hence making them ideal targets for persecution.

At the time, the largest Jewish community in Europe lived on the Iberian Peninsula (present day Spain and Portugal). Here Jews had been treated better than in any other part of the Christian world, with only isolated incidences of anti-Semitism occurring over the centuries. Jews served in leading positions in Spanish society, as tax collectors, managers, apothecaries, physicians and interpreters. However, the era of Black Death ended such tolerance abruptly. Why? Because it was believed that Jews had brought on the dreaded Black Death by poisoning the wells and local drinking water.

This was in fact an old idea, which was simply revived in 1348. Just over two decades previously in 1321, a group of lepers had been accused of fouling the drinking water in the Languedoc, France. Minutes before their execution they loudly cried out that the town's Jews had encouraged their foul deed. Unfortunately, these accusations came back to life again in 1348, when a Jewish physician in the German town of Neustadt confessed under torture, to poisoning the local well. Although he was doubtlessly innocent, he broke – literally – under the rack. Word spread from Germany and pogroms erupted wherever Jews resided. They were rounded up and burned, or drowned in marshes. Persecutions only ended when deaths from the plague began to decline.

In Spain the excuse of the wells was not even necessary; Jews were especially vulnerable, due to their great wealth. Although the kings of Aragon and Castile swiftly moved to protect their Jewish subjects, three-quarters of the Iberian Jewish community had been disseminated by the time that normal judicial authority had been re-established.

Medical pronouncements on the outbreak

In response to a request by the King of France, Philip VI, in October 1348, the faculty of medicine at Paris University issued *A Compendium of Opinion on the Black Death*, which was considered the most up-to-date authoritative medical information on the causes of the plague outbreak.

Their pronouncements were divided into three chapters: one cause was listed as 'up above and in heaven', the second as ' lower and on earth' and the third as 'prognostications and signs, which are connected to both'.[17]

Their primary explanations for the outbreak of the Black Death was deduced from astrology '...a certain configuration in the heavens [...] the lining up of three higher planets in Aquarius [...] being the present cause of the ruinous corruption of the air that is around us'.[18] As this indicates, astrology was firmly linked to medicine in medieval times, a fact which Church authorities had no difficulty in accepting – after all, the universe and consequently planetary configuration and influence, were God's creation.

When authorities related the outbreak of the Black Death to the position of various heavenly bodies, this made perfect sense within contemporary medical theory: the signs of the zodiac were associated with certain elements, which were linked to the four humors, and to the various body parts and organs. (See chapter 2, Humoral bodies – a healthy balance)

Astrologers and physicians traced the beginning of the epidemic, to a lunar eclipse, which occurred on the evening of 18 March 1348.[19] Others, among them the Italian doctor Gentile of Foligno, conjectured that the disaster was caused by a particularly unfortunate conjunction of Saturn, Jupiter and Mars in the sign of Aquarius that had occurred on 20 March 1345. This conjunction resulted in hot, moist conditions, which caused the earth to 'exhale' poisonous vapours, which when breathed in and out, spread plague.[20] [21]

'Poisonous vapours' were in fact the conventional premise offered by medieval doctors for the outbreak of plague epidemics and other diseases. Traditional hypothesis held that diseases such as malaria, cholera and the Black Death were caused by *miasma*,[22] a noxious form of 'bad air' or 'poisonous vapours'. Miasmic theory, the substantial change in air quality, was first advocated by Hippocratic writers and further advanced by Galen.

In modern times miasmic theory lingers on in the belief regarding the health benefits of 'fresh country air'. Miasmic or 'poisonous vapours' were thought to contain suspended particles of decaying matter, characterised by their foul smell. This is why malaria was originally so named – from the Italian *mala* 'bad' and *aria* 'air' – as evidence of the disease's suspected miasmic origins.

Accordingly, diseases were seen as the product of environmental factors such as contaminated water and foul air and *not* as passed between individuals: 'Almost every fourteenth century doctor took it for granted that the corruption of the atmosphere was a prime cause of the Black Death'.[23] And in view of the many poor, filthy, foul-smelling neighborhoods that tended to be the focal points of disease and epidemics, miasma theory made perfect sense.

'Noxious vapours' caused by social and hygiene factors

In order to understand this hypothesis we have to imagine living conditions during the Middle Ages. In this context it is primarily important to accept the different mind-set, and widely differing sensibilities of people of past centuries. What modern people would find offensive, shocking, and intolerable, once formed a part of everyday living. In general, medieval life for the vast majority of the population was not clean and sweet smelling by modern standards.[24] Open sewers, filth, blood and gore were very much a part of everyday existence; it was not uncommon to see the decapitated heads of enemies, or decaying human bodies hanging on gibbets outside city gates; medications included the most vile ingredients – as discussed in the chapters on Sewer Pharmacology and Corpse Medicine; excrement was not only attributed therapeutic qualities until the mid-eighteenth century, it was also used in aromatic preparations[25] – again a question of changing sensibilities when considered from a modern perspective.

Medieval towns and cities were cramped, the houses small and standing close together. Fetid odours were an accepted fact of life. Large parts of medieval cities smelled of sewage, human faeces, urine, and rotting matter. For instance, Walbrook stream running down through the centre of London, '…seems from early times to have been used as an open sewer, in which people got rid of much dung and other filth and rubbish from their stables and houses'[26] during the fourteenth century.

Although many of the larger medieval cities *did* have public sanitation systems, these were rudimentary and not ubiquitous. Monasteries, castles and palaces,[27] as well as many wealthy establishments around Europe, occasionally had running water,[28] and generally housed 'privies', which jutted out over rivers. But it was a different scenario when privies projected over a ditch or a shallow flowing stream – one can only imagine the horrendous 'build-up'. Records document several public latrines in London during the early fourteenth century, for use by the general population.[29] Especially the latrines on London Bridge, all draining into the Thames, were of considerable importance, servicing the general populace, as well as the proprietors of about one hundred and thirty eight shops situated on the bridge in 1358.[30]

However, most residents were not as fortunate to avail themselves of their own 'privies' and in many parts of medieval Europe, sanitation legislation simply required homeowners to shout 'look out below' three times, before dumping the contents of full chamber pots and slop buckets into the street below.[31] Very often '…filth and garbage of all kinds was thrown into the streets and left there until the town officials made a fuss, when it was carted away and dumped into the river or some other convenient place'.[32] This is given credence by King Edward III's complaint in the mid-fourteenth century that '…the smells of York were worse than those of any town in the kingdom'.[33]

Similarly, although many medieval towns and cities had sanitary regulations in place, shopkeepers often dumped their refuse in the streets. Some streets had open gutters to carry waste, but often there were no drains to take away dirty water and rotting sewage. All this was paradise for flies, flitting from faeces to food. Fly-, germ- and rodent-infested rubbish, bringing disease-carrying ticks and fleas into human contact, would often stay in the streets until it was eventually removed or washed away by heavy downpours.

However, citizens and authorities were not indifferent to such conditions and attempted to clean up the streets by instituting compulsory sewers and cesspools. Public outcry was especially aimed at the outdoor slaughterhouses in cities and towns. Butchers would slaughter their animals in the streets, and leave bloody entrails and offal to pile up, which resulted in swarms of black rats that lived off the filth. Hence, a royal instruction by King Edward III during the time of the Black Death, regarding '…putrid blood running down the streets […] the air in the city very much corrupted and infected, whence abominable and most filthy stinks proceed'.[34] The royal decree forthwith ordered butchers to dump all offal directly into the Thames – a river, which already had all private and public privies draining into it.

In England the first national Sanitation Act, which applied to all towns, was passed in 1388 – many years after the Black Death – by a parliament sitting at Cambridge.[35] This Sanitation Act seems to have had its genesis due to the peculiarly filthy condition of that borough. The Act consisted of a general prohibition of the pollution of rivers, ditches and open spaces, thereby giving parliamentary support to the by-laws on that subject, which already existed in all the larger towns. Unsavoury, polluting trades, such as tanners, fishmongers, and brick burning, were then banished to the outskirts of the town.[36]

It is disturbing to note that by the early fourteenth century '…so much filth had collected inside urban Europe that French and Italian cities were naming streets after human waste. In medieval Paris, several street names were inspired by *merde*, the French word for 'shit'.[37] For instance, to name but a few: the Rue Merdeux, Rue Merdelet, Rue Merdusson, Rue des Merdons and many others. These were the smelly, unsanitary facts of life during those times – leaving no doubt as to the facilitation of the spread of pestilence.

No wonder, miasma theory or 'deadly vapours' were advocated by physicians to explain disease. And it made pefect sense for centuries to come, which is why miasma theory was still used to explain the spread of cholera in London and Paris during the 1850's. Eventually, in the nineteenth century, sanitary reformers realised that by removing the causes of bad smells, thereby often inadvertently removing disease-causing bacteria, levels of disease were seen to fall. But during the Black Death outbreak no such conclusions had as yet been drawn. Therefore, when the Black Death arrived in England in 1348, Edward III ordered London to be '…cleaned of all bad smells, so that no more people will die from such smells'.[38] What is however interesting, is how these 'bad smells' were cleared. Canons were fired repeatedly to 'clear' the air and bells were rung to dissipate the 'corrupt airs'.[39]

Another school of thought advocated fighting the 'noxious vapours' that were allegedly spreading the plague, with foul odours, much like the motto of 'fighting fire with fire' or 'like influencing like'. It had been noticed that attendants cleaning out latrines and other 'malodorous places' often seemed immune to infection. Therefore, '…it was not unknown for apprehensive citizens of a plague-struck city to spend hours each day crouched over a latrine absorbing with relish the foetid smells'.[40] Some people considered this infallible protection.

Recommended medical treatments

Medicine, firmly rooted in Galenic principles, dismally failed to respond successfully to its greatest challenge – the Black Death. In many respects, physicians in fact harmed rather than helped as they did not understand the causes of infectious disease or how it spread. Preventive measures were frantically sought. Although doctors clearly lacked confidence in their ability to keep the plague at bay and doubted their ability to cure it once it had struck, this did not deter them from putting forward a host of remedies. Doctors especially recommended purges by way of laxatives, diuretics, cautery and bleeding.

Once the incredibly painful hard black buboes appeared on the neck, under the armpits and in the groin of those infected, doctors treated them with cautery and incision. They believed that the buboes were a sign of the body putting up a fight, by expelling 'evil' humors to the surface. It was therefore essential to squeeze out the corrupt matter. In desperation many victims themselves tried to cut out the pestilent carbuncles under the most excruciating pain, even driving red-hot pokers into the sores, in the futile hope of eradicating them.

Within the perspectives of medieval physiology, phlebotomy or bleeding was a rational precautionary measure and treatment. When the plague attacked, body juices were thought to stop flowing and air to stop circulating through the body – the person died. Because the heart was seen as occupying a central position in the body, and because body 'juices' flowed through it, veins close to the heart were bled to treat plague victims. As particular veins were seen as linked to certain organs, which in turn were influenced by astral signs and humors, bleeding these veins was thought to lead to a desired change in the course of body fluids and body heat.

Body heat was considered of utmost importance if the person were to maintain good health. Generally physicians treating the plague followed the position of the Parisian Medical School, linking a lack of natural body heat to inadequate air circulating through the lungs. Body heat was also considered essential to eliminate all 'noxious vapours' spreading the plague. Therefore, Pope Clement VI, living at Avignon at the time of the plague, was recommended by his surgeons to sit between two large fires, in order to heat the body and breathe pure air.[41] As the plague *bacillus* is actually destroyed by heat, this may have been one of the few truly effective measures taken.

Another defensive measure involving heat, was a recipe containing sulphur, arsenic and antimony. These ingredients, mixed together were to be thrown into the fireplaces of homes. This recipe may have had beneficial effects, as sulphur '…is now recognised as being destructive to bacteria, as well as to rats and flees. The other compounds had the minor merit of making the usually smelly medieval house a little more agreeable to live in'.[42]

The question remained, as to why some people escaped infection while so many others died. The answer given by most doctors at the time lay in humoral balance. The reason people succumbed to the plague was thought to be an imbalance in the body's humors or fluids – a theory already going back over a thousand years at the time of the Black Death. Emotional, dietary, seasonal or other external factors were deemed to cause humoral imbalance which resulted in illness and death.

Physicians advocated that persons of moist, hot temperament were most likely to succumb to the plague, which is why the medical establishment regarded the previously mentioned conjunction of Jupiter, Saturn and Mars in the sign of Aquarius on 20 March 1345, as especially important. To physicians this conjunction was plausibly explicable within the recognised humoral theory: Jupiter was seen as warm and humid, while Mars was held to be hot and dry, therefore setting those elements aflame in humans. Saturn was another matter altogether, as no one quite knew what Saturn's characteristics actually were. Nevertheless, it was firmly held that anything associated with this planet negatively affected the body's humors. (See chapter 2 on humors)

Although most physicians endorsed miasma theory, others thought that all severe southerly winds carried the deadly vapours of the plague – a theory already advocated by the great polymath Avicenna who suggested that most epidemic disease came from the equator. This is why the famous Montpellier medical school advised all doors and windows to face in a northerly direction – in other words away from the equator – in northern Europe.

Physicians also believed that the air was at its deadliest in summer and early autumn, when heat opened the pores and made individuals more susceptible to assault by diseases. As we have become aware in more modern times, certain weather conditions influence rodent and insect life cycles and could therefore be considered factors in the frequency of pandemic plague, giving some merit to the 'deadly summer and early autumn air' idea.

While the precise cause of the plague was not completely understood until the beginning of the twentieth century, it is surprising that medical observers failed to make a connection in 1348 with the epidemic outbreak and the overabundance of dead rodents seen beforehand. This oversight is especially significant because Avicenna had noted centuries before that one of the signs of pestilence was that '…mice and subterranean animals flee to the surface of the earth and behave as if intoxicated'.[43]

To avoid contracting the plague, medical wisdom of the time and for centuries to come recommended staying indoors with all windows tightly shut. Also, bathing was to be avoided at all costs as it softened skin and widened the pores, thereby allowing diseases to penetrate the body. Hence, physicians denounced baths as dangerous, an outlook advocated by the medical faculty of the University of Paris. The faculty advised people to avoid baths except perhaps just prior to bleeding, when hot water could loosen bad humors and so expel them.[44] Hands and feet could however be washed with vinegar and rose water.

To bathe or not to bathe

In view of the terrible outbreak of pestilence, this raises the important question of personal attention to physical cleanliness and hygiene during these times. As it is of relevance, this question has been discussed in some detail. Utterly opposed views are given by distinguished medieval scholars regarding the frequency of bathing during the Middle Ages and beyond.[45] While some historians categorically denounce that people took baths,[46] others advocate that the practice of warm-bathing prevailed in all classes of society and was very much a part of medieval life[47] owing to the number of public bathhouses in the large European cities.[48]

The answer, in all probability, lies somewhere in between, and it can be assumed with certainty that the poorer classes did not have access to regular water resources for bathing. People were often covered with '… foul eruptions, exacerbated by rough woollen clothing and the constant presence of dirt, ticks and fleas'[49] – ideal conditions for the spread of pestilence. Owing to the lack of personal cleanliness, skin diseases were rife.[50] An early thirteenth century English chronicle, describing the Danish invasion, dwells on the fact that the Danes bathed on Saturdays. As the chronicler mentions this twice in a dozen lines, it seems to suggest that weekly bathing was something highly unusual in his own experience.[51]

While castles and palaces often housed baths [52] during medieval times, personal 'hygiene' amongst the general populace was restricted to the bare essentials. Cleanliness seems to have been a matter of appearance, washing the visible parts of the body and not scratching one's fleas too obviously.[53] Medieval books on etiquette insist upon the duty of washing hands and face every morning, but say nothing on the subject of bathing,[54] except to do so occasionally on therapeutic grounds.

A popular medieval health text, the *Secreta Secretorum*, gives elaborate advice regarding the specific seasons suitable or unsuitable for bathing. In other words, baths were not a frequent occurrence.[55] Detailed accounts of King John's (1166-1216) household indicate that the monarch indulged in a bath every three or four weeks'.[56] King

'Edward III scandalised London when he bathed three times in as many months'.[57] Although Louis XIV of France had six *cabinets de bain* installed in Versailles, he '...disliked bathing and rarely took one'[58] – in fact, some sources quote Louis XIV as only having taken two baths in his lifetime.[59] An English chronicler wrote that '...vermin boiled over like water in a simmering cauldron',[60] when Archbishop Thomas à Beckett (c.1118-1170) was stripped naked after his assassination.

Preventive measures and remedies

Apart from actively discouraging baths of any kind during the time of the Black Death, physicians recommended that all forms of exercise be avoided, as fatigue made one more susceptible to the plague. In addition, exercise introduced more air into the body, hence, through the air, more poison or miasma. Doctors also advised on sleeping habits: never should one sleep on one's back as this allowed plague-ridden noxious airs to slip into the body; too much sleep was ill advised, especially during the day or after meals; when sleeping it was important to shift from side to side frequently in order to aid digestion and maintain a healthy humoral balance.

Preventive measures also included the burning of aromatic woods such as juniper, cypress, pine, laurel, and ash, as well as herbs such as rosemary, aloe and musk to disperse noxious plague fumes. In fact, anything aromatic was deemed of value. As a result people carried nosegays of blossoms or little bags filled with crushed herbs and flowers pressed over their noses – but to little effect.[61] Another ineffective protective measure against the Black Death was to sprinkle perfumed water on clothes to keep the air around one's person pure. A survivor of one particular 'plague water' is still in use today – Eau de Cologne. All perfumes in fact were thought to act against noxious miasmic air by '...attacking and transforming the very essence of unpleasant odours'.[62]

Although most physicians fled from towns to the countryside, those who stayed behind protected themselves with fragrant substances. Physicians distinguished themselves by wearing the square hat typically worn by them at the time, as well as outlandish long beaked masks.

The long bird-like beaks, through which they breathed, were filled with aromatic herbs, believed to ward off the dreaded disease. The eyeholes were covered with glass, to keep the 'noxious vapours' out and the thick wax-coated, long leather garments served the same purpose. In addition, they wore platform soles to prevent them from stepping into anything suspect. To complete the outfit they habitually carried a wooden cane, which was used in giving directions to family members regarding patients or to keep those infected at a distance.

One of the countless remedies recommended by physicians at the time and for centuries to come was theriac, popularly known as 'Venice Treacle' by English apothecaries. Theriac was one of *the* most expensive medications available, containing sixty-four different ingredients, the most prized being viper flesh. Other highly recommended antidotes were 'Plague Water' as well as 'Plague Pills', all sold at considerable cost to the desperate populace. In his *Letter and Regimen concerning the Pestilence*, written in 1348, Alfonso de Córdoba, associated with the medical school at Montpellier, advocates especially 'pestilential pills' and theriac, to '…preserve one from infected air'.[63]

In addition, specific remedies were recommended for the rich, such as powdered horn; and for the poor such as garlic, butter and onion plasters, thought to effectively suck out the contagion. Pepper and saffron, onions, leeks and garlic, taken during the day, were recommended as prophylactic measures, as well as the consumption of fowl, fish and beef, all cooked in rainwater.

It is interesting to note, that sixteenth century plague remedies promoted by physicians were still much like those of the fourteenth century. For example, Thomas Vicary (1490-1561), chief surgeon to King Henry VIII,[64] advocated many 'goodly and present' remedies to cure the plague: 'Because the evil humors that bee in mans body do easily receive the corruption and infection of the aire, it is good to keepe the stomacke and the head cleane purged, not to overlade it with eating and drinking'.[65] He recommended avoiding 'grosse meates', heavy meals and regular purging to stay clear of the plague. To treat the hard buboes appearing in those infected, he prescribed poultices or 'plaisters' made from burnt ashes, clay, oil of roses and 'hennes dung', claiming that he had successfully treated numerous plague victims in this manner. The poultice would successfully draw forth all poisons 'without any other help'. However, it was important to 'keepe this as a secret'.[66]

Another specific therapy advised to simply transfer the disease by taking a hen and plucking the feathers 'from her arse, and from the place where she layeth her egges'. The rear end of the hen was then to be placed on top of the pestilent buboes, and the hen held *in situ* for a while. Vicary continues: 'Then you shall see that the saide Henne will have drawn all or at least some of the poison and infection and shortly after she will die'. This treatment was to be repeated successively with several hens to draw all poison out efficiently.[67] The notion of transference of disease to an animal or another human being was once universally popular.

In spite of the many notions based on ignorance and superstition – when seen from a modern perspective – many logical, objective observations were drawn. For instance, it seemed clear that the plague was most likely to appear in summer or early autumn. It also appeared to strike more often in the poorest, most crowded neighbourhoods, which is why avoiding contact with the sick, or moving from infected towns, was deemed the best defence. Wealthy families often hired special servants to watch over their sick, while the rest of the family moved away. In addition, the well to do could afford to avoid crowded markets or other public venues, as they employed servants to do their bidding. This resulted in a reduction of infection amongst those most likely to be able to isolate themselves. Unfortunately, it also reinforced the idea that the poor were morally and physically predisposed to sickness in general.

Social ramifications of the Black Death

Finally, the year 1351 brought an end to the terrible Black Death – it had run its dreadfully destructive course. But, what were the social ramifications around Europe? Beyond the immediate symptoms of utter devastation of human life, the effects were manyfold, shaping European life in the years that followed. The direct consequences to such incredible loss of life were deeply psychological. Diverse aspects of human conduct were affected and feelings were ambivalent. On the one hand the all-pervading likelihood of a sudden and painful death increased religious desire for penitence. On the other hand this also evoked a panic-stricken aspiration for amusement and hedonistic behaviour while it was still possible.

The clergy stressed that people should go to sleep every night as if it were their last, that their bed was their coffin – a comforting thought to an already psychologically stressed populace. Hence, the horrors of the times were culturally assimilated throughout Europe in the fervent outcry *memento mori*, a Latin phrase meaning 'remember your mortality', 'remember you must die'. In modern times this outcry refers to a widely varying genre in artworks, which all share the same purpose: to remind people of their mortality.[68] The most obvious places to find expression for this genre were in funeral art and architecture. Funerary monuments and death masks were relatively scarce before the advent of the Black Death, even amongst the nobility. But then suddenly they became common. Perhaps the most striking examples of funerary monuments are the cadaver tombs or *memento mori* tombs, which were particularly characteristic of this time.[69] Also at this time German woodcuts called 'The Art of Dying' appeared – linked panels showing the painful, drama of death. Paintings portrayed gruesome aspects of pain, and Death was illustrated not as a skeleton, as in pre-plague art, but as a cloaked old woman with talons, snakelike hair and clawed feet, collecting her victims.[70]

While the face of art and sculpture changed as a result of the Black Death, commercial institutions, as well as religious belief structures also came to be severely challenged. The Black Death has been linked to the downfall of feudalism. After the epidemic, newly prosperous peasants and merchants now confronted aristocrats and churchmen, who had dominated pre-plague Europe through property control. Whole families had died, with no heirs, their houses standing empty. Because plague destroyed the general populace and not possessions, a drop in population was accompanied by a corresponding rise in per capita wealth.

The sudden, overwhelming shortage of peasant labour gave those who survived a bargaining power unimaginable in previous centuries. Workers who remained alive could now earn up to fivefold what they had earned before the outbreak of this dreaded disease, while profits for landlords and merchants declined as they found themselves having to pay higher wages. As a result, governments attempted to regulate the price of food, as well as the wages paid to labourers, trying to hold them at pre-plague levels – King Edward III passed ordinances in 1349, to attempt at keeping wages at pre-plague levels. Similar statutes were passed in various parts of France, Germany, and Italy, leading to unrest and revolt amongst labourers in most parts of Europe during the second half of the fourteenth century.

While the plague had no permanent effect on the course of politics, it did take its toll. All parliaments were adjourned when the plague struck, but later reconvened. Even the Hundred Years' War (1337- 1443) was suspended in 1348 because so many soldiers had died of the plague – but it started up again, soon enough. Amongst the nobility King Alfonso XI of Castile (1311-1350) was the only reigning monarch to die of the plague. However, many lesser nobles died of the contagion, including Eleanor of Portugal who was Queen of Aragon (1328-1347), Joan of Burgundy, Queen consort of France (1293-1348), Joan of England (1333-1348) daughter of King Edward III. But, since they were isolated from crowded towns, not as many nobles died as people amongst the peasantry.

Certain professions had suffered a high mortality, especially those whose duties brought them into contact with the sick, such as the clergy and doctors. Although the Church prospered in the aftermath of the plague – the newly rich, more than willing to make large contributions in gratitude for being spared – the plague was nevertheless to have a lasting impact on ecclesiastical affairs. Literally thousands of clerics had been killed by the plague, which brought about a reduction of church control. It has been theorised that this allowed Latin, the official language of the Church, to be replaced by local dialects around Europe.

Effects on the development of medicine and health care

Generally historians are not in agreement about the effects of the Black Death on the development of medicine and medical practices in Europe. While some historians minimize its effects or even omit the Black Death's influence on medicine completely, there are those who credit it with revealing the general failure of medieval medicine and hence creating the impetus for reassessment and reformation of medical practices. Others, place the effects of the Black Death on the future of medicine between these two extremes.

One of the most important changes brought about by the Black Death was that it helped shape medicine's course of development, thereby gradually leading up to the slow beginnings of its modern successor. In 1348, Europe's medical community was characterised by rigidity and what would be perceived as blatant incompetence from a modern perspective. Medical practices were based firmly on the ideas of Hippocrates (c.460-c.370 BCE), Galen (129-c.200/216 CE) and Avicenna (c. 980-1037). Although these physicians had written about plagues, none of them had any first-hand experience with infectious diseases and had based diagnosis firmly on humoral imbalances. Hence, medieval doctors stressed reasoned argument and debate around classical theories, laid down more than a thousand years before.

What the Black Death made glaringly obvious and highlighted, were the shortcomings of the existing medical system, in which physicians were unable to successfully treat plague victims. Medieval chroniclers of the Black Death generally accused doctors of the times of impotence, cowardice and above all greed.[71] One Florentine chronicler, Matteo Villani (died 1363), critically declared that '...for this pestilential infirmity [of 1348], doctors from every part of the world had no good remedy or effective cure, neither through natural philosophy, medicine [physic] or the art of astrology. To gain money some went visiting and dispensing their remedies, but these only demonstrated through their patients' death that their art was nonsense and false'.[72] However, despite such criticism, many doctors, succumming to the disease themselves, did in fact give their lives in service to plague victims.

But changes, however they may be evaluated, were to come. Firstly, because leading theoreticians, writers, practitioners and university lecturers of the old medical establishment had died of the plague.[73] In 1349 for instance, there were vacancies in every single chair of medicine, at the University of Padua in Italy. Naturally, this paved the way for new people with new ideas – fertile ground for novel thoughts to take hold.

Although rules for the isolation of lepers already existed in Old Testament times, it was not until the Black Death outbreak of the fourteenth century that Venice established the first formal system of quarantine, requiring ships to lie at anchor for forty days before mooring.[74] At the same time, again in Italy, health boards and systems of public health services developed. Both quarantine measures as well as health boards seem to have been set up on advice and under the guidance of physicians.[75]

At first, health boards were temporary creations to deal with the plague, but soon they became permanent and were subsequently instituted in most major cities around Europe. The first task of the board was to report an epidemic; the second was to isolate it – usually by quarantine. However, as medieval society followed the traditional theory of miasma contagion, with quarantines only segregating infected persons and their goods, this did not solve the rodent and insect problem. Therefore, quarantine measures were not successful where the Black Death was concerned.

By the sixteenth century, quarantines were common throughout Europe and governments created medical boundaries or *cordons sanitaire*, between their countries and the areas to the east from whence epidemics came. Ships coming from the Ottoman Empire were now forced to wait in quarantine before passengers and cargo could be unloaded. All who attempted to evade medical quarantine were killed. While the plague continued to affect the areas of the eastern Mediterranean, it disappeared in the West – the medical border seems to have been effective.

Another important transformation in the field of medicine related to medical texts. Until the 1340's almost all medical books were written in Latin, as this was the exclusive language of the medical elite. But by 1400 this had changed and texts were being written and translated into the vernacular language. This meant that everyone who could read now had access to such books, including apothecaries, non-professional practitioners, laymen and women. Pre-plague texts and theses were now finally demystified.

A further post-plague change applied to the rise of surgeons and their craft, especially in view of the fact that university-based medicine had dismally failed the general populace. Surgeons now came to challenge the position of physicians and to assert their own authority as medical practitioners. Hence the Black Death was instrumental in causing a shift toward greater emphasis on practice, as opposed to just theory, which of course intensified the struggle for status between surgeons and physicians. Universities came to recognise the need for new ideas and Paris University soon encouraged surgery and anatomy in their medical program.

Until this time, physicians had been poor anatomists, given that Galen had based his anatomical findings on animals. Although Bologna University had welcomed surgeons since the twelfth century, their surgical *curricula* were intensified after the Black Death. Dissections now took place regularly, even in summer, despite the more rapid decomposition of bodies. As a result anatomy texts slowly evolved with more accuracy. At the end of the fourteenth century various books on surgery were widely read – functional books, based on experience, dealing with treatment and care as opposed to theoretical medicine.

Yet another post-plague development was the new role of hospitals – to cure the sick. Before the Black Death hospitals had been institutions to isolate, to keep the sick away from the mainstream of people so that they would not infect or offend the healthy. A further step in the evolution of medicine came with the advance in public health and sanitation. Public health laws, which first developed in post-plague Italy, spread from there to the rest of the Continent. By the sixteenth century public health was a recognisable phenomenon in most European cities.

However, in spite of new ideas there was no breakdown of the existing medieval medical system – the works of Hippocrates and Galen continued to be taught in universities. In this context it is interesting to note that the same notions about humors, contagion, and quarantine were again at first used to fight cholera when that disease appeared in Europe in the 1830's.

In the aftermath of the plague the towns of Europe were nearly deserted, with many European cities loosing half or all of their population, some even disappearing altogether. All major cities were forced to create mass graveyards where the dead could be buried. Although the population losses could have been quickly made up, new epidemics prevented a return to the high population levels of the period before 1348 and European population only began to grow again in the last decades of the fifteenth century.

In modern times plague outbreaks around the world have become erratic and isolated, kept under control by modern surveillance techniques and international regulations mandating the control of rats in harbours and the endorsement of rat proofing on ships. In addition, the advent of antibiotics and routine vaccinations have made large-scale quarantines a thing of the past.

LEPROSY – DISEASE OF THE SOUL

The title of this chapter refers to a disease, which in past centuries was viewed as an accursed blight associated with vice and moral corruption. Conversely, this dreaded ailment was regarded as a special gift of God's divine favour and sanctity. The disease in question is leprosy – Hansen's disease, as it is known today.[1]

Leprosy or Hansen's disease, as it is known in modern times, is produced by the *mycobacterium leprae*, which was not scientifically identified until 1874. The bacterium multiplies very slowly and may lie dormant in its host for many years without symptoms. Although the bacterium exists in only one strain, the disease can in fact appear in several forms – depending on the host's immune defences. Even though *leprae* bacteria spread from person to person, through prolonged close contact and transmission by nasal droplets, disease does not necessarily follow. This is due to the bacteria not being particularly virulent and because most people have a natural resistance to the disease.

If left untreated, which of course was the case in medieval times, leprosy can be progressive, causing permanent damage to the skin, nerves, limbs and eyes. In modern times it is known that those at highest risk of contamination live in endemic areas and are subject to poor conditions, polluted water, insufficient diet and other diseases which compromise the immune system. Before the leprosy outbreak in medieval Europe the plague had just raged through the Continent and all of the other aforementioned conditions conducive to leprosy were similarly present. Leprosy was never a great killer and its demographic impact not remotely comparable with the terrible plague or syphilis and smallpox epidemics.

The symptoms of leprosy are particularly confronting. In the later stages of the disease victims are so hideously defaced and mutilated, that they become a dreaded sight indeed. Leprosy is a chronic infection, which develops slowly over many years, and by itself rarely kills its victims. However, it causes decades of severe pain and distress for the sufferer.

Medieval lepers infected with lepromatous leprosy, typically bore the horrendous signs of decay and putrefaction of this disease: facial features which slowly rotted away, until the countenance became a formless mass; numb and deteriorating limbs, the extremities of sufferers slowly decomposing over time; nose, fingers and toes literally falling off, leaving only short stumps. To make matters worse, rancid breath, a raspy, fading voice, festering sores, which were host to worms and insects, and foul odours emanating from gangrenous body parts – a terrifying, distressing scenario not only for those afflicted, but for onlookers as well. Believed to be highly contagious, it is not surprising that leprosy was one of *the* most feared diseases throughout the ages – associated with extreme stigmatisation.

The spread of the disease

In ancient times leprosy was widespread throughout Asia, Egypt and in the Greek and Roman world. Although leprosy was not uncommon in India as far back as the fifteenth century BCE, Egypt has always been seen as the starting point for its spread into the Western world – probably due to Galen's statement that leprosy 'flourished' there, during the first century.[2] From Egypt, leprosy spread to Palestine, Syria, and Asia Minor. Eventually the various campaigns of Roman armies disseminated the disease in the Roman colonies of Spain and Gaul. Ultimately, leprosy travelled north as the Roman Empire expanded its borders and mercantile traffic increased, the disease reaching Britain in the fourth century CE. After the eighth century, references to leprosy in European annals are rare and almost disappear from West European sources – that is, until the High Middle Ages.

After the year 1000 CE until the 1300's, Western Europe witnessed an unprecedented outbreak of leprosy. Again, it was as a result of an immense movement of people through religious pilgrimages and war, which spread the scourge. Most historians agree that Crusaders, contracting the disease in Palestine and the Middle East, brought its return to Italy, France, Germany and England.[3] This would explain the concentration of the disease in France, the prime recruiting ground for 'Soldiers of Christ' against Islam. The disease then remained endemic throughout Europe, declining slowly and disappearing almost entirely in the early 1500's.[4]

The Old Testament view on leprosy

In ancient times leprosy was deemed a tainted, unclean disease validating the moral impurity of its victims. However, although leprosy is vividly described in the Old Testament, it was certainly not the disfiguring condition caused by the *mycobacterium leprae*, but a milder form of skin ailment – the Hebrew word for leprosy, was used at the time to describe most skin conditions.[5] In fact, archaeological exhumations of hundreds of skeletons in Palestine found no human remains evidencing true leprosy.[6]

The Old Testament[7] propagates that lepers were singled out for divine punishment because of sinful behaviour. The undefiled leper was described as impure, unholy, and hence removed from God – whereas purity was seen as synonymous with holiness, hence closeness to God. The Book of Leviticus states: 'Now whosoever shall be defiled with the leprosy, and is separated by the judgement of the priest, shall have his clothes hanging loose, his head bare, his mouth covered with a cloth, and he shall cry out that he is defiled and unclean…'.[8] Furthermore: 'And if he see the leprosy in his skin, and the hair turned white, and the place where the leprosy appears lower than the skin and the rest of the flesh: it is the stroke of leprosy, and upon his judgement he shall be separated'.[9] In other words, the Law of Moses cast lepers out, removing them from society because of their impurity – moral as well as physical – to live in segregation.

In the *Midrash Rabbah*, a collection of Old Testament interpretations, numerous sins are associated with the cause of leprosy. Whilst the various commentaries do not necessarily agree on the type of sins, there is nonetheless consensus that this *is* a sinner's disease. The annotations on Leviticus 14:2 contain a list of seven sins which result in leprosy: 'Proud eyes, a lying tongue, hands that shed the blood of the innocent, a mind full of evil schemes, feet running towards wrong, a false witness breathing out lies, and one who stirs up quarrels between brothers'.[10] Tragically, the idea of lepers as symbols of spiritual and emotional corruption continued over many centuries.

A Christian perspective

So how did Christian society view leprosy, and how were victims of this disease treated in early and medieval Europe? The traditional prevailing view amongst medical historians has been that the Christian world depended on the Jewish Old Testament for its understanding of leprosy, and that this notion dominated early and medieval Christian thinking. In other words, Christian interpretation of Mosaic Law relied on '…the conviction that leprosy was God's punishment for sin'.[11]

Consequently, past scholars and historians[12] frequently represented medieval Christianity's response to leprosy as an attempt to punish victims of the disease, rather than to assist them in their suffering. Leprosaria – leper hospitals – were in fact often portrayed as veritable detention centres for those afflicted with the disease. The theory has also been postulated that medieval leprosy was partly a 'construct' disease, often fabricated by those in power to safeguard their political, cultural, and economic interests.[13] In other words, leprosaria also served as detention centres for those whom local church and lay rulers considered potential trouble-shooters whereby informants with malicious intent would report such people as having contracted leprosy. Consequently, they would be 'tried' by a panel consisting of local church and secular authority, and subsequently incarcerated in leprosaria.

However, the contention that the medieval leprosy 'outbreak' was just a means of political oppression is not widely accepted. This is due to credible archaeological evidence of the numbers of lepers buried in leprosaria cemeteries that were identifiable by the tell-tale skeletal signs attesting to the disease: corroded, scarred bone around oral and nasal cavities, and around finger and toe bones.[14] What's more, leprosy may have been far more prevalent than osteo-archaeological indication bears out, as not all those infected with lepromatous leprosy develop destructive bone lesions,[15] and those stricken with tuberculoid or borderline leprosy are not subject to any mutilating symptoms. Thus, modern historians[16] cast a different perspective on leprosy and its consequences for sufferers.

Across the cultural spectrum in Europe, the all-pervasive influence of the Bible presented leprosy as a '...dramatic affliction, whose only cure was by miracle'.[17] A fitting example is the 'cleansing' of the ten lepers in the Gospel of Luke [18] – the perfect metaphor for tainted souls in search of spiritual health.[19]

Therefore, what was the reaction of Christian society to this dreadful disease? Were lepers reviled, cast out and segregated by Christian society, or did the Church advocate charity and compassion towards these unfortunates? The answer seems to lie somewhere in-between – Christian attitude towards leprosy was one of ambivalence and dichotomy. [20]

Numerous sources of early Christian writers portray the care of lepers as the greatest act of Christian charity, endeavouring to raise an awareness of kindness and empathy for the leprous. As Palestine, Syria, and Asia Minor became predominantly Christian after Emperor Constantine declared toleration to Christianity in 312 CE, church leaders in these areas were forced to address the rapid spread of leprosy. Predictably, a disease with such horrendous physical manifestations, resulting in banishment for its victims from populated areas, would prove to be a great challenge for early Church leaders – after all, this faith was based on a creed of love and compassion. Hence, 'Christianity constructed a rather ambiguous but nevertheless plausible moral theory based on ideas and practices depicted in the Old and New Testaments'.[21]

The disease was deemed a blessing as well as a curse – a 'gift from God' and His way of calling the ailing to a life of holiness.[22] Due to their obvious suffering, the leprous were seen as going through the pains of purgatory here on Earth – an existence of living hell – which, in the eyes of many, transformed their misery and pain into something almost sacred, in line with hermits. Many believed that these individuals would ascend directly to heaven after their demise. After all, death to the world was the highest vocation one could possibly aspire to. Hence, lepers should be viewed with sympathy and compassion, especially deserving of love and assistance.

On the other hand, the leprous state was also seen as a symbol of spiritual degeneration and moral corruption, representing a vice-ridden soul – therefore the ailment was often referred to as the 'disease of the soul'. The '...association between leprosy and sin was varied and complex'[23] and the general populace frequently reviled those afflicted, as bearers of disgusting pollution. Various repulsive characteristics such as malevolence, deviousness, deceit, uncontrolled anger and a burning sexual desire, were associated with this 'tainted' condition. Lepers were often represented as a threat to society not only because of the danger of infection, but also due to their perceived corrupt, licentious conduct. The main focus generally centred on the professed uncontrolled sexual appetite of the leprous. Certainly this prejudice was totally unfounded, as the severe weakened physical condition of medieval lepers would have diminished their sexual desire altogether.

First century Greek physician Aretaeus of Cappadocia, was the first writer to provide an accurate – although incomplete – description of leprosy symptoms: he referred to blotches and fissures of the skin, a discoloration of skin texture, and the loss of appendages. Furthermore, Aretaeus stated that lepers suffered a long debilitating state between life and death – a kind of living death, which started in the remote parts of the body causing the hair to fall out and fingers and toes to drop off.[24]

Fourth-century Christian writer Bishop Gregory of Nazianzus (c.329-c.395) later adopted this particular image of a 'living death', to arouse sympathy for lepers. The bishop's wide-ranging treatise on lepers, and their infirmities, stressed Christian obligation to all sufferers of the disease. He preached that God did not send leprosy as a punishment, but rather as an example of how even righteous people sometimes have great tribulations to bear.[25] As the writings and utterances of Gregory of Nazianzus were very popular at the time, later Byzantine and Latin writers embraced his compassionate representation of leprosy.[26] In other words, the idea that leprosy was a form of living death to be treated with mercy and empathy – and not the typical Jewish Old Testament rejection of lepers – was prevalent in Christian Europe.

In 370 CE, Bishop Gregory of Nyssa (c.335-c.395 CE) delivered an intriguing sermon on the disease. Apart from stating that leprosy had become widespread in Cappadocia, he offered added symptom indicators of the disease, which neither Galen nor Aretaeus had identified before him, such as a hoarse voice, and partial or complete loss of feeling in affected body-parts, which later became the key distinguishing-factor for leprosy from other skin conditions. In his address, Bishop Gregory of Nyssa also emphasised that true followers of Christ should show compassion and love to these most dejected members of society, and in doing so ensure their own salvation.[27]

Through the centuries, the Church regulated in favour of lepers, providing widespread care and shelter. At a synod held in the French city of Orleans in 539, bishops approved, amongst other canons, one specifically stating that each French city provide lepers with food and clothing from the funds of the local church. Many years later, at a synod held in Lyons in 583, bishops confirmed that lepers should be assisted, but only in the cities where they had permanent residence – in other words they should not roam from city to city – thus enacting the first restrictive directive against lepers.[28] By the end of the sixth century, permanent establishments to house and feed lepers had been set up in Gaul and other European countries.

While sixth and seventh century sources from Frankish Gaul occasionally refer to leprosy, mention of the disease almost disappears from West European sources up until the outbreak of the eleventh to fourteenth centuries – this outbreak is generally described by prominent medical historians.[29]

Outbreak of the eleventh to fourteenth centuries

Leprosy was not restricted to the poor; many aristocrats and knights returning from the Crusades harboured the disease. The most illustrious sufferer was no doubt the future King of Jerusalem. Chronicler of the Crusades, William of Tyre, who was physically and actively present in the Holy Land at the time, graphically describes the onset of the nine-year-old prince's disease in 1170. Chronicler William of Tyre (c.1130-1186) was tutor to Prince Baldwin, the son of Amalric (1136-1174), King of Jerusalem at the time. One day William watched the young prince playing a rough game with his friends. They were digging their nails into each other's arms to see who could endure the most pain. Prince Baldwin appeared to be the undisputed winner, as no amount of pain seemed to cause him any discomfort. However, tragically it turned out that his insensitivity was not due to bravery but the dreaded leprosy.

This is a famous example of the then widespread and accurate concept regarding loss of sensation at the nerve ends, which is one of the early and reliable indications of leprosy. When King Almaric died four years later '...the crown of Jerusalem passed to Baldwin IV (1161-1185), who by now was a thirteen year old sickly leper'.[30] Crusader knights infected with leprosy were required by a legal code – the *Livre au Roi*, set up in 1198 – to join the order of the brethren of St. Lazarus, which cared for them.

As returning crusaders and pilgrims brought the disease to the attention of European society, '...their trained eyes seemed to detect similarly affected individuals at home'.[31] A new climate of dread and hostility towards urban lepers rapidly took hold, and in many European cities lepers were made scapegoats for various calamities befalling the general population. For instance, in 1321 a group of lepers were accused of fouling the drinking water in the Languedoc, France, and summarily executed for spreading disease. In this new climate of fear, reports of concealment and deliberate infection of healthy individuals spread, and people were encouraged to denounce someone suspected of harbouring the disease, to relevant authorities.

Medical assessment of symptoms

Medieval law required anyone thought to have contracted leprosy to report his or her condition. But, '...the factors that played a role in suspecting, reporting and judging a person of "leprosy" were as complex as the repercussions were far ranging'.[32] Since the Church was responsible for upholding the moral definition of the disease, it also created procedures to officially identify and diagnose the leprous. But, how this was handled before the early fourteenth century is unknown as no trial evidence seems to have survived.[33]

From the early fourteenth century onwards, evidence from France documents that panels to investigate and administer the diagnostic process of those potentially infected, comprised of medically untrained personages. These panels consisted primarily of priests and members of the clergy, as well as town magistrates, townspeople or villagers, and often lepers themselves. 'Witnesses known to be trustworthy citizens of the community, or countrymen of the accused, were allowed to be present and explain their reasons for their presumption'.[34] Only during the fifteenth century were medical men added to such panels or juries.

In the mid thirteen hundreds, Guy de Chauliac, personal physician to Pope Clement VI at Avignon in 1348, listed the distinctive marks and signs of leprosy, thereby providing the diagnostic tool for identifying true lepers. Individuals undergoing medical assessment by the panel were required to undress. Then, in front of all assembled, a meticulous examination of the body would follow – usually starting with the face. But, what *were* the '...fateful manifestations that pointed to the most stigmatised condition in medieval society'? [35] Certain diagnostic precursors were sought: a change in the shape of the eyes and the lips, changes in skin colour, the loss of eyebrows and lashes – in fact, hair loss in general – nasal enlargement or malformation, areas of thickened or shiny skin, loss of sensation, stinking breath and voice changes. A hoarse or raspy voice, implying a lesion in the palate, was suspect and directly investigated further by having the person sing.[36] Furthermore, muscular weakness, more specifically the subject's grip, was tested.

In some countries the evaluation ended with a 'blood test': a barber extracted sufficient blood to fill several cups. The blood was then scrutinised for colour: dark, motley blood pointed to leprosy, while thick, oily blood was also suspect. Lastly the coagulating blood was subjected to a test formulated in the thirteenth century by physician Theodoric of Cervia (1205-1298): three grains of salt were added to a small quantity of the blood, in order to observe how quickly the salt dissolved in it – a 'speedy' dissolution was seen as indicative of the early stages of leprosy. Although Theodoric surely had not observed any concurrence between these 'signs' in the blood and leprosy, he 'may have persuaded himself of it. This capacity of combining fact and fantasy',[37] being typical of medieval medicine.

Apart from taking all these points into consideration, the panel also tended to take into account the suspect's libido. Intense sexual drive and activity was deemed one of the tell-tale symptoms of leprosy – evident here is the deeply ingrained link in Christian thinking between sexuality, sin and consequential disease – even amongst 'learned' physicians. Another association considered by the panel and physicians in their evaluation of suspected lepers, was a propensity towards melancholia, violence, aggression, anger and mood swings in the accused – even recurring nightmares were suspect.

All these characteristics were attributed to humoral imbalance, and therefore highly suggestive in someone accused of harbouring leprosy.[38] Tragically, many tried to cover-up and hide the ominous signs such as the discoloured white skin spots. To achieve this, a mixture of honey and red madder root would be employed. But, in spite of such camouflage, the disease would relentlessly advance until the dysfunctional, crippling signs became inescapably clear for all to see.

It is safe to assume that the afore-listed clinical symptoms would have allowed, or required, a high degree of subjectivity in diagnosis. As leprosy is difficult to diagnose *per se*, and the laity initially made such diagnoses, a variety of disfiguring diseases were probably often identified as leprosy.[39] In addition, many of those classified with leprosy did not necessarily exhibit any of the symptoms, which have since been identified in modern times. In its most extreme form, the disease causes terrible disfigurement, but in a more moderate manifestation, such as tuberculoid or borderline leprosy, the condition can easily be confused with other skin diseases. Hence, panels and physicians undoubtedly made diagnostic mistakes.[40]

However, it should be taken into consideration that medieval physicians perceived the disease from a different perspective to the modern position, and having no perception of prolonged incubation periods, anyone with unsightly skin lesions and infections could be suspected of harbouring leprosy. Medieval illuminations, woodcuts and manuscripts, depict lepers with countless spots representing the lesions on their bodies – marking the emblem of leprosy rather than the actual physical appearance of living lepers. Diseases such as syphilis, smallpox and a selection of chronic skin conditions, presenting as sores, ulcers and scabs, were initially often thrown into the 'leprosy hat'. Medieval medicine therefore turned the already existing fear of leprosy into an unnatural horror.

The 'ritual of separation'

Regulations were soon set up in all European towns and cities to deal with those afflicted by this dreadful condition. There was nothing more terrifying than a diagnosis of leprosy – not only was this a death-sentence, as the person was to be physically segregated forever from family and loved-ones, but death would also most certainly be '…a long time in coming'.[41] By law, lepers had no rights and were stripped of all ownership and the right to inheritance. Upon formal diagnosis, lepers were considered dead to society, banned from all public places, markets, churches, inns and taverns. One of the most devastating consequences was that these unfortunates would forthwith be unemployed, dependent on charity, often homeless, and unwanted by society.

At the Third Lateran Council in 1179 it was suggested that a ceremony take place to formally separate lepers from 'the company of persons'.[42] Although this separation ritual varied from place to place, it had certain common procedures: once a leper had been formally diagnosed, the victim was brought to either a graveyard or a church, where the ceremonial could take place. There the 'ritual of separation', attended by all interested members, would be officially read out to the sufferer. Sometimes the victim was even made to stand in an open grave while a priest read the mass out loud, probably one of the most touching in ecclesiastical liturgy:

'I forbid thee ever to enter a church, or a monastery, or a market, or a mill, or a procession, or the company of the people.

I forbid thee to appear out of thy house without thy lazar-dress, so that thou mayest be known; or to appear barefooted.

I forbid thee ever to wash thy hands or anything that thou wearest at a bank or a fountain, or to drink there; and if thou wishest to drink some water, draw it in thy own barrel or thy own porringer.

I forbid thee to touch anything that thou sellest, or that thou buyest until it is thy own.

I forbid thee to enter any inn. If thou desirest wine, either by buying it or having it given thee, let it be poured into thy own barrel.

I forbid thee to dwell with any other woman than thy wife.

I forbid thee, if thou walkest along the roads and meet any person that speaks with thee, to answer before thou hast placed thyself away from that side whence the wind is blowing.

I forbid thee to walk by any narrow lane, so that if thou shoudst anywhere meet a person, he may not be the worse thereof.

I forbid thee, if thou goest through any passage, to touch a well or the rope, unless thou hast put on thy gloves.

I forbid thee to touch children or to give them anything.

I forbid thee to drink from any vessels than thy own.

I forbid thee to eat or drink with any other persons than those of thy own sort'.[43]

After these fateful, soul-destroying words, the leper would be considered symbolically dead. The leprous person was then given specific attire and utensils, all individually blessed. Forthwith, he or she was required to wear this distinctive garb, as well as the gloves and shoes at all times. In addition, lepers carried a stick used for touching objects, a begging bowl, and a wooden clapper or bell, which they would sound when approaching settlements – to warn the healthy to keep their distance.

Leprosaria – safe-houses for the infected

Because a cure for the disease was unknown, segregation seemed the only course of action. Leprosaria – leper hospitals or houses – have a long history stretching back to the Greek Church Fathers of the fourth and fifth centuries. In Lombardy and Gaul, lepers were first recognised during the fifth century, and in England a century later.[44] Initially, lepers continued to have contact with family and members of their parish. A letter issued by Pope Gregory II (669-731) in 726 permitted lepers to take evening meals with healthy members of their community, providing they did not touch anyone.[45]

Centuries later, the leprosy epidemic of the High Middle Ages resulted in considerable numbers of leprosaria springing up in most of the larger towns of France, Germany, Spain, and England. English Benedictine monk and chronicler, Matthew Paris (1197-1259), roughly estimated the number of leper-houses in Europe at 19,000, during his lifetime. Although this exact figure is doubtful, the number of leper houses would nevertheless have been considerable. By 1220, the city of Paris alone is thought to have had at least forty-five leprosaria,[46] while a number of two thousand leprosaria is estimated in France as a whole during this century – a significant number, given the fact that the entire population of France at that time is estimated at twenty-two million.[47]

Leprosaria were generally built near rivers and streams, thereby ensuring a fresh water supply. In addition, they were usually built downwind from nearby towns and cities, and situated close to well-travelled routes to facilitate the obligatory institutional begging for inmates.

Leper communities and leprosaria were funded by public taxes, tolls and donations. As numerous nobles had contracted the disease in the Holy Land, leprosaria also benefited from their generosity, ensuring that lepers in the care of such institutions enjoyed a relatively comfortable life. In addition, large endowments to leper houses were made by the wealthy – such open-handedness strengthened by the Church's assurance that all charitable acts would be rewarded in the hereafter by a remission of sin.

Ecclesiastical authorities, the founders of leprosaria in most western European countries, ran these centres patterned on monastic convention – prayer and work. Numerous documents regarding the regulation of leprosaria survive from the twelfth and thirteenth centuries. They provide detailed information on how lepers went about their daily lives, and how those infected with the disease were treated. While charters regulated all matters of conduct in detail, health care and health related subjects are not mentioned in the care of sufferers in these institutions.

Some of the oldest surviving leprosaria regulations originated in the town of Montpellier in southern France and date back to 1150. The rules state that lepers who wished to take up residence in a leprosarium were to give up their material goods upon entering the community. The *leprosarium regulae* stated that lepers should wear a habit similar to that worn by monks and initially serve as novitiates before attaining official acceptance to remain within that community.

If they chose to leave, their property was returned to them and they were free to re-enter the secular world – where they were however segregated, and severely restricted. If they chose to become members of a leprosarium, lepers were obligated to take modified Augustinian vows of obedience and celibacy.[48] They were also required to attend daily church services and to pray for the patrons of their community. In exchange for 'board and lodging' they were obligated to beg for institutional alms in nearby towns. The statutes further mention that lepers were referred to as 'brothers' and 'sisters', again substantiating the religious nature of this confinement, but also giving an indication that men as well as women were accepted by these hospices.[49]

Often leprosaria consisted of dormitories with several beds, or small separate huts or 'lazar houses', with inmates sharing communal meals once a day. Habitually leprosaria developed into veritable 'monastic estates', housing granaries, workshops, gardens, and livestock on arable land. In 1179 the Third Lateran Council, decreed that leprosaria throughout Europe should also include chapels and cemeteries – thereby reinforcing segregation of the leprous – and that lepers be exempted from paying tithes to the local bishop.[50]

Within the leprosaria all major decisions were made by a collegium, which had been elected by the 'brothers' and 'sisters'. Leper priests ministered to the inmates. Policy mandated regular fasts and prayers, as well as disciplinary expulsion from the community for nonconformity and misconduct. In most leprosaria, lepers were not permitted to leave without prior permission being granted. Overnight absences, especially if these involved nocturnal conjugal visits, resulted in expulsion, and celibacy was enforced at all costs.

Those refusing to abide by the rules were forced to leave – in other words, lepers were not strictly confined to leprosaria. Many lepers in fact opted to forego the relative safety and comfort of community living, choosing to live a life of vagrancy, living off the land in forests. They would frequent urban centres only to beg. However, because their condition was thought to be highly contagious, certain requirements had to be observed when lepers were not within the walls of leprosaria: they were required to stand downwind from all healthy people, forbidden to frequent narrow footpaths, or to drink from public water sources, wash in streams and rivers, or to engage in sexual intercourse, even with their own spouse.

On the whole, life in the leprosaria must have been tolerable, perhaps even moderately comfortable. Surrounded by fellow sufferers to varying degrees, friendships must have been forged, resulting in companionship, care, and support for each other. At least they were assured of being looked after as their disease progressed and became increasingly debilitating – a disgusting, repugnant task for fellow sufferers. According to monastic principles, life was well ordered, quiet and disciplined. However, separation from society, as well as physical discomfort, pain, and the enforced strict monastic rules, often resulted in frustration, occasional violence, quarrels and brawls. Methods of punishment included fasting, penance, or expulsion.

After the rapid decline of leprosy in Europe during the early 1500's, empty leprosaria were converted to hospitals, or used for the poor, for incurables, madmen, or those afflicted with syphilis, which was virulent and raging throughout Europe at the time.

Medical theories on transmission, causes and cures

Regarding transmission, causes, and cures for leprosy, various medical theories and notions abounded. As such, '…public opinion concerning leprosy was based on a hodgepodge of religious beliefs and observations of physical corruption, medical theories about the nature and transmission of this disease were equally inconsistent'.[51] Like with all other diseases, medieval physicians viewed leprosy within the structure of humoral theory. Hence, Avicenna's *Canon of Medicine* (1025) and Guy de Chauliac's *Chirurgie* (1363), which both stressed humoral imbalance, remained the principal medical sources on the disease.

Thirteenth century physician Theodoric of Cervia, like all other physicians, accepted the humoral theory and distinguished four different types of leprosy, all based on the corruption of blood: Elephantine leprosy, the result of an imbalance of black bile in the blood; leonine leprosy from bile corrupting the blood; alopecian leprosy from contaminated blood and tyrian leprosy from phlegm polluting the blood. Related to the element of fire, leprosy was characterised by causing the body to become 'hot and dry' – hence ingesting anything 'cold and wet' would re-balance the humors.[52]

Because humoral imbalance could not be passed on, leprosy in itself was therefore not seen as contagious. Rather, physicians thought the disease was transmittable through miasma or atmospheric poisons, which is why sufferers were always to stand downwind from healthy people. Benedictine monk Constantinus Africanus (1020-1087) especially emphasised the widely held theory that leprosy could result from sexual contact with adulterous females during their menstruation[53] – here again the moral causal element.

Various orthodox attempted cures included phlebotomy, dietary prescriptions, bathing routines as well as external and internal mercurial ointments and potions, although nothing seemed to halt the progression of this disease. Popular cures were based on the 'doctrine of signatures' and sympathetic theories. The doctrine of signatures [54] was founded on the belief that God 'marked' specific objects, be they animals or plants, with a sign or 'signature' for their intended purpose. Especially in the case of plants, this implied a systematic method of discovering their medicinal use based on their external appearance, which was thought to resemble the disease they would cure.

In other words, each plant was believed to carry its use and purpose clearly marked upon it. For instance, all red flowers were prescribed for disorders of the blood and yellow ones for those of biliary secretions. Therefore, treatment was not based on observed therapeutic benefits, but solely on the colours associated with the condition.

On the recommendations of physicians, this even extended to bed coverings and hangings, which is why John of Gaddesden (c.1280-1361), physician to King Edward II (1284-1327) of England, directed his patient the king's son, suffering from smallpox, to be wrapped up in scarlet sheets, while red bed-coverings were employed to bring the pustules to the surface of the body.[55] Queen Elizabeth I also received the so-called '…red treatment, that people once thought cured smallpox',[56] during the second half of the sixteenth century. Similarly, as late as the mid-eighteenth century the Holy Roman Emperor Francis I (1708-1765), when infected with smallpox, was by order of his physicians wrapped in scarlet clothes.[57] According to the doctrine of signatures not only the colour, but also the shape of objects was of importance. For example, a heart-shaped leaf was meant to cure heart disease and seeds containing a dot resembling the pupil of the eye, such as the herb 'eye-bright' were deemed beneficial for the eyes – hundreds of such examples exist.

For the cure of leprosy, herbs from the *fumaria* family, especially 'bleeding heart', were a popular 'signature', their red, black and purple blossoms signifying the leprous lesions. Similarly, the white hellebore plant, already recommended by Pliny the Elder for 'leprous sores', was popularly used during the Middle Ages to treat leprosy.[58]

According to sympathetic theory the consumption of vipers was especially recommended as a cure for leprosy. As vipers shed their skin, the ingestion of their flesh was thought to sympathetically promote a cleansing action in the leprous. Vipers were already regarded as an important medicinal agent in Galen's times. For medicinal purposes they were dried and pulverised or boiled and the resulting mixture ingested. In fact, snakes in general were once considered essential in medical cures in western European countries and constituted a profitable trade item throughout the Middle Ages until the nineteenth century.[59]

Alternatively the sufferers of this dreaded disease were advised to bathe in the blood of virgins and children.[60] This was accredited with special healing powers. During the Middle Ages blood from a virgin was regarded as a certain cure for leprosy, a theme which is central to the Middle-High-German epic *Der arme Heinrich* (written circa 1195). The tradition of healing leprosy with the blood of innocent children is seen in many texts of the Middle Ages, as well as in early Hebrew biblical commentary. As leprosy was thought to stem from moral impurity and sin, it was perceived that the antidote or cure could only be one of high moral purity – to bathe in the blood of a virgin or young child.

The practice of using blood – not necessarily human – for healing purposes was still recorded in many parts of Europe as late as 1891[61] Pliny the Elder describes the use of blood as a well-known cure for leprosy in Egypt: 'Leprosy is endemic in Egypt. When kings contracted the disease it had deadly consequences for the people because the tubs in the baths were prepared with warm human blood for its treatment'.[62] It is almost certain that the belief that human blood cured this dreaded disease was also prevalent in ancient Greece and Rome, as well as being popularly believed during the Middle Ages.[63]

In closing, it may be concluded that even if the leprous had *never* been condemned for their supposed moral defilement, they would nevertheless have been regarded with aversion and disdain, simply on account of their horrendous physical deformity.

By the late fifteenth century, leprosy had become somewhat rare in many parts of Europe '...and soon confusion arose between its manifestations and those of an ailment to be known as the "pox", a condition eventually equated with venereal syphilis'.[64] The following chapter deals with one of the most virulent and deadly infections in the history of medicine...

THE FRENCH POX – NOT JUST FRENCH

One and a half centuries after the Black Death had wiped out a third of Western Europe's population, and the widespread incidence of leprosy throughout Europe was slowly declining, a new pestilence swept across the Continent – the Great Pox or venereal syphilis. This disease did not kill rapidly, like the plague before it, but endured in victims' bodies for many years, causing weeping sores, horrific disfigurement, and excruciating pain, before ultimately ending in an agonising death. The Great Pox was to devastate European society for four hundred and fifty years and changed the field of medicine considerably. It lead to new ideas and produced a quantity of medical literature second only to that of the Black Death. The availability and effectiveness of penicillin in 1943 to cure venereal syphilis finally put an end to its proliferation.

The origins of venereal syphilis in Europe

There is very little consensus amongst researchers and historians as to the origins of venereal syphilis in Europe. While scholars may never come to an overall agreement about where syphilis originated, and how it came to the Old World, the most widely held theory propagates that Christopher Columbus' (1450-1506) return from the New World – more specifically the island of Hispaniola[1] – in 1493 was the conduit through which the venereal form of this disease arrived on the shores of Europe.

This theory has not gone unchallenged over the decades. Various researchers and historians have argued that syphilis bacteria had long been present in Europe, and that unknown circumstances triggered the deadly outbreak in the late fifteenth century. Proponents of this theory point out that fifteenth century doctors in Europe would not have been able to distinguish syphilis from disesases which exibited similar symptoms, and that skeletal evidence showing the tell-tale syphilitic lesions pre-dates Columbus's epic voyage. Archaeologists have found numerous ancient skeletons evidencing the telltale signs of syphilis in England, Italy, and several other locations, indicating that syphilis could have been around in Europe for a much longer time. However, this is not irrefutable proof: syphilitic infections cause thickening of lower leg bones and pitting in the skull – but so do other diseases,[2] especially leprosy, which was prevalent in Europe at the time.[3] In addition, dating methods used on skeletal evidence have since been found to be questionable.[4]

After numerous intensive studies, modern researchers[5] have come to the overall conclusion that evidence for an Old World origin for syphilis remains absent, and that syphilis originated in the New World as a non-sexually transmitted disease, which then mutated into a venereal form after it arrived in Europe in the 1490's.

The notion that syphilis originated from the New World was given prominence with the twentieth century concept of the 'Columbian Exchange', which resulted from Christopher Columbus' first voyage to the Americas in 1492. The Columbian Exchange is generally defined as the widespread trade of animals, plants, ideas and culture. But, there was a sinister and deadly side to the 'Columbian Exchange', namely the exchange of communicable diseases, between the Old and New World.[6]

Although the exchange of plants and animals on the whole had favourable outcomes, Europeans introduced 'Old World' diseases, such as smallpox, measles, typhus and cholera to the Americas, depopulating many of their cultures, as these were diseases to which the indigenous peoples of the New World had no natural immunity. Waves upon waves of repeated epidemics followed each other resulting in more deaths among Native Americans than any wars with the Spanish invaders ever claimed.

Spanish soldiers did far less to eradicate the Incas and Aztecs than smallpox, measles, typhus and other communicable diseases from the Old World did – for instance by 1600 at least two million people had been killed by typhus alone in the Mexican highlands.[7] But, syphilis was a different matter. The Amerindians, had immunity to this disease, as syphilis is estimated to date back at least 7,000 years in the Americas. The Amerindians thus experienced a much milder form of syphilis than that, which Columbus brought to Europe after his return. When Columbus made transatlantic contact, it caused epidemiological havoc in Europe, where there was no immunity to the mutated syphilis bacterium *Treponema pallidum*.

The people of the Iberian Peninsula were perhaps more immunologically fit than any other people on earth. After all, not only had Portuguese and Spanish explorers united the Old World with the New, they had been in touch with the outside world for centuries. Spain and Portugal had been a melting pot of invading Arabs and incoming Jews, Christians and Crusaders. The Iberians traded from the North Sea to the Mediterranean, not to mention their voyages of discovery to Africa, South America and India.

Hence the cities of Spain and Portugal, especially those with harbours, were clearing houses of diseases and a haven for specific conditions conducive to infection and the spread of disease: living conditions during the Middle Ages were not clean by modern standards – foul odours were an accepted fact of life. Although many of the larger medieval cities had public sanitation systems and sanitary regulations in place, sizeable parts of these cities smelled of sewage and rotting matter. Rivers were habitually used as open sewers, and shopkeepers would often dump their refuse in the streets,[8] until ordered to clean up their mess. This created a paradise for flies and vermin. By the early fourteenth century so much filth had accumulated in certain parts of the larger European cities that various French and Italian cities were naming streets after human waste.[9]

Owing to the lack of personal hygiene, skin conditions were common amongst the poorer classes,[10] aggravated by rough woollen garments and the presence of ticks and fleas.[11] It may therefore be taken for granted that survivors of such conditions must have been equipped with highly robust immune systems – but, they had no immunity to the mutated bacterium *Treponema pallidum*,[12] or syphilis.

Columbus's log reported no 'serious' illness among his crew. But this may simply be explained by the fact that syphilis does not necessarily exhibit symptoms for years – while those infected may haplessly spread the disease in the meantime.[13] In addition, any symptoms the crew may have had would have been construed as resulting from the adversities of such a long and gruelling voyage – hence, no need for Columbus to account for them. On his second voyage in September 1493, Columbus' journal does however note that he became ill, experiencing intermittent high fevers and subsequent delirium for several weeks.

After his return to Spain, five months of illness followed. He recovered enough to embark on his third voyage, which was however again marked with 'grave illness', as he noted in his journal.[14] Whatever his illness may have been, 'Columbus became sick in the New World and complained for fifteen years about incurable ailments'.[15] Before his death he believed that he was on a mission from God and spoken to by angels.[16] A diagnosis of syphilis would explain his progressive mental derangement, which is why various researchers [17] have entertained the speculation that Columbus himself may have been among the first European victims of what was to become known as the dreaded pox.[18], [19] From the Iberian Peninsula the new disease rapidly spread due to the mobility of armies crossing over into different European countries.

The outbreak of syphilis

However baffling the origin of the *Treponema pallidum* bacterium and its connection to humans may be, history *does* record a specific event as the genesis of the global syphilis outbreak in the late fifteenth century – an outbreak which was to last for several centuries. In August 1494, King Charles VIII (1470-1498) of France led an army of fifty thousand soldiers into northern Italy. The soldiers were mostly mercenaries, coming from Spain, Italy, and Flanders. The French king's objective was to take over the kingdom of Naples from Alfonso II (1448-1495) in order to expand his kingdom. After crushing all resistance, the French occupied Naples. Once provisions in the city had run out, numerous prostitutes crept over to the besiegers' camp, and offered their services to the French soldiers. These Neapolitan prostitutes were hungry for food, while the French soldiers were starved for womanly comforts, hence indulging in long bouts of celebration and debauchery.

Within a short period of time it became apparent that a terrible disease had struck the French soldiers. Unbeknown to everyone, they had been infected by the Neapolitan prostitutes, who in turn had contracted the new disease from Columbus's sailors, many of whom were Neapolitan mercenaries, who seem to have been laden with more sickness than gold. Coming back from the New World, thinking that their symptoms were due to the hardships of such a long and arduous voyage, they had first spread the disease around Barcelona and then infected the prostitutes of their native city, Naples, which was under siege by the French.

But the French siege did not last too long: the speed and power of the French army's advance had frightened Italian rulers, as well as the Pope. This prompted the forming of an anti-French coalition, the League of Venice, which defeated Charles at Fornovo in July 1495. Charles lost nearly all the booty of the campaign, as well as several hundred men. On his retreat back to France, many soldiers were desperately ill.[20] When the army of mercenaries disbanded and the soldiers returned to their respective homelands, the scourge rapidly spread. Hence the famous quote by Voltaire: 'On their flippant way through Italy, the French carelessly picked up Genoa, Naples and syphilis. Then they were thrown out and deprived of Naples and Genoa. But they did not lose everything – syphilis went with them'.[21]

After the French siege, Italian chroniclers began to record a disease, which they recognised as new, repugnant, and deadly [22] – they called it *Mal Francese*, 'French sickness', or by the Latin term *Morbus Gallicus*. Similarly, the English and Germans called it the 'French Pox', while the French assiduously called the new scourge the 'Neapolitan Disease'. In fact, during the time of widespread syphilis outbreaks in Western Europe, the disease was generally known by the origin of one's current enemies.

As the infection spread, it was therefore identified as the French, the Neapolitan, the Spanish, the German, or the Polish malady, while the Turks blamed Christendom in general for the terrible outbreak. The Arabs on the other hand called it the 'Christian Malady', the Japanese called it the 'Chinese pox', and in Africa and India, to where syphilis was spread by Portuguese explorers, it became known as the 'Portuguese Sickness'. The term 'syphilis', coined by Italian physician Girolamo Fracastoro (1476-1553) in 1530, only came to be used during the late eighteenth century – it was a popular term, because it did not connect the disease with any specific nation.

As is obvious from the various names of the disease, the infection spread rapidly from country to country. By the end of 1495 the epidemic extended throughout France, Germany, and Switzerland, reaching England and Scotland in 1497. Then the contagion moved swiftly to the Scandinavian countries, as well as Southern and Eastern Europe. Europeans took the disease to India in 1498, and by 1520 it had reached Africa, the near East, China, Japan and Oceania.[23]

Although the 'pox' was a new scourge in fifteenth century Europe, sexually transmitted diseases were not unknown, and certainly not uncommon. Gonorrhoea had in fact been a problem since antiquity and was later erroneously thought to be the first stage of syphilis, once this disease started to become widespread – which is why the great Renaissance physician Paracelsus (1493-1541) called it 'French Gonorrhoea'[24] instead of 'French Pox'. Symptoms of what may have been gonorrhoea were already described in the Egyptian *Ebers Papyrus* and *Kahun Papyrus* and appropriate treatments recommended.[25] Similarly, the Israelites seemed to have known this sexually transmitted disease. The *Book of Leviticus* warns the children of Israel to avoid contact with any man or woman who 'hath a running issue' (discharge) or who is 'unclean'.[26]

In medieval England gonorrhoea was referred to as the *brennynge* or the burning, reflecting the symptom of painful, burning, sometimes-bloody urination. Correspondingly, the French knew the condition as *chaude pisse* or 'hot piss', which was just as apt a description for gonorrhoea. Polite society in England called the disease by its French name, *chaude pisse,* until the sixteenth century when it became generally known as the 'clap' – probably derived from the Old French term *clapier*, meaning brothel. When syphilis first made its appearance it was not immediately recognised as something new and different, and therefore was also initially known as the 'burning'. The erroneous link between syphilis and gonorrhoea, namely that they were both the manifestation of the same, but different phases of the disease, persisted to the end of the eighteenth century.

The pox had appeared in Naples seemingly from nowhere, and initially no one knew where it had come from. Its sudden appearance perplexed physicians and made them despair of ever finding a cure. The new disease was so lethal that those who contracted it were considered incurable. Generally chroniclers and records of past centuries describe a disease of much greater virulence, far greater severity, and higher mortality, than anything seen in modern times – possibly because it was a novel disease and the population had no immunity against it.[27] In modern times however, even in third-world countries, the disease is seldom allowed to progress without the intervention of antibiotics.

Symptoms of the disease described by chroniclers

The variety of symptoms described by chroniclers in the fifteenth and sixteenth centuries '…underlines the need to avoid adopting too rigid a picture of the disease'.[28] Initial signs of the pox varied so greatly that the German seventeenth century physician, Tobias Knobloch (1596-1641), boasted to have seen at least three hundred diverse 'species' of this disease; and others despairingly proclaimed that it seemed that all diseases were indeed contained in the pox.[29] Syphilis was in fact generally known as the 'great imitator', as it mimicked so many diseases.

Chroniclers of the disease generally mention specific symptoms: genital ulcers, rash accompanied by fever, and severe joint and muscle pains. In 1519, the great German reformer, Ulrich von Hutten (1488-1523), wrote a book titled *De morbo gallico*, 'On the French disease'. He graphically describes therein his own experience with syphilis, and the treatments he underwent for the last fifteen years of his life until the illness finally ended his days. According to von Hutten, sufferers were covered with acorn-sized boils that emitted foul, dark green pus, a secretion so vile that the horror at the sight of their own bodies was even more troubling to victims than the burning pains of their sores. But this, according to von Hutten was only the beginning. The onward bitter march of indisputable syphilitic symptoms included foul-smelling abscesses and sores, or 'pocks', which developed into deep ulcers that dissolved skin, muscle, bone, palate, even lips, noses and genital organs. These horrible, filthy looking and stinking abscesses eventually appeared all over a victim's body and racked the sufferer with pain – the flesh ultimately rotting away over a long period of time, slowly killing the person.

Chroniclers tell us that '...sometimes the pain was so intense that patients screamed day and night without respite, envying the dead themselves'.[30] Many were driven to suicide. Italian chronicler Matarazzo describes how bodies rotted inside, as well as on the outside. He cites the example of a merchant who was so consumed by the sickness between his torso and thighs that a great big hole had been gouged in his body.[31] Sometimes, mercifully, early death occurred.

The repulsion, anguish, and suffering caused by the pox, were incontrovertible. German artist Albrecht Dürer pleaded: 'God save me from the French disease. I know of nothing of which I am so afraid ... Nearly every man has it and it eats up so many that they die'.[32] In a similar vain, sixteenth century German court historian, Joseph Grünpeck, commented that the new disease was '...so cruel, so distressing, so appalling that until now nothing more terrible or disgusting has ever been known on this earth'.[33] After he fell victim to syphilis, Grünpeck lamented that '...the wound on my priapic gland became so swollen, that both hands could scarcely encircle it'.[34]

However, not everyone seems to have been affected as badly, and the disease appears to have had many forms. In this context the observations by fifteenth century professor of medicine, Nicolò Leoniceno (1428-1524), at Ferrara in Italy, are especially useful because they were based on the autopsy results of victims who had died in Naples during the initial stages of the spread of the pox. Leoniceno identified two forms of the disease, one displaying horrific external sores, while the other caused intense pain in joints and nerves with no outward signs of the disease. Autopsies of those free of external lesions revealed internal abscesses, which had caused the tormenting pains.[35]

Presumed causes and origins

Naturally, numerous theories surrounded the cause and origin of such a dreadfully disfiguring disease: an astrological conjunction of the planets; punishment by a wrathful God disgusted by fornication; and, as some suggested even then, an entirely new disease brought from the New World by Columbus's men and '...fermented in the loins of Neapolitan prostitutes'.[36]

Humanist scholars fervently sought astrological causes for the scourge. Unsurprisingly, a seemingly acceptable and valid explanation was soon found. Court historian to the Emperor Maximillian, Joseph Grünpeck, based his rationalisation for the origin of the French pox on classic Arab astrology, the 'Great Conjunction' of Saturn and Jupiter, which foreshadowed natural calamities and turmoil by corrupting the air.[37] Contagious diseases during medieval times were generally blamed on foul or corrupt 'airs', which is why the lighting of herbal aromatic fires was recommended for cleansing the atmosphere and staving off syphilis. Even though the Great Conjunction of 25 November 1484 had taken place as much as a decade before the arrival of the pox, it was nevertheless deemed by physicians, astrologers, and scholars, to be a fitting and satisfactory explanation for this scourge.

Unfortunately, according to Joseph Grünpeck, the Great Conjunction was not the only astrological calamity at the time. What was apparently exacerbating the dire pox situation was the additional unfavourable aspect of Mars in its own house. He speculated that all those affected by the new disease were most susceptible to this specific unfavourable aspect: acute disease linked to Mars, and a chronic long-lasting malady connected to Saturn. German artist Albrecht Dürer graphically portrays this widely accepted clarification in a woodcut: the pox-stricken, pustule-covered nobleman standing below a representation of the zodiac showing the year 1484 – the year of the Great Conjunction, more than ten years before the first recorded case of the pox.

Perhaps more than any other disease before or since, syphilis provoked a widespread moral panic in Europe. The fundamental nature of the disease was seen as a manifestation of God's displeasure in humankind – a view many doctors shared. Syphilitics were condemned from church pulpits and from chairs in university medical schools. Promiscuity in medieval society was too widespread to initially appear as a suspect in the transmission of such a foul disease. In this context, twentieth century historian Claude Quétel (born 1939) fittingly states that '… nothing is more revealing of a society than the history of its diseases, particularly the "social" diseases'.[38] Soon, most people came to associate syphilis with the sins of the flesh, more specifically sexual contact. Moralists immediately seized upon this fact as divine punishment for the rampant licentiousness of the age. While the influential Italian Dominican friar, Girolamo Savonarola (1452-1498), called for strict moral change, reformer John Calvin (1509-1564) railed against the sin and debauchery, which had given rise to the French pox.[39]

Syphilis was attributed to the sin of lust, which was certainly a logical assumption as soldiers and prostitutes traditionally associated with sexual license and moral disorder, were amongst the first victims. The connection with moral failings became even closer when people noticed that the first outward signs of the disease in the form of sores often appeared on the genital organs. Such disgusting symptoms were taken as a sign that those so repugnantly afflicted housed similarly debauched and sinful souls. In keeping with such sentiments, French physician Jacques de Bethencourt (1477-1527) – who naturally rejected the term 'French pox' – fittingly introduced the term *morbus venerus*, the 'malady of Venus' in 1527, since the pox was deemed to have arisen from illicit love.[40], [41]

Once syphilis was associated with sexual activity, the blame was swiftly and irrevocably transferred to the 'weaker sex'. Commentators on the malady were exclusively male. Hence, women, especially prostitutes, were undeservedly presumed to be the cause, while men were cast as helpless victims instead of the actual contaminators. It was thought that women only carried the disease – not contracting it themselves, but transmitting it to men. In fact, it was popularly held that syphilis made women insatiable in their sexual ardour. Ulrich von Hutten conspiratorially declared: 'This thing as touching women resteth in their secret places, having in those places little pretty sores full of venomous poison, being very dangerous for those that unknowingly meddle with them'.[42] Similarly a sixteenth century court doctor from Ferrara boldly stated: 'Men get it from doing it with women in their vulvas'.[43] Chronicler Giovanni Portoveneri of Pisa declared that '...it is spread through having sex with women who have these sicknesses, and especially with prostitutes'.[44]

A malady for rich and poor alike

The infection of syphilis was passed on swiftly in a deadly spiral: men communicated it to prostitutes, who then passed it on to their next client, who in turn contaminated other prostitutes or their own wives. Tragic consequences of the new disease were innocent children who were infected through their own mothers or wet-nurses. Wet-nursing was a significant and widespread cultural practice in European countries. As breast-feeding was linked exclusively with the lower classes since medieval times, the practice was deemed an 'inappropriate' activity for upper-class women. Therefore, wealthy married women hired wet nurses as a matter of course, while working-class mothers breast-fed their own babies.[45] Unfortunately thousands of babies were thus infected with the deadly pox.

Shakespeare refers to the disease as the *pox* in ten of his plays. In *Measure for Measure*, first staged in 1604, three Viennese citizens openly discuss venereal disease, which was rife during these times. Lucio, upon seeing a brothel madam approaching, exclaims: 'I have purchased . . . many diseases under her roof".[46]

The disease was widespread in the courts of Europe. Many royals and prominent figures in the European courts had syphilis. Unfortunately, the French King Charles VIII was the first of many monarchs to contract the disease. He fell ill shortly after the siege of Naples, which was to be the beginning of the global syphilis outbreak in the late fifteenth century. A historian from the House of Burgundy specifically records Charles's persistent malady as the pox '...a violent, hideous and abominable sickness by which he was harrowed; and several of his number who returned to France were most painfully afflicted by it [...], it was called the Neapolitan sickness'.[47]

The pox also affected English royalty. Second husband to Mary, Queen of Scots, Henry Stuart Lord Darnley (1545-1567), was described by his own wife as a 'pockish' man. 'There seems little doubt that Mary's second husband, Darnley, and probably her third, Bothwell, had syphilis'.[48] Initially Darnley was thought to have had smallpox, but given his medical history, this was more likely to have been syphilis.[49] After Mary had visited him on his sickbed she uttered: 'I thought I should have been killed by his breath: and yet I sat no nearer to him than in a chair by his bed and he lieth on the further side of it'.[50] At a later date, she noted that his rash had faded somewhat, that he had large bald patches on his head and was receiving special baths. These were most likely mercury treatments, which characteristically cause the hair to fall out, while the foul mouth odour is typically associated with sufferers of the pox.

Some time later, Lord Darnley sent Mary a letter which caused her to declare in desperation: 'I wish I were dead'.[51] Then she consulted her physician and remained in his care for some weeks. In view of the fact that Darnley in all probability had syphilis – Darnley's skull, preserved in the Royal College of Surgeons, London, was judged to be syphilitic [52] – there have been many suggestions regarding the contents of the letter. Perhaps Darnley informed her that he had syphilis '…and perhaps even accused her of being its source'.[53]

At the baptism of her son James VI of Scotland (1566-1625), the future King James I of England, Mary Queen of Scots refused to allow Archbishop Hamilton, to use his spittle to anoint the child, as was customary during baptism at the time, for fear that he would infect the infant. She was adamant that she would not allow a 'pockie priest' with 'stinking breath' to 'spit' on her son.[54] Syphilis eventually deprived all its victims of dignity and decorum, no matter what their station in life. This included George II of England (1683-1760) who, suffering from an aneurism resulting from syphilitic infection, died '…unbecomingly while sitting on his privy stool in his closet'.[55]

Sexual mores in Europe at the time were no different for courtiers, commoners, and ecclesiastics. Even the highest echelons of the priesthood were not exempt from the pox. Corruption in the Church was manifest, and celibacy clearly unenforceable. The tell-tale 'purple flowers' – as repeated bouts of syphilis were euphemistically known – adorned the faces of cardinals, bishops and priests.[56] Cardinal Francesco Soderini

(1453-1524) was rumoured to be suffering from the pox in 1510, and in fact several sources confirm this.[57] Cesare Borgia (1475-1507), one of the illegitimate sons of Pope Alexander VI (1431-1503), and brother to the famous Lucrezia, was reared for the Church and made archbishop of Valencia – a position he later discarded. Cesare contracted syphilis in Naples, and as the disease progressed, he was forced to wear a black mask to hide the disfigurement of what was once a most handsome face.

Nose patching, condoms and codpieces

Together with distinctive sunken eyes and the dreadful stench of rotting flesh, the absence of the nose was one of the most horrific features of syphilis. For many, this was the most outward visible stigma resulting from the dreaded pox – an affirmation of corruption and debauchery. The disintegrated or missing nose was known as a 'saddle nose'. Consequently, the end of the sixteenth century provided many opportunities for plastic surgery on the face and saw the beginning of a new era in nose 'patching'.[58]

The spread of syphilis led to the first 'imitation' nose, created by Italian physician Gasparo Tagliacozzi (1546-1599) who is widely considered the 'father of modern plastic surgery'. The only problem was that his initial constructed nose could in fact fall off, if the recipient blew through it too hard. Later Tagliacozzi perfected his highly acclaimed operative procedure, which was accomplished in six sessions over two months. A skin pedicle from the inner upper arm was swung up and affixed to where the nose ought to be – perhaps inspired by the old Indian method of rhinoplasty – while the arm was tied to the patient's head for several days. Eventually the graft healed, was severed from the arm and a nose of sorts had thus been created.

Nose 'patching' was not the only consequence of syphilis. As the disease epidemic spread across Europe it gave rise to the first published account of the condom, described in contemporary slogans as an 'armor against pleasure and a cobweb against infection'. Initially, condoms were used solely to prevent infection and disease rather than to function as birth control, as their efficacy in preventing pregnancy had simply not yet been recognised. In the mid-sixteenth century, anatomist Gabriele Fallopius (1523-1562) claimed to have invented the 'sheath of linen', which was wrapped around the penis to protect men against syphilis. Alternatively, condoms made of sheep's gut were also widely obtainable, tied around the scrotum by means of a ribbon. These condoms were expensive to buy, hence often reused several times – not ideal under any circumstances, especially when the ultimate aim was to contain the spread of syphilitic infection.

However, condoms did not become common until the eighteenth century, and even then they were not easy to come by outside of London or Paris. As with the disease itself, names for the protective sheath revealed national antipathies: the French rogue, Casanova, referred to them as 'overcoats from England', while they became known as 'French letters' by the English, and 'capote Anglais', meaning 'English cloak', by the French.

In a society where sexual license and gratification, especially in the upper classes, were commonplace and the resultant effects of promiscuity fully recognised, there was an acceptance of the pox as something which, although most unwelcome, was nevertheless unavoidable. Through fashionable style the disease was even effectively covered up. Thus, pancake makeup and painted-on beauty spots were a response to recurrent attacks of syphilis as well as smallpox.

Even court fashion became part of the story: during the early sixteenth century, male dress style of the higher classes in Europe was revolutionised by the introduction of the 'codpiece' to the male tunic – 'cod' being an old English term for scrotum. As may be observed from various court paintings the codpiece at times assumed proportions which can only be described as grotesque. Historians have speculated about the codpiece, describing it as a statement of virility, which is indeed confirmed by various royal portraits. One has only to look at Holbein's representation of King Henry VIII: with arms akimbo, wide shouldered, the oversized codpiece thrust forward, he appeared as the embodiment of a lusty male.

However the question has been raised whether the origin of the codpiece coincided with the rapid spread of syphilis at the time, and may in fact have been a disguise for underlying disease.[59] Perhaps this fashion developed out of necessity, rather than a whimsical fashion sense. The new disease, which swept across Europe from 1495 onwards '…caused foul and large volumes of mixed pus and blood to be discharged from the genital organs and the swellings in the adjacent groin tissue'.[60] The resulting 'mess' would necessitate bulky woollen wads to be applied, hence distorting the entire genital area. What better way to hide this unfortunate state than by a generally accepted fashion accessory?

The codpieces were invariably painted a 'vivid' scarlet, which is an interesting fact. The popularly topical ointment of mercuric oxide and sulphite, known as cinnabar[61] – applied to syphilitic ulcers – was deep red in colour and was known to 'stain the linen'.[62] Again, the codpiece presented the ideal cover-up. Once the fashion of codpieces had been established, many men may have followed suit simply to be in *vogue*. The question of whether they were victims of fashion or victims of disease remains speculative.

As the scourge of syphilis spread in the early sixteenth century, people were horrified and revolted. In many instances, those afflicted were driven out of town for fear of contaminating innocent people. Panicked townsfolk barred their city gates against syphilitics. Within two years of the first reported cases, cities stretching from Geneva to Aberdeen expelled the pox-ridden. The disease was perceived as being such a threat in Scotland, that James IV signed a decree ordering all those suffering from syphilis to leave Edinburgh.[63] The Scottish 'Ane Grandgoret' Act of 1497 ordered all those infected with the pox 'this contagius seikness',[64] to be taken by boat to the island of Inchkeith – the island can be seen from Edinburgh Castle. Any failure to comply with this order was punishable by branding on the cheek, so that the sufferer would be henceforth recognisable to everyone.

The Burgh of Aberdeen had issued a similar regulation, a year earlier, in 1496. Clearly both acts recognised the venereal aspect of the disease. The Aberdeen Act specified that 'all light (loose) women' should 'dicist from thair vices and syne of venerie'[65] and rather work for their support on the pain of being branded. The pox had thus already claimed its victims in Scotland by 1496. In that same year, the Paris parliament issued a decree giving syphilitics twenty-four hours to leave the city – failure to do so was punishable by hanging.

Repeatedly, city elders blamed prostitutes for the disease. Prostitutes came under special attack as they were seen as the agents of contamination. Ironically these women were condemned far more harshly than the men who habitually used their services and, in all likelihood, were the initiators of the spread of the disease. As fear of the dreadful malady spread, a tightening of control over places where the disease could be spread was evident throughout Europe. Bathhouses were closed and abandoned, innkeepers refused entry to anyone possibly infected with the pox, and calls went out to close brothels.

However, attempts to suppress or control prostitution were slow to follow through – too many wealthy and influential personages, among them the clergy, profited handsomely from these establishments. A well-known example of such moral rectitude was the Bishop of Winchester, who '…derived a substantial income from the Bankside brothels, which were known colloquially as Winchester stews. So notorious were prostitutes from the stews that the term "Winchester Goose" became a widely used euphemism for syphilis'.[66] In his play *Troilus and Cressida*, Shakespeare has Pandanus utter: 'Some gallad goose of Winchester would hiss: Till then I'll sweat and seek about for eases, and at that time bequeathe you my diseases'.[67] Eventually in 1546, King Henry III took decisive steps to close these brothels.

Similarly, Paris brothels were shut down and the pope endeavoured to stamp out prostitution altogether. In spite of such measures or perhaps because of them, vice was not exterminated, but simply driven outside the bounds of regulation. Decrees against prostitution were renewed from time to time until the pox became so widespread that there was no point in pursuing these strict measures.

Incurabili hospitals and 'lazar houses'

As the disease spread, calls arose in the early sixteenth century for the foundation of hospitals – the *incurabili* hospitals – to accommodate pox-sufferers. One of the first *incurabili* hospitals, built in 1521, the church-hospital complex of *Santa Maria del Popolo degli Incurabili* still stands today as a refurbished modern medical facility in Naples. Such charitable institutions were eventually to be found in virtually every major European city. Although hospitals in medieval Europe were benevolent institutions, designed to provide care and shelter to the ailing poor, as the disease continued to spread like wildfire, infirmaries soon refused to admit syphilitic patients.

The most famous of such hospitals was the Paris *Hôtel-Dieu*, which was known to boast about the scope of its generosity towards poor, destitute and ailing sufferers. This hospital even took in plague victims. But there was one exception – those inflicted with the pox. Such reluctance and extreme prejudice to let pox-victims into the general hospital wards was widespread throughout Europe. However, increasing numbers of debilitated syphilis sufferers were lying in the streets begging, covered in terrible sores, and surrounded by the foulest of odours. Even in those days, when any knowledge about hygiene was sorely lacking, pox sufferers were considered a threat to all healthy passers-by. But, pox victims could not be left to pollute the streets.

A partial solution was to put those afflicted with syphilis in the now empty 'lazar houses', attached to medieval hospitals. These hospitals had been founded in the twelfth and thirteenth centuries for the segregation of lepers. But the decline in this terrible disease had made the lazar houses redundant after the 1350's. Generally hospitals in the larger cities followed the example of the *Hôtel-Dieu*, by turning away pox sufferers and sending them to the deserted, ghostly leper houses.

By the eighteenth-century hospital admission conditions had not changed much. In Paris for instance, only a small number out of fifty hospitals and clinics, admitted and treated pox sufferers. Marginal and poor people, and those infected with syphilis, were instead sent to prison hospitals like *la Salpêtrière* and *la Bicêtre*, where the pox-ridden were locked up with '...felons and petty criminals, some of whom were diseased and some of whom were not [...] little effort was made to provide any treatment'.[68] For 'moral purification', especially female inmates of *la Salpêtrière*, irrespective of whether they had the pox or not, were disciplined into confession thrice daily. They slept six to a bed; lived on bread and water; and spent their days in fetid rooms, which had five-foot high ceilings. Similar conditions prevailed at *Bicêtre*, where the pox-ridden were locked up with the mentally insane, criminals and the poor, who had nowhere else to go.

Medical theories on the pox

Not only were health authorities challenged with institutional problems posed by the new disease, but medical professionals were equally confronted. While modern medical research takes place in a laboratory, doctors living during the Renaissance would consult books in medical libraries to see what the ancients had said. Indisputably, Renaissance medicine still continued to rely on the theories and practices of Hippocrates, Galen, and Avicenna. But they had never described anything in their writings even similar to the syphilitic cases suddenly appearing in increasing numbers. However, physicians refused to accept the notion that the pox could be a new or independent disease and continued to evaluate this disease through the acknowledged hypothesis of humoral balance.

Hence, in the 1620's German physician, Tobias Knobloch, clearly distinguished in his writings four kinds of 'French pox': the melancholic, phlegmatic, choleric and sanguine pox. He claimed to be able to diagnose each specific type by smell, colour, size and appearance of the physical symptoms presented by each individual. For instance, he claimed that the choleric pox could be easily identified by the hard red boils, covered by a yellow lid, which spread all over the body,[69] while the melancholic type rarely covered the whole body and was identifiable by large blue or greyish cones. Other physicians similarly described four general types of the disease, but varied the typical symptoms for each one. Although the medical establishment avoided going into too much detail regarding the various symptoms of the French pox, all associated excruciating pain with this disease – resulting, according to humoral theory, from the rapid change of the body's material configuration.

According to the theory of humors a distinct predisposition to the French pox existed with regard to the sexes. The male body was perceived as being warm and dry. Women on the other hand were seen as being cold and moist, as the elements of water and phlegm were thought to be dominant in women. In addition, through monthly bleeding and the production of breast milk, women's' bodies regularly purged themselves of tainted bodily fluids. However, this process was not available to men, leading to an accumulation of noxious matter in their bodies, which in turn made them far more susceptible to the pox than women.

Reputable physicians warned that obstructions and deficiencies in liver and gall bladder were the '…root cause for an accumulation of the poisonous matter of the dreaded pox' [70] in the blood. Others associated the cause of 'pox matter' with irregularities in spleen or lung function. Although there was disagreement with regard to which organ was responsible, physicians generally concurred that the '…coagulated matter of the French pox', resulted from an '…unnatural excess of black bile and/or phlegm', thus unbalancing the humors.[71] It was thought that the various body parts drove this 'morbid matter' into the skin, resulting in the poisonous scabies known as the 'pox'.

In his book *A useful regime against the French Pox*, German physician Alexander Seitz (1470-1540) warned against any foods, in which the '…complexional composition came close to that of the pox matter'.[72] In other words, foods, which were moist, cold and acidic. He thus furnished readers with long lists of balanced, pox-preventing meals as well as food-items to be avoided at all costs. Forbidden foods for instance were the meats of all fish and birds dwelling or standing in stagnant waters; game such as deer, geese and cranes; all legumes; all radishes, onions, garlic and mustard, thought to block the pores in the skin.[73]

A further contention by the medical establishment was that emotions such as anger, fear, or shock contributed to the physical causes of disease: anger was believed to overheat all humors, resulting in fevers and inflammation; fear and shock caused fainting, weakness, and slowing pulse. Therefore, violent emotional swings could be as much the causes of the pox as eating contaminated food or sharing one's bed with a pox sufferer.

Various 'mild' medical remedies

But, what treatments did physicians and the medical establishment offer? It was soon observed that traditional methods of drawing out the corrupted humors, such as bleeding and purging, as well as chicken broth and other dietary prescriptions, had no effect in alleviating the suffering of those inflicted with the 'pox'. In fact, it was not entirely clear whether physicians of old had *anything* constructive or helpful to offer. Many warned of the dangers of sex with prostitutes, and some even proposed preventing the pox by washing the genitals in hot vinegar or white wine before and after intercourse. But, such remedies, while doing no harm seemed to do little good. Within the framework of Hippocratic-Galenic theory concerning the quality and quantity of body fluids, there was however general consensus amongst physicians that the greatest danger lay in direct contact with the contaminated bodily fluids of pox-sufferers. Body fluids such as saliva, sweat, urine and semen were considered by-products of 'nutritional blood' which, once corrupted by poisonous pox matter, could be absorbed by the open pores of a healthy person (See Chapter 2 on 'Humoral bodies – a healthy balance').

New methods had to be found to expel the gruesome matter unbalancing the humors. So-called 'mild' remedies quickly gave way to treatments the patient could physically 'feel', which at least indicated that doctors were doing something to help their patients – after all, had not Hippocrates already taught that 'desperate diseases needed desperate cures'?[74] Initially high temperatures were a novel approach. Sores would be cauterised and patients subjected to dry heat to induce sweating. This was achieved by seating the hapless victim in a wooden barrel, surrounded by sand and hot stones, in a small confined space. The patient was left there to steam for as long as possible, a treatment recommended twice daily for about a week. During this time, no food was given to the sufferer, in case noxious matter built up in the body again.

In another type of cure, patients were repeatedly bathed in herbs, wine or olive oil. Disconcertingly, it seems that these liquids were in fact often reused several times. A declaration by the Health Board of

Venice in 1498, specifically forbade the reuse of olive oil, which had been infested with revolting scabs, filth and muck from a long line of previous patients.[75] Another agonising method of dealing with one of the disease's symptoms, specifically the racking headaches, was by trepanation – the ancient practice of boring holes into the skull. A part of this treatment included cauterising oozing ulcers in skin and bone with fearsome, white-hot irons.

Mercury treatments – the cure that killed

In addition to bleeding, bathing, cauterisation and herbal applications, physicians increasingly fought syphilis in two ways: firstly with mercury and the secondly with *guaiacum*. Mercury, which had already been used for hundreds of years in the treatment of scabs, leprosy, psoriasis and other skin conditions, became the treatment of choice for syphilis and remained so for over four hundred years. It was used externally as an ointment, painted onto the sufferer's lesions, or used in conjunction with heated mercury fumes to be inhaled by the sufferer.

In his book, *De morbo gallico*, 'On the French disease', written in 1519, Ulrich von Hutten describes the appalling mercury vapour treatments he underwent – eleven extensive treatments in nine years – until the illness finally ended his life: patients would be smeared from head to toe with a mercury-based ointment. Then while seated or made to lie down, they would be swathed in thick blankets and shut in a small steam room. While perspiration poured from their skin, patients often fainted from the intense heat, but suffered silently, believing that the hotter the steam room, the quicker they would be cured. During this ordeal, large sores appeared on cheeks, tongues, throats and mucous membranes, and vile secretions discharged from their mouths and noses, causing an overwhelming stench to surround the suffering patient.

Facing such horrendous prospects, there were many who decided to rather die from the disease than undergo the 'cure'. However, many also died while undergoing treatment from kidney or heart failure, or because their throats had swelled so much from mercury poisoning that they were unable to breathe. Von Hutten cites one example, where a medical practitioner had killed three men in a single day by overheating the steam room. He laments that '...very few there were that got their health, if they passed through these jeopardies, these bitter pains and evils'.[76]

Treatments with mercury had severe side effects, such as kidney failure, uncontrollable shaking spells, corrosion of the membranes in the mouth resulting in painful gum ulcers and a loosening of the teeth, as well as a relentless deterioration of the bones, and loss of all hair. But such results were in fact desired by '...medical practitioners and patients alike. It was believed that such effects were the excretion of the morbid matter of the pox and had to be endured'.[77]

Another specific side effect of mercury treatments was copious perspiration and salivation, both of which could be considerably increased by augmenting the amounts of mercury used. In fact, numerous eighteenth century French and English physicians specifically advocated a strict regime of 'salivation' or ptyalismus, to treat syphilis. Excessive salivation, induced by increased amounts of mercury, was thought to expel the disease.

Before confinement to the small chamber in which the patient sat on a perforated stool, the patient would be thickly covered with a mercurial unction to bring forth the venereal poisons through extreme salivation. Desired salivation constituted at least four to six pints of saliva daily. In 1736 English physician Daniel Turner (1667-1741) claimed to have successfully treated hundreds of patients with a mild to stubborn pox in this way. If patients did not sufficiently salivate, Turner used a mixture of mercury and sulphur in the fumigation chamber. Various prominent physicians, among them English physician John Douglas, in his *Treatise on Venereal Disease* (1737) were opposed to excessive salivation and started advocating less harsh regimes, although mercury continued to be used as the prime medication.

Mercury treatments would be maintained at intervals for years, until all stubborn symptoms of the pox had been effectively erased. Physicians believed that if even *one* symptom remained, the poison still contained within the body could again redistribute itself. Such ruthless treatment regimes gave rise to the expression: 'A night with Venus, a lifetime with mercury'.[78] Mercury treatments also gave rise to the term 'quack' used in modern times to depict a medical doctor of dubious qualifications. Derived from the German word 'quacksalber', for quicksilver or mercury, the word 'quack' was originally used to describe those who poisoned their patients with mercury.

Charlatan cures and orthodox drugs

Inevitably there was an immediate, insatiable market for any mixture that might cure the pox, without the harmful and unpleasant side effects. In 1720, an acclaimed remedy, advertised as antisyphilitic 'vegetable essence' appeared in the *Journal de Paris*. Six bottles of the dubious mixture were assured to be sufficient '…for a recently acquired bout of venereal disease'.[79] Other charlatan cures included various prophylactic ointments and antivenereal aphrodisiacs. Throughout Europe, the selling of these cure-alls depended on effective marketing. In London signposts and pamphlets posted and distributed throughout the city allowed the pox-inflicted to choose from numerous advertised remedies or those hawked in the streets by local self-acclaimed healers.

While questionable 'practitioners' marketed their equally questionable remedies, the orthodox medical establishment debated their own cures and practices, and who in fact should be administering them. As far back as the sixteenth century, English surgeons were already giving written practical instructions on treating syphilis. Traditionally orthodox surgeons dealt with external manifestations of disease, while physicians treated internal disorders. During the eighteenth century surgeons and physicians were still arguing as to which practitioner should deal with the pox. Amongst medical practitioners syphilis was identified and diagnosed mainly on its external manifestations. Hence, surgeons argued that it slotted into their area of trade (See Chapter 1 on 'Medical practitioners of the past). Records show that surgeons were indeed '…accustomed to manually administering long labour-intensive treatment'.[80]

While physicians remonstrated that only members of their eminent organisation should rightfully deal with venereology, and surgeons argued that they alone had the practical training to deal with the pox, countless drugs and treatments flooded the market. In France alone, between 1772 and 1782, more than fifty requests for permission to test new drugs were approved[81] by the ill-fated Bourbon monarch, Louis XVI. Unfortunately, the most common place for experimentation with these drugs was the *Bicêtre*, where the pox-ridden poor had been sent. Here, pox sufferers were singled out for harsh 'medicine', before new drugs could be administered. Moral purging or whipping was brutal and ruthless, thought to 'open' the body for healing. After that patients were bled, purged and bathed for several days,[82] before oral and external treatments began.

Guaiacum – 'holy wood'

As indicated previously, physicians increasingly fought syphilis in two ways; with mercury and *guaiacum*. Consequently, apart from mercury the only other treatment considered effective by the medical establishment was the wood of the Central American *guaiacum* or *lignum vitae* tree. *Guaiacum*, which first arrived in Europe in 1517, was championed by many as less deadly and more effective than mercury. *Guaiacum*, also known as 'holy wood', a dark hard wood – considered to be the same wood as the wood of the Cross on which Jesus had been crucified – soon became the widespread wonder drug for syphilis during the early sixteenth century. It was reasoned that a medication from the New World must surely be supremely effective against what was essentially perceived as a New World disease, especially when it became known that indigenous inhabitants of the West Indies themselves used *guaiacum* to treat the 'pox'.

The House of Fugger, a wealthy German merchant and banking family from Augsburg – the Rockefellers of their day – imported *guaiacum* wood and bark into Europe at astoundingly high prices. The Fugger family, the '…richest merchant and banking family of the time, immediately requested monopoly control for import of *guaiacum* wood from Emperor Maximilian. He granted it in return for having his huge debt with the Fugger Bank waived. Besides the gold and silver robbed from the Aztecs and Incas, the Spanish galleons now carried masses of *guaiacum* wood to Europe',[83] where it was sold to apothecaries.

The wood, which soon became known as 'pox wood', was ground to a fine powder, soaked in eight times its volume of water and then boiled until it had been reduced by half the volume. The resultant scum was removed, dried and applied on pox sores, whilst the liquid was given to the patient to drink. But the drink was only to be taken after the sufferer had been starved, purged and sweated in a heated room for several days. This remedy, hailing from an untainted land, with no association to university-trained doctors, was greatly propagated by the German reformer Ulrich von Hutten. The reformer's zeal in advocating the 'holy wood' had a personal motive, as the 'conventional' mode of treating his own case of the pox, namely mercury treatment, had been unsuccessful. Another great believer in *guaiacum* was the Italian sculptor Benvenuto Cellini (1500-1571) who by his own admission caught the pox around 1532 from '...a fine young servant girl I was keeping'[84] while working on a commission by Pope Clement VII (1478-1534).

By 1520 the Italian towns of Bologna, Ferrara, Genoa, Rome, Naples, Florence, Venice and Padua had established Incurables hospitals.[85] Admission procedures to these hospitals were posted on the doors of city churches. Those admitted were seen twice a day by medical staff, who examined their urine, and advised appropriate food and drink to treat the patient.

As surviving records attest, the Italian *Incurabilis* hospitals were large consumers of *guaiacum* from the mid-sixteenth century and the 'pox-wood' was even distributed for free to thousands of sufferers, at great costs to these hospitals.[86] Even though *guaiacum* treatments were highly recommended by orthodox physicians, it was in fact totally ineffectual against the pox, apart from inducing severe perspiration in the patient. The eccentric Paracelsus astutely commented that the Fuggers were the only people who benefited from the use of *guaiacum*. But, physicians generally continued to be convinced of the curative effects of this 'wonder-wood', many, such as noted London physician, Thomas Sydenham (1624-1689), known as the 'English Hippocrates', combining it with mercury treatments.

Unfortunately for patients, the varying cures for the pox were often far more excruciating than the symptoms. Although sufferers received differing medical care depending on their status in society – all cures at the time were problematic. The syphilitic rich consulted physicians whose assorted treatments ranged from being totally ineffectual to deadly noxious. The wealthy either suffered through lengthy mercury treatments with lethal side effects, or were made to sip guaiacum-cocktails and starved of all other nutrients, while being installed in small heated spaces where they had to sweat for weeks.

Meanwhile, the middle classes had the option of hiring barber-surgeons to torture them with knives and drills or searing hot cauterisation irons, while the poor, if they were lucky, gained admission to charity hospitals and leper quarters. Once admitted they were housed and fed in these institutions but received little medical help for their ailment. A refusal of entry meant that they would suffer and die in the street, scorned and abhorred by all, or be hounded out of town or city. It is hard to determine which must have been worse: to literally rot untreated, as syphilis ate its way through the body's organs, or to be poisoned and tortured by painful therapies. Syphilis was indeed an agonising torment and a tragedy for rich and poor alike.

Syphilis – the malady kept secret

It is estimated that at the end of the nineteenth century approximately fifteen percent of the population of Paris was infected with syphilis,[87] but very little was written about it at that time – as this was considered a dark secret, a secret malady. In Vienna, during the early 1900's one or two out of every ten young men were given the dreaded diagnosis and many chose the revolver rather than perish from the disease.[88] Numerous prominent nineteenth century figures were infected with syphilis: painters Vincent van Gogh (1853-1890) and Paul Gauguin (1848-1903); authors Oscar Wilde (1854-1900), Charles Baudelaire (1821-1867), Gustave Flaubert (1821-1880) and Guy de Maupassant (1850-1856); composers Franz Schubert (1797-1828) and Robert Schumann (1810-1856) and philosopher Friedrich Nietzsche (1844-1900) along with many other historical figures.

Well-known artist Paul Gauguin contracted the disease in Paris and subsequently passed it on to many of his beautiful Polynesian lovers, who would come to his 'bed every night as if possessed'.[89] Once Gauguin developed running sores, which did not respond to any form of treatment, he became less attractive to Tahitian women. Although he longed fervently to return to his native France, he died on his island paradise in 1903. Years of agonising pain, misery and relapsing illnesses are also true of three of the best known French writers, all of whom had syphilis: Charles Baudelaire, Gustave Flaubert and Guy de Maupassant.[90]

The question of how the disease may have affected the creative talent of writers, artists and composers is a thorny one, difficult to establish. While Van Gogh painted skulls towards the end of his life, Schubert's powerfully grandiose last works are impregnated with the awareness of death. A clinical manifestation of tertiary syphilis, which may appear anywhere between five and twenty years after the first manifestation of the disease, is 'paralysis of the insane'. In some cases literary masterpieces may have come about, corresponding to a peak of creativity, which is sometimes associated with 'paralysis of the insane'. This may have been the case with both the philosopher Friederich Wilhelm Nietzsche as well as writer Guy de Maupassant.

Nietzsche's great masterpieces were written during his decline into the dementia of tertiary syphilis. His intense '...reflections about his dreadful health are well known, and yet how often has his excruciating pain, so poignantly revealed in his remarkable correspondence and in his public work, been considered as a possible manifestation of the disease that was to send him into madness'.[91] Although some of his symptoms would also be consistent with schizophrenia, it is a known fact that he was initially infected with syphilis as a young man, when he regularly played the piano at a brothel, where he also habitually sampled the 'wares'.

Some wore their illness as a badge of pride. Author Guy de Maupassant boasted: 'I've got the pox! At last! Not the contemptible clap... The majestic pox...and I'm proud of it...I don't have to worry about catching it any more, and I screw the street whores and trollops and afterwards I say to them, "I've got the pox"'.[92] But, in spite of such triumphant words, flaunting the consequences of sexual license, he died fifteen years later '...in an asylum howling like a dog and planting twigs as baby Maupassants in the garden'.[93]

Others were secretive about their condition, helped along by the fact that syphilis in its later stages mimics so many different diseases that it was easy to hide the truth. In Oscar Wilde's work *The picture of Dorian Gray*, the face of the debauched hero retains its youthful beauty, while his body reflects the ravages of syphilis. Only in death does Dorian Gray's corpse reveal the despicable, repugnant decay brought on by his depraved way of life. Similarly, Erik, known as the 'Phantom of the Opera' hides his disfigured face behind a mask in Gaston Leroux's 1911 novel. When reading a description of Erik we can understand why he kept his face covered: His 'eyes are like two big black holes in a dead man's skull'…his skin 'is nasty yellow…' and his nose 'you cannot see it side-face'.[94]

The pox ravaged society for over four hundred years and in spite of the horrendous side effects, mercury was considered the only effective form of syphilis treatment until 1910. In April that year Paul Ehrlich, a German doctor, announced to the tightly packed Congress for Internal Medicine in Wiesbaden that he had discovered a compound that was effective against the notorious microbe *Treponema pallidum*. This compound had secretly and successfully been tested in the hospital wards of St. Petersburg, as well as in several German hospitals. Ehrlich named the compound 'Salvarsan', from the word 'salvation'. But the drug was popularly known as the 'magic bullet' – 'magic' for its specificity and 'bullet' for its capacity to kill.[95] Ehrlich had proved that '…diseases were just pathological locks waiting to be picked by the right molecules'.[96]

However, Salvarsan contained arsenic which, over the protracted course of treatment eventually led to arsenic poisoning. After the discovery of penicillin in 1928, lengthy trials with this drug ultimately confirmed its effectiveness in the destruction of *Treponema pallidum* in 1943 – even decades later syphilis remains sensitive to this drug. Easily treated in modern times with antibiotics, syphilis has progressed from being a deadly curse to a relatively rare ailment in western countries.

The following chapters discuss aspects of medical history relating solely to women's physiology, bound up in firmly held biases and misconceptions, entrenched in societal fabric and the medical establishment for millennia.

HYSTERIA – THE WHIMSICAL, WANDERING WOMB

From ancient times until the late eighteenth century the internal workings of women's sexual organs were governed by numerous misconceptions firmly held by the orthodox medical establishment. This chapter discusses specific conditions, such as hysteria, the 'wandering womb', 'suffocation of the mother' and the 'green sickness', all of which were once associated only with female physiology. These ailments were firmly anchored in the discrimination against women, the social oppression of women, and dominant male opinions.

Condescending and prejudicial attitudes towards women, which were to resonate for over two thousand years, were already represented in ancient times. According to classical Greek belief women were not only fundamentally different from men, but also decidedly inferior to men.[1] Women were in fact regarded as defective versions of the male species. This was clearly stated by Aristotle in the *Generation of Animals,* where he described the male as the '...properly formed result of generation' and declared that '...we should look upon the female state as being a deformity' – his unquestioning implication being that the male is naturally superior.[2]

Females were seen as the result of a 'generative occurrence not taken through to its ultimate conclusion'[3] and in chronological terms, women, the *genos gynaikon* or 'race of women', were even thought to be created at a later time than men.[4] In this context Plato (428-348 BCE) put forward the notion that before the creation of women, and '…in the second generation of humanity, men who acted in a cowardly or unjust way in the first generation are reborn as women'.[5]

Flawed female physiology

In the second century CE, Galen propagated that female reproductive organs were a reversed version of the male reproductive tract, turned inward instead of projecting outward – the uterus corresponding to the scrotum and the neck of the uterus to the penis. Views of an inherently flawed physiology were strengthened by the mysterious female conditions of puberty, pregnancy and childbirth, all of which involved periods of pain and sickness, even leading to postpartum mental illness, while menopausal women acted highly temperamentally and unpredictably. For over two thousand years these varying symptoms were seen as caused by an anomaly found only in women – the womb.

The notion of a 'wandering womb', was first described in the *Hippocratic Corpus* [6] dating back to the fifth century BCE. In this context, the Greek philosopher Plato put forward the idea that the womb was a separate living creature, living an independent existence inside a woman's body. He stated that the womb could 'become vexed' and begin wandering throughout the body, 'blocking respiratory channels' and 'causing bizarre behavior'.[7] First century medical writer Aretaeus of Cappadocia described the womb as '…lying in the middle of the flanks of a womans female viscus, closely resembling an animal; for it is moved of itself hither and thither in the flanks, also upwards […] to the right or to the left, either to the liver or spleen; and it likewise is subject to prolapse downwards. […] on the whole, the womb is like an animal within an animal'.[8]

The concept of a wandering womb was strengthened in ancient times by the fact that the internal physiology of women was pictured as a tube, in which the womb was free to move from its normal position '… blocking passages, obstructing breathing and causing disease'.[9] The idea of the internal physiology of women as a tube is confirmed in Hippocrates' *Aphorisms*, where he implies a connection between orifices on both ends of a woman. For instance, in order to ascertain whether a woman is capable of conception she should be fumigated from below and '...if the odour, pervading the body, be perceptible at the nose and mouth, it is an evidence that her non-conception proceeds from no impotence on her part'.[10] In other words, if there were no blockages present to impede normal conception, odours would pass through a female's body from one end to the other unimpeded.

In the *Hippocratic Corpus* as well as in *Timaeus*, descriptions of the wandering womb phenomenon allude to symptoms of 'madness and illness'[11] caused by this condition. Unfortunately, the ancient idea that the female gender was more prone to irrationality, and specific behaviours, linked to their reproductive organs persisted through the centuries. Eventually the concept of a pathological, wandering womb, gave rise to the term 'hysteria' derived from the Greek word for 'uterus'.[12]

Contrary to firmly held perceptions of the past,[13] the diagnosis of hysteria was not made by the ancient authors of the Hippocratic texts, but by a nineteenth-century translator of the *Hippocratic Corpus*. The misleading notion that hysteria is described and given its name in the *Hippocratic Corpus* is due to an error in translation and can be traced back to Émile Littré (1801-1881), who published the first volume of his French translation of the *Hippocratic Corpus* in 1839. 'Littré read the Hippocratic Corpus in the context of the mid-nineteenth century, in which hysteria was a recognized condition of debated aetiology; he expected to find hysteria in the text, duly found it, and drew it out in the headings [...] for the various sections'.[14] The diagnosis 'hysteria' was never utilised in the ancient texts. Instead, the word *hysterikos*, 'hysteric' is used, but with the explicit denotation as 'coming from the womb' or 'suffering due to the womb'.[15] In other words, the Greek *hysterikos*, 'from the womb', is solely a physical description of cause, denoting the body part from which other symptom originate.

What caused the womb to 'wander'

Hippocratic texts advocated that movement of the womb was initiated by menstrual suppression, a deficient diet, physical exhaustion, sexual abstinence, as well as dryness or lightness of the womb. Hence, suggested curative treatments were marriage i.e. intercourse, pregnancy, aromatic therapy, irritant pessaries, and different herbal mixtures administered by mouth, through the nose, or into the vulva. Intercourse and pregnancy, due to their beneficial physical effects formed part of advised treatment protocol in the ancient texts. Not only did intercourse moisten the womb, hence discouraging it from relocating elsewhere in the body to seek moisture, but intercourse also roused the body, hence aiding the passage of blood within it. Regarding pregnancy and childbirth, it was held that these conditions broke down the flesh throughout the body, hence creating extra space to harbour excess blood.

Regular menstrual bleeding, outside of pregnancy and before menopause, was regarded as essential to female health and was seen as central to Hippocratic gynaecology. This viewpoint was closely connected to the perceived qualities of female flesh: generally woman's flesh was considered to be of softer and of looser texture than that of a man. This notion was especially applicable to women who had already given birth, a process thought to 'open' internal channels, thereby facilitating menstruation. As women were 'loose-textured', they naturally retained moisture, and also absorbed more fluid from the digestive process. Thus Hippocratic texts describe women as 'wetter' than men. Women therefore needed regular menstruation to purge them of excess fluid-build-up.

Childless women, those who had not given birth, and those who abstained from the moistening activity of sexual intercourse, were thought to have firmer, denser flesh; hence fewer spaces in the body where moisture could be stored. In this case the womb would be deprived of sufficient moisture, causing the dry, light womb to move upwards in search of moisture and 'throw itself'[16] on the liver, because this organ was perceived as being saturated with moisture. Such movement of the womb would interrupt the breathing process through a woman's belly, cause symptoms of suffocation, and '…the whites of the eyes are turned up, the woman is cold, and her complexion is livid; she grinds her teeth and has excess saliva'.[17] Soranus and Aretaeus of Cappadocia, gynaecological writers of antiquity, named this condition not 'hysteria' – the word hysteria was not used in this period – but *hysterike pnix* or 'suffocation caused by the womb'.[18]

A 'wandering' womb was thought to be attracted back to its usual location by sweet and rank odours, introduced into the vulva or the nose. Aretaeus of Cappadocia stated that the womb '...delights also in fragrant smells and advances towards them; and it has an aversion to fetid smells and flees from them'.[19] Pungently sweet smelling fumigations and vaginal suppositories were applied 'below', to attract the womb downwards: 'The sick were made to sit astride the smouldering herbs, so that the smoke rose into the vagina'.[20] Similarly, to drive the womb away from the upper parts of the body, foul, putrid smelling substances were administered to the nostrils. The ingredients to be inhaled were diverse and unappealing in nature: '...cow dung, dried cypress, goat horn, gall and frankincense. A speciality was oisype, soiled goat wool from the anal tract'.[21] In addition the woman was advised to ingest various disgusting and repulsive ingredients also thought to force the womb 'southwards', away from the lungs and heart.

Galen refuted the idea that the womb really could move, but despite the fact that Galen was *the* Greco-Roman medical writer with the most powerful overall influence on medieval and Renaissance medicine in Europe, the idea of the 'wandering womb' continued amongst physicians for centuries. Galen held that the womb was stationary, rather suggesting that abnormal sexual functioning led to hysterical suffocation of the womb. He maintained that when the womb was disfunctional, either because of retention of menses or non-release of semen, such failure poisoned the body. The resumption of normal sexual function was seen as a difinitive cure for this malady.

The perception of uterine suffocation caused by 'emptiness' due to a lack of intercourse and failure to fall pregnant served as the most striking evidence that women suffered from a specific set of illnesses of their own and that their health was reliant on their reproductive functions.[22] According to Aristotle's and Galen's ideas on woman, the female '...is characterized by deprived, passive and material traits, cold and moist dominant humors and a desire for completion by intercourse with the male'[23] – a perception '...by which the imperfect should desire the perfect'.[24] Such notions of male superiority were firmly integrated into Christian thought centuries later.

'Woman is the gate of the devil'

In early Christian times the Church strengthened existing dissenting attitudes towards women, but with the added connotation of sinfulness and deviousness with regard to women. With regard to female sexuality, varying messages were extant: women were expected to be 'fruitful', but doctrine also decreed that the distress, pain and danger of childbirth were allotted to women, due to an Edenic myth, laying the culpability for humankind's immutable sin on Eve. In addition, women were expected to reproduce abundantly, especially male heirs, yet also remain chaste.

Key archetypes of womanhood, set by the Church, were the virtuous, immaculate Virgin, the prostitute and the witch.[25] Ignorance regarding women's physiology was fuelled by a dichotomous attitude towards the assumed weakness of their sex – women were necessary instruments for procreation, but at the same time an aura of mystery surrounded them. In the fourth century St Augustine unequivocally declared that the only reason for sexual intercourse was procreation. But, the Church also propagated that women were to be feared as child-bearers. Since they were traditionally viewed as deceptive, no man could be absolutely sure that the children he was raising were his own – an anxiety which stemmed from men's dependency on women for the line's survival.[26]

Furthermore, it was thought that chaos would ensue if women were to have the fear of childbirth removed from them. Hence, it was deemed essential that they view sex with the utmost apprehension – a joyless act, nothing but a marital duty, which invariably led to suffering and even death in childbirth. In the sixteenth century Martin Luther bluntly expressed the views popularly held at the time: 'If women die in childbirth that does no harm. It is what they were made for'.[27]

The church father Tertullian (c.160-235), although himself married, condemned sexuality as illicit and referred to women as 'gateways to the Devil'.[28] St. Jerome (c. 340-420 CE), who could probably be aptly described as the 'patron saint of misogynists',[29] speculated whether women were in fact entirely human. He summed up the existing mindset by declaring that '…women's love in general is accused of ever being insatiable; put it out and it bursts into flame; give it plenty, it is again in need; it enervates a man's mind and engrosses all thought except for the passion which it feeds'.[30] But, his most damaging declaration for all women and for centuries to come, pronounced that '…woman is the gate of the devil, the path of wickedness, the sting of the serpent, in a word, a perilous object'.[31]

The elements of misogyny were further strengthened when St. Augustine (354-386 CE) declared that women were morally and mentally inferior to men, while Thomas Aquinas (1225-1274) regarded women as a temptation into evil. The feminine role was not blessed but cursed. Sex was to be endured, not enjoyed, while menstruation, pregnancy and childbirth were seen as shameful states – because they were not physiologically understood.

An indication of how ancient medical notions were mingled with religious beliefs is a Christian medieval formula to exorcise the 'wandering womb'. In it, the priest directly commanded the womb to desist in tormenting the suffering woman: 'I conjure you, womb, by our Lord Jesus Christ…not to harm this maid-servant of God…nor to hold onto her head, neck, throat, chest, ears, teeth, eyes, nostrils, shoulders, arms, hands, heart, stomach, heart, liver, spleen…but to quietly remain in the place which God delegated to you, so that this hand-maiden of God…might be cured'.[32]

The green sickness 'peculiar to virgins'

Apart from the 'wandering womb', another condition firmly linked to female physiology was known as the 'green sickness'.[33] Although this condition was already described before 1554 as a digestive disorder affecting all ages and both sexes, German physician Johannes Lange (1485-1565) allotted the English green sickness as 'peculiar to virgins' and transformed it '…to a condition found only in young women'.[34] He determined that *morbus virgineus* was caused not by digestive blockages, but specifically because virginity blocked the normal flow of blood through the body.

Decades later, Jean Varandal, professor of the faculty of Montpellier, in 1620, coined the term 'chlorosis', from the Greek word *chloris*, meaning 'pale green' or 'pallid', and established the term into pathology. After the introduction of this new description, diagnosis of the green sickness was increasingly based on colour: the pale or green-yellow tinged skin colour of sufferers, pale colour of the urine and faeces, as well as body parts which would suddenly become 'blanched', remaining thus for several hours. *Aristotle's Masterpiece*, published in 1684 states that '… the greene-sickness is so common a distemper in virgins, […] showing itself by discolouring the face, making it look green, pale and of a dusty colour, proceeding from raw and indigested humors […] arising from several inward causes'.[35]

As late as 1887, in an article published in the *Lancet*, by Sir Andrew Clake, titled *Anaemia or Chlorosis of Girls, Occurring More Commonly between the advent of Menstruation and the Consummation of Womanhood,* the condition was still firmly linked to female reproductive organs.[1], [2] The 'green sickness' gripped the imagination of the European medical establishment with lightening speed – proof that Hippocartic/Galenic medical tradition and associated attitudes about women amongst medical practitioners and the general populace, were still very much in evidence.

Suffocation of the womb

By the beginning of the seventeenth century, various medical conditions linked to a woman's womb, were still firmly embedded in medical literature. Physician Edward Jorden (1569-1633), learned member of the Royal College of Physicians, noted that '…the passive condition of womankind is subject unto more diseases and of other sorts and natures than men are' and held the 'suffocation of the womb' as chiefly responsible for all female ailments.[3] Suffocation of the womb was thought to cause symptoms of choking, a suffocating sensation, insensitivity of the skin, seizures, convulsions, contractions, eating disorders and mood swings.

Unfortunately, all of these could easily be interpreted as stemming from demonic possession, bewitchment and being in league with the Devil. These were times when some of the most notorious witch trials, exorcisms, and executions were still taking place across Europe – witch-trials only started declining in most parts of Europe after 1680. Who knows, how many innocents were thus convicted during the witch craze, which engulfed most of Europe from the thirteenth to the late seventeenth century – estimates given by modern scholars run into tens of thousands.[4] Several historians have in fact linked the condition of hysteria to witchcraft. In the early eighteenth century French philosopher Pierre Bayle (1647-1706) thought it '...very possible for a woman to persuade herself that someone has put the Devil into her body', resulting in the belief that she was possessed, hence producing symptoms of screaming and convulsing.[5]

In his treatise *A Briefe Discourse of a Disease Called the Suffocation of the Mother,* written in 1603, Jorden aimed to demonstrate that symptoms previously attributed to the Devil, were in fact caused by 'suffocation of the womb'. Jorden's treatise deals with an incident involving an accusation of possession: fourteen-year-old Mary Glover, suffered from recurring fits thought to be explicit proof of possession. Suspicion immediately fell on a family acquaintance, Elisabeth Jackson, who was subsequently tried and condemned to prison and pillory for bewitching her – had her trial been held one year later in 1604, she would have been sentenced to death. Jordan maintained that Mary Glover's symptoms were due to natural causes, specific to women [6] and supported his position in court with his treatise *A Briefe Discourse of a Disease Called the Suffocation of the Mother.*[7] Elisabeth Jackson appears to have been released.[8]

Henceforth 'suffocation of the womb' or 'suffocation of the Mother', as this condition was known in England, became widely accepted amongst orthodox physicians. The Mother, meaning literally the 'womb', was thought to rise or swell in the body, thus disturbing the function of other organs.[9]

In her book *The Midwives Book: or the Whole Art of Midwifery Discovered*, published in 1671, Jane Sharp mentions 'fits of the Mother' caused when 'monthly courses' were interrupted or when 'the Seed' of the woman was corrupted.[10] Furthermore, she reiterates the Hippocratic belief already held two thousand years earlier, when she speculates that it was '...strange that the womb should discern between sweet and stinking scents and to be so diversly affected with these smels'.[11] Although she reasons that a sense of smell belonged only to the nose she states that '…Sweet scents are pleasing to all womens wombs, and ill savours offend, but not in all women alike'.[12] As to why the womb 'chuseth sweet smels' and refuses the contrary, she admits that 'I know not why it is so'.[13]

Aristotle's Masterpiece, probably the most widely reprinted book on a medical subject in the seventeenth and eighteenth centuries, states that suffocation of the Mother was due to 'a retraction of womb towards the midriff and the stomach' thereby impeding respiration.[14] The manual advocates that suppression of the menses or the seed could be cured ' by a good husband',[15] in other words intercourse. Decades later, the varying symptoms produced by 'suffocation of the Mother', were regrouped under the term 'hysteria'.

Theories of female imperfection continued

In the seventeenth century attitudes towards women had not changed much. Women were still fundamentally seen as walking wombs – slaves to their biology. Theories of female imperfection continued to be widely accepted, not only by the general populace but also in medical circles. In his work *De usu partium corporis*, published in 1625, physician Kaspar Hoffman (1574-1648), comments that women being colder than men took longer to form *in utero*, had smaller veins and arteries, reached puberty earlier, aged faster than men, and above all lacked moral strength, honesty and courage.[16]

Another ancient notion which still remained in the seventeenth century was that the inadequacies of women already began in the womb. Published in 1684, the marriage and midwifery guide *Aristotle's Masterpiece* – written by an unknown author claiming to be Aristotle – succinctly stated that not only was gestation considered far longer for females, but it also took more time for a girl to fully form and start moving in the womb.[17] Prominent English physicians argued that ten, sometimes eleven months were needed for the completion of a daughter, on the ancient grounds that females were weaker even in the womb.[18], [19] At the beginning of the seventeenth century, physician Edward Jorden noted that '…the passive condition of womankind is subject unto more diseases and of other sorts and natures than men are'.[20] He held 'suffocation of the womb' as chiefly responsible for all female ailments.

Hysteria and the 'vapours'

William Harvey described the uterus as '…insatiable, ferocious, animal-like', and drew parallels between 'bitches in heat and hysterical women'.[21] Furthermore, he queried: 'How many incurable diseases, are brought about by unhealthy menstrual discharges?',[22] a question echoed by most medical practitioners at the time. The effects of hysteria in women were thought to cause garrulity and an excessive desire for coitus, which was being called *furor uterinus*, a clinically entrenched term amongst doctors.[23] This so-called 'furore of the uterus', embodying women's gross carnal appetites was thought to govern the entire sex, determining their words and deeds.

Renowned seventeenth century English physician Thomas Sydenham, was the first to assert that hysteria afflicted both men and women, regarding hysteria as a function of civilization – the wealthier and influential the person, the more likely he or she was to be affected. But in spite of such insights, Sydenham claimed that women were more subject to hysteria than men, because '…their anatomic nervous constitutions were weaker'.[24] With this notion, he firmly entrenched the concept of the weak, nervous, feminine constitution, a belief that was to play a determining role in 'European hysteria' for the next two hundred years.

To be hysterical became synonymous with being nervous. Fortunately, due to the partial de-sexualization and de-mystification of hysteria much of the shame associated with this condition, was shed and sufferers were perceived as the victims of a delicate nervous system, crumbling under demanding societal and work pressures.

During the nineteenth century hysteria became an almost fashionable condition frequently overlapping with general nervousness, nymphomania and insanity, although these conditions were still often adversely linked mainly to women. For most writers of the mid-nineteenth century, hysteria was '…rooted in the very nature of being female'[25] and towards the end of that century, in 1883 prominent politician Auguste Fabré (1820-1878) stated that '…all women are hysterical and . . . every woman carries with her the seeds of hysteria. Hysteria, before being an illness, is a temperament, and what constitutes the temperament of a woman is rudimentary hysteria'.[26]

Intriguingly, the condition seemed to change gender after the First World War when male 'hysterics' were identified as suffering from shell shock. In the twentieth century, views about an organic female biology that produced hysteria mutated into psychological representations and Viennese women who were treated by Sigmund Freud (1856-1939) for hysteria, in a sense initiated the 'talking cure', or psychoanalytic treatment method.

Ideas and notions of diseases change throughout history. Modern medical professionals have substituted the condition of 'hysteria' with the more specifically defined diagnostic categories of 'conversion disorder' and 'somatisation'. In modern times, hysteria is defined as the 'physical expression of a mental conflict', a state describing uncontrollable emotional excesses, which may be experienced by any person regardless of age or gender.[27] In conclusion it may be said that the demise of hysteria, as it were, and its association with female biology, has come about, not through medical enterprise, but through cultural and social changes, which have brought about greater understanding, knowledge and insights.

WOMEN'S WOES – FERTILITY, CONCEPTION AND MENSTRUATION

From ancient times until the late eighteenth century the internal workings of women's sexual organs were governed by numerous misconceptions, firmly held by the orthodox medical establishment and the general populace. The following chapter aims to highlight some of the fallacies and notions once associated with fertility, conception, and menstruation.

The multi-chambered womb

Early medieval anatomical drawings depicted the womb as a mysterious organ with seven chambers – the three chambers on the right were thought to bring forth boys, the three on the left to produce girls, while the chamber in the middle was held to create hermaphrodites '...a monster, halfe a man, and halfe a woman'.[1] It was thought that, as the right side of the womb was associated with warmth due to its proximity to the liver, it tended to form male children while the left, associated with coolness from the spleen brought forth female offspring. This particular notion of right and left used in a positive and negative association, dates back thousands of years and is part of a tradition found worldwide of associating male gender with the right side and female gender with the left.[1] The differentiation of male and female into the opposites right and left originated with Pythagoros (570-495 BCE) and was written down in his *Table of Opposites*. This valuation gave clear preference '…to the right over the left and therefore included a sex-polarity framework in its foundation'.[2]

First century Roman scholar and naturalist, Pliny the Elder, confirmed this belief, stating that boys are usually carried on the right side and girls on the left.[3] In addition, such differentiation once not only applied to the womb, but also to the ejaculated seed. In the first century CE Plutarch recorded '…that when ejaculation from the right testes falls into the right side of the womb, males are formed'.[4] Similarly, females were formed through ejaculation from the left testes falling to the left side of the womb.

While twelfth century anatomists in Salerno still incorporated the notion of the seven-chambered womb into their general anatomical tracts, the idea was only slightly modified much later, when physicians argued for the theory of five rather than seven chambers. This was owing to the firm belief that a woman could not possibly give birth to more than quintuplets.[5] However, although not accepted by the majority of physicians, the notion of a multi-chambered womb nevertheless persisted in medical circles throughout medieval times and beyond.

During the sixteenth century Elizabethan astrologer, occultist and practicing physician Simon Forman,[6] as well as many others, still acknowledged the seven-celled womb or 'matrix'.[7] Similarly, at the end of that century, Thomas Vicary, chief 'chirurgion' to King Henry VIII, and other royals such as Edward VI, Queen Mary and Queen Elizabeth I, made numerous references to 'womens chambers'[8] in his comprehensive medical treatise *The English Man's Treasure*. Many university-educated medical practitioners during this century however disdained the idea of a multiplicity of uterine chambers. In *The Byrth of Mankynde* (1545), physician Thomas Raynalde stated this belief to be '…but lies, dreams and foolish fantasies' and goes on to say that '…the woman's matrix [9] is […] as strong as a bladder, having in it but *one* universal hollowness'.[10] *The Byrth of Mankynde,* was an immensely popular book, between 1545 and 1655, offering invaluable information on pregnancy, birth and other women's 'issues' to physicians and midwives alike.

Female seed – retained or released

From ancient times, and for many centuries to come, the question of human conception was dominated by mistaken beliefs and confusion. Hippocrates and Galen described human conception as taking place from two 'seeds', male and female,[11] although they differed on the relative importance of each of these. According to Galen, female reproductive organs were an inverted, imperfect version of male generative organs – hence they were seen as homologous anatomical structures. Female generative organs projected inwards instead of outwards, with the uterus corresponding to the male scrotum and the neck of the uterus to the penis.[12] For Galen, female seed stored in the womb in no way elevated women to an equal position with males, since female seed was regarded as naturally inferior.[13] Only the male body was thought capable of producing the '…procreative spirit […] that is distributed as sperm […] to the woman's womb'.[14]

Galen propagated that it was crucial for the woman to 'ejaculate' her seed for conception to be successful, and the only way to 'release' female seed was through the female orgasm, which was therefore considered essential. In fact, female seed was believed to turn venomous if not discharged through regular intercourse.[15] Retained seed would decay, leading to anatomical and humoral imbalance affecting the rest of the female body. Galen compared the effects of retained seed to the bites of venomous creatures, causing dramatic if not fatal symptoms.[16]

Galen's teachings, that orgasm was necessary in order to conceive, was to have long-lasting consequences in a social context. The contention was that if a woman was brutally raped, deriving no physical pleasure from this experience, she should and would not conceive. Although there were specific statutes in medieval and later times, declaring rape a crime, if a woman fell pregnant as a result of rape, she was automatically deemed to have physically enjoyed the incident – therefore technically no rape had taken place.[17]

The belief that 'retained' or 'corrupted' female 'seed' would cause 'fits of the Mother',[18] and other conditions of the womb, lingered for centuries and is still mentioned in Jane Sharp's *Midwives Book*, of 1671. As in ancient times, the advocated cure was intercourse, or as Jane Sharp put it more aptly, a 'good husband'.[19] In other words, motherhood was regarded as a socially mandated approach for women to preserve their health and wellbeing. Those women who remained unmarried, straying from the feminine norm, '…were considered more susceptible to illness, both mental and physical',[20] which is why prevailing medical theories of the time regarded reproduction as a matter of essential importance to women's overall health.

During the Middle Ages physicians questioned the physical derivation of 'seed' or semen, in men and women. The medieval mind, working by association, linked the whiteness of semen to the whiteness of the brain, with the spinal cord providing a physiological link between the two. In regard to determining the sex of a foetus, Galen's notion that heat was vital in this process, was still firmly held more than one and a half thousand years later. In the late seventeenth century, the marriage and midwifery guide, *Aristotle's Masterpiece*[21] advised that after coitus '…let the woman repose herself on her right side […] that by sleeping in that posture […] on the right side of the matrix, may prove the place of conception: for *therein is the greatest generative heat*, which is the chief procuring cause of male children'.[22] Predictably, as stipulated at the beginning of this chapter, the recommendation continues '…for a female child, let the woman lie on her left side'.[23]

Female testicles containing diverse eggs

Female ovaries, as yet not 'decoded', were still described as 'testicles' in the sixteenth, seventeenth and eighteenth centuries, and even beyond. Intriguingly, *Aristotle's Masterpiece* (1684), described what came close to the female ovary: '…testicles, so called in women, afford not any seed, but are two eggs, like those of fowls and other creatures neither have they any office as those of men, but are indeed the ovaria, wherein the eggs are nourished […] the truth of this is plain, for if you boil them, their liquor will be the same colour, taste, and consistency, with the taste of birds eggs'.[24] The text also describes the 'testicles' of women as containing 'diverse eggs'.[25] But, whether female 'testicles' generated any 'creative' material corresponding to that of the male remained a matter of controversy. The widely accepted theory was that male seed was the source of fertility in the womb, while female eggs merely provided the raw material for the sperm's development.[26]

Therefore, a particular discovery by William Harvey during the seventeenth century was astounding and at odds with contemporary views. One of King Charles I's closest courtiers and appointed as one of his doctors in 1639, renowned William Harvey had been permitted to pick specimens of deer during rutting time '…when the Females are lusty and admit the Males'[27] in order to dissect their genital parts. He ascertained that during the early stages of pregnancy the womb of impregnated does did not contain any traces of the stags' 'seed' or semen – a confounding discovery. Therefore, if no male semen was present, how could the does have become pregnant?

The king and his medical team were sceptical of Harvey's findings. Harvey himself was baffled and unable to clarify his results. In fact, he remained undecided about the role of the male seed and female egg for the rest of his life. In his book *De Generatione Animalium* (1651), in which he published his findings on the king's deer, Harvey reflected whether the process of fertilisation might in fact be something lying dormant in the body for some time, before producing its symptoms.[28] Although the Greek physician Herophilus (335-280 BCE) had already discovered the ovaries in the third century BCE,[29] their function was not understood until the twentieth century.

Menstrual blood – the 'curse' or the 'flowers'

Similar to the perceptions of fertility and conception, attitudes to menstruation and menstrual blood were equally diverse and ambiguous. In the past, the menstrual process was enveloped in a cloud of mystery and the regular, monthly discharge of blood from a perfectly healthy woman's womb was universally regarded by most cultures as an act of pollution. Revulsion and the stigma of uncleanness were once the characteristic reactions not only to menstrual flow, but also to pregnancy and childbirth.

Although Galen described menstruation as a 'benign excrement' [30] regulating the female body and providing raw material to form and nourish the foetus, the popularly held notion of impurity in regard to menstruation persisted for centuries. It is important however to stress, that no fixed, mainstream belief about menstruation and menstrual blood, was extant within European society, but consisted of a range of beliefs instead.

During the first century CE, Pliny the Elder [31] implicitly warned that the touch of a menstruating woman would blight crops, kill seedlings, rust iron, turn wine to vinegar, dim mirrors, blunt razors, kill bees, and generally cause misfortune in all ventures.[32] Similar extreme views were championed by Archbishop Isidore of Seville [33] during the sixth century, and were also contained in later medieval works such as the *De secreta mulierum*, or Women's Secrets. This book, essentially about reproduction, depicted women as lascivious and evil, and remained popular even during the Elizabethan period.

Extreme attitudes of contaminating menstrual flow were strengthened by the teachings of the Church – teachings which were no doubt based on the Biblical Old Testament declaration of Leviticus, stating '…if a woman have an issue of her blood … she shall be unclean' and '…if any man lie with her at all, and her flowers be upon him, he shall be unclean'.[34] During the seventh century, Archbishop Theodore's *Penitential* [35] forbade women to enter a church or receive communion during their monthly 'courses'. The same ruling applied to pregnant women until forty days after childbirth. The Christian practice of 'churching' therefore had the purpose of purification, as well as reintegrating the new mother into the religious community.[36]

Amongst the general populace, menstruation and the pains of childbirth were generally seen as a 'curse' on womankind – the majority of women were sinners who deserved their lot. Why else did menstruation not seem to occur in pious, reclusive and ascetic 'holy' women? This was perceived as an undeniable sign from God attesting to the saintliness of nuns as opposed to the worldliness of other women – although in all probability the exceptionally meagre diets of such devout and virtuous women were to blame. Lacking the appropriate nourishment, their bodies were no longer able to sustain the reproductive process, which is why their menses stopped. To further strengthen the notion of the saintliness of cloistered women, numerous wealthy medieval women turned to a secluded, cloistered religious life of contemplation in their later years, hence they may have been post-menopausal, thus accounting for their lack of menses.

During the Middle Ages menstruation was still firmly associated with pollution, as well as with certain harmful physical effects. It was for instance believed that menstrual blood in many cases involved the transmission of diseases such as leprosy and smallpox.[37] Sixteenth century physician and astrologer, Simon Forman stated that lepers could in fact be begotten, if conceived '…by a woman when she had her course'.[38] Such perceived malignancy of menses chronicled by ancient medical texts was unfortunately reproduced in the attitudes of some Renaissance writers.[39] However, most physicians – Thomas Raynalde for instance – declared such ideas as '…lies, dreams and plain dotage',[40] and by the end of the sixteenth century, the majority of medical texts represented menstruation as a 'harmless excrement',[41] which is exactly as Galen had described it one and a half thousand years earlier.

The ambivalent notions and beliefs about menstruation and menstrual blood are clearly reflected in the variety of expressions used to refer to this condition.[42] In England, as in other European countries, menstruation was known by several names and euphemisms. For example, it was known as Latin *menstrua*, because '…once a month they happen always to womankind after 14 or 15 years of age passed'[43] or, in English as women's '…terms because they return likewise at certain seasons, times and terms'.[44] If however, the monthly flow endangered a woman's health through excessive loss of blood, it was termed 'woman's sickness'.[45] When menstruation was described as the means to achieving pregnancy, it was known as the 'flowers'[46] or generally as 'women's courses'.

Menstruation was of crucial concern to ancient, medieval and Renaissance physicians, as it indicated fertility and was considered vital to a woman's health. The regular purging or discarding of superfluous blood rid the female body of ill humors, hence resulting in a cooling of the heightened emotions regarded as specific to women. Galen had in fact stated that women did not suffer lethargy, spasms and melancholy, *because* of the cleansing action of their menses[47] – a process of natural phlebotomy not available to men. Therefore an absence of menstruation was considered dangerous, especially for young, otherwise healthy women. 'Tudor physicians viewed abnormal stoppage of menstruation as very serious, leading to […] fevers, obstructions, evil habits, loathing, dropsy, heart-ache, cough, short breathing, fainting, sore eyes, madness, and the like'.[48]

Hence, concern for regular menstruation led physicians to advise and implement a number of remedies to bring 'down the courses': sexual intercourse, as well as hot baths, pessaries and fumigations; mixtures of ground metal to be taken orally. More drastic measures were bloodletting, cupping, scarification of the breasts or venesection of a woman's thighs,[49] as bleeding from a vein or any other part of the body was considered the same as menstrual bleeding – a means of removing the dangerous excess.[50]

Menstrual blood – nutrition for the foetus

In the context of becoming pregnant, menstrual blood was seen as favourable and helpful. Galen's notion of the role of menstrual blood in conception, wherein menstrual blood provided nutrition to the foetus, was still widely accepted during the seventeenth century. In 1603, physician Edward Jorden, learned member of the Royal College of Physicians, noted that '…blood is that humor wherewith we are nourished: without which the infant in the mothers wombe could neither grow and increase … and therefore it was necessarie that those that were fit for generation, should be supplied with sufficient store of this humor'.[51] Several decades later physician Thomas Raynalde similarly stated that without menstrual blood, the conceived seed '…cannot thrive, but wastes away and issueth forth again for lack of nutriment',[52] in other word conception could not take place, without proper nourishment for the foetus.

As much as menstrual blood was thought to supply sustenance for the formation of the foetus, so university-educated physicians viewed breast milk as converted menstrual blood. In other words, once conception had taken place during pregnancy, menstrual blood would be redirected to the mother's breasts and converted to a new form of sustenance for the infant in the form of milk. For centuries, both female semen and breast milk were thought to derive from blood, which had undergone a series of purifications during which they lost their colour.[53]

During the sixteenth century, anatomist Vesalius described at length the suppression of menstrual flow during pregnancy as due to the diversion of this blood via the intricate connections of various blood vessels and ducts to the breasts, which therefore became enlarged and converted the menstrual blood into milk.[54] Most Elizabethans seem to have agreed that menstrual blood originated from the vena cava and that breast milk was '…engendered of the Terms'.[55]

The notion that the body converted menstrual blood into breast milk is also discussed at length in *The Byrth of Mankynde*, a popular work during the sixteenth and seventeenth century.[56] Similarly, this idea is reiterated in the late seventeenth century by Jane Sharp in her manual *The Midwives Book*,[57] which was well received and consulted by doctors as well as midwives at the time. In discussing menstruation, she states that '…after the birth, this blood comes not hither but goes to the Breasts to make Milk; but at all other times it is cast out monethly what is superfluous […]. It is not only blood is voided by the Terms, but multitude of humors and excrements'.[58]

It is interesting to note, that it was not until 1831 that French physician Charles Négrier (1792-1862) suggested that menstruation controlled ovulation. In 1877 the notion that menstruation was dependant on ovulation was challenged by Mary Putnam Jacobi (1842-1906), the first female member of the American Academy of Medicine, in her book *The question of rest for women during menstruation*,[59] and the realisation that woman menstruated because they had failed to conceive took hold some years later. However, it was only in 1901 that the endocrine cause of menstruation was demonstrated by Joseph Halban, while our modern understanding of the connection between ovulation and menstruation was eventually attained in the 1930's.[60]

WOMEN'S WOES CONTINUE –
CHILDBIRTH AND 'WITH-WOMEN'

From ancient times, throughout the medieval era and for centuries to come, a woman's greatest fear was childbirth – and with good reason, as those who survived this ordeal would live to 'bear a child every year for ten to fifteen years'.[1] It was therefore no wonder that women were thought of as weak, since they were either continually pregnant, or else recovering from childbirth, or dying during the process.

The following chapter highlights the complexities of childbirth, a formerly exclusively female concern; it also places special emphasis on the once crucial role of the midwife or 'with-woman', and the many, often grossly mistaken, beliefs surrounding her person and vocation. It should be emphasised at the outset that until the time of science-based male-dominated obstetrics[2] – although it was not known as obstetrics at the time – in the early seventeenth century, childbirth was not considered a category of medicine.[3] Rather, the birthing process formed a part of everyday life – hence, it fell entirely into the sphere of female experience. Hidden in a woman's lower extremities childbirth was regarded as taboo or too unseemly to be dealt with by male practitioners – an attitude which prevailed for centuries.

The power of imagination

As indicated in the previous chapter, the internal workings of women's 'private' organs were once governed by numerous misconceptions, resolutely held by the medical establishment and the general populace until the late eighteenth century. Diverse beliefs and notions not only applied to fertility, conception and menstruation, but also to pregnancy and childbirth.

For example, during medieval times and centuries later, doctors especially stressed the power of the mind exerted on the uterus and the growing child therein. The power of imagination was in fact once held entirely responsible for phenomena, which were later to be explained in terms of genetics, embryology and other scientific disciplines. It was firmly believed that conjuring up the 'wrong' mental images could result in deformities, stillbirths and birthmarks[4] – one can only imagine the tremendous psychological burden this must have placed on expectant mothers.

A comprehensive denunciation of the 'power of imagination' notion only occurred in 1727 with the publication of *The strength of imagination in pregnant women examined*, by physician James Augustus Blondel, a member of the Royal College of Physicians. The book prompted controversy and debate for decades, with many medical practitioners continuing to adhere to the theory that the expectant mother's mental imaginings affected the shape and form of the foetus.

Misconceptions about the foetus

Another misconception held for centuries concerned nourishment of the foetus. As late as the seventeenth century, physicians, including the eminent William Harvey, still subscribed to the idea that the foetus ingested sustenance from surrounding amniotic fluid through the mouth, whilst much thinner fluids were thought to travel through the umbilical chord. In fact, Harvey seemed unusually perplexed by the function of the navel, pronouncing in one of his lectures to the College of Physicians in the 1630's that 'women experienced sexual pleasure through the umbilicus'.[5] This unusual notion – even for those times – was however refuted by renowned seventeenth century herbalist and medical reformer Nicolas Culpeper, who named the source of female pleasure as the clitoris: 'In form it represents the yard of a man and suffers erection and falling in that doth; this is that which gives lust in women and gives delight in copulation'.[6]

Varying ideas were also extant with regard to how the unborn child was clasped within the womb. During the sixteenth century, the ancient notion that the foetus was held in position through the presence of suckers persisted. Therefore the birth process was thought to depend on the efforts of the child to 'break free' from the womb, aided by lubrication of the amniotic waters. A century later it was still generally unknown, even by distinguished physicians,[7] that contractions of the womb provided the thrust for birthing. Because it was thought that the unborn child could literally be 'stuck to the spine',[8] and that the foetus needed assistance in 'fighting' its way into the world, such misconceptions once resulted in much tugging and violent pulling by those assisting in the birthing process.

Gossips in the birthing chamber

In medieval times the event of childbirth was experienced and witnessed exclusively by women. The birthing or lying-in chamber was a closed female space for up to a month – a space from which men were categorically barred. This was an area where women were brought together, where they discussed women's issues, and where they escaped marital authority. Because this area was closed to men, they in turn viewed the lying-in chamber with a mixture of superstition and fear.

Routinely, those present in the birthing chamber consisted of a midwife and six or seven other women. These attending women, specifically invited by the expectant mother to her 'birthing event', were known as 'gossips' – the old English word *godsibb* originally referring to 'godparent'.[9] Growing unease about such exclusively female gatherings in birthing chambers eventually resulted in the negative implication of the word 'gossip', linking it to unrestrained speech amongst women.

Apart from experienced females supporting and helping the mother-to-be in her hours of need, the gathering of women in birthing chambers also served another important purpose: there were numerous witnesses to the birth. Therefore, if the child died, these women could attest to the mother's innocence in not having caused its death – something that was not unknown to happen, especially if it was an illegitimate child.

Childbirth – 'the pains of Hell and snares of death'

In the past, pregnancy and childbirth were fraught with danger. An Anglican Prayer Book of 1662 alludes to the 'pains of Hell' and 'the snares of death' afflicting women at this time.[10] Infant mortality was at its highest during the first few days after birth – a time also when the mother could succumb to childbed fever. Therefore, a successful birth was an occasion for great celebration, commemorated by various sacraments and rites such as baptism and churching, as well as by specific ritual objects.[11]

Childbirth was always followed by a lengthy, obligatory lying-in period – which is why most women did not attend the baptism of their newborn child. Besides, women were only allowed to re-enter a church after their 'churching'[12] ceremonies. This observance took place forty days after the birth of a child. Motivated by the ancient, universal fear of pollution by uterine blood, as well as by the 'Christian notion of defilement by the gestation of an unconsecrated being',[13] the churching ceremony served the purpose of purification. Wearing a veil, her eyes demurely downcast, a lighted candle in one hand and the obligatory offering for the priest in the other, the new mother 'knelt before the church to be purified before she might re-enter it'.[14] Under Protestantism the ceremony was progressively altered over the centuries into one of Thanksgiving.

The role of the 'with-woman'

Throughout the childbearing process, as well as during the various Christian rituals that followed, one specific person featured prominently.

It was she, who delivered the child, she who often carried the infant to the baptismal font, and she, who together with the 'gossips', was present at the churching of the mother. This specific person, who featured so notably in the expectant and new mother's life, was none other than the midwife – hence also termed the 'with-woman'. The term midwife, is derived from Middle English *midwyf*, *mid* meaning 'with', and *wyf* meaning 'woman' – not necessarily 'married woman'. In other words the midwife was someone who was 'with' a woman during childbirth.[15]

Midwives have played an integral part in childbirth for millennia and several Old Testament Books mention these 'helpers' of women in their darkest hour. For example, the book of Exodus[16] states: 'God dealt well with the midwives: and the people multiplied, and waxed very mighty'.[17]

Midwives occupied an exclusive role with specific authority in European society. Until the fifteenth century, the official religion in Western Europe was Roman Catholicism. For centuries Church authorities actively controlled a wide range of human activities, especially sexual morality. Because of her close association with female illness, pregnancy and childbirth, the midwife' character, moral disposition, and religious orthodoxy were of crucial concern to ecclesiastic authorities. As a result, she filled several vital roles in law enforcement: since a woman's chastity – if not continual, then at least outside of marriage – was one of the Church's foremost tenets, and the midwife was explicitly forbidden 'to perform any act which might shield from discovery and punishment those falling short of this standard'.[18] Therefore she was expressly prohibited from aiding or assisting in miscarriage, or conspiring to conceal a birth resulting from an illicit relationship. She was also obliged to force the mother of a bastard child to name the father, so that he would not 'evade his duty to maintain his offspring, nor escape the punishment that could be inflicted for his offence in fathering it'.[19]

The midwife's further responsibilities included: examining women charged with procuring a miscarriage; scrutinising unmarried women claiming to have been raped; testing for virginity in prospective brides; asserting impotence in potential or actual husbands; and certifying infant deaths.[20] Midwives were also bidden by church authorities to ascertain pregnancy in those condemned to death who 'pleaded their belly'. The midwife's pronouncement of pregnancy would then either diminish punishment or at least suspend it until after the birth.[21]

The possibility of death during the birthing process, for both mother and child, was very real, and expectant mothers generally confessed their sins before going into labour. According to Christian doctrine, every child born was imbued with 'original sin'. This meant eternal damnation of the immortal soul, unless this sin was removed by baptism. Therefore, it was imperative that any infant thought likely to die should be baptised as soon as possible. Apart from being allowed to touch a woman's genitals, midwives were formally instructed by the Church in infant baptism – to ensure a child's place in heaven. The deliverance of an infant's soul was so crucial to the Church that a midwife was required to extract the infant by Caesarean section in the event of the mother's death. It is in fact well known that the Church 'always preferred saving the child to saving the mother'.[22, 23]

Stillborn children were a different matter altogether. According to Christian tenets, these children were seen as a 'powerful source of evil: unclaimed by baptism from original sin, they remained children of the devil and unfit for burial in consecrated ground'.[24] Midwives were required to bury these little infant bodies secretly and 'in such a manner that they should not be discovered by man nor beast'.[25] Midwives were also obliged to report the birth of deformed children, once believed to be the devil's offspring, to church authorities.

Witch-midwives

'Christianity was a male-centred, sex-negative religion with a strong misogynistic tendency. The very fact that it was male-centred and suspicious of sex would lead to a suspicious attitude towards women'[26] – and especially towards midwives. Prompted by the Papal Bull of 1484, the control of midwifery by urban authorities in Europe became more common from the fifteenth century onwards.[27] But, how did the Papal Bull affect the control of midwives? Spurred on by the Bull the most damning book on the subject of witchcraft, the *Malleus*

Maleficarum, written by Dominicans Heinrich Krämer (1470-1501) and Jacob Sprenger (1468-1494), appeared in Germany in 1486. Those faithful Christians who could read were now given formal authority to all the fables and phenomenal assertions allegedly collected about witches and their craft. In addition, the book especially singled out midwives, levelling various dreadful accusations against them.

An entire chapter in the *Malleus Maleficarum* was devoted to 'witch-midwives' committing the most appalling crimes, killing newborn infants and devouring them, 'murdering babies in the womb, roasting them at Sabbaths or offering them to the Devil'.[28] Unfortunately, midwives, deemed to have knowledge and control over sexuality and fertility – subjects which were veiled in mysterious secrecy – could easily be accused of sorcery, especially if anyone bore them a grudge. By the nature of their work they also had the greatest access to unbaptised children, which according to the *Malleus Maleficarum*, were used for nefarious purposes. These were wicked accusations indeed – by the nature of their profession, midwives were mandated by non other than the Church to discard all stillborn foetuses.

'In sorrow shalt thou bring forth'

In addition, the Church considered the very fact that midwives knew how to alleviate the pain of birthing a threat. Throughout medieval times and centuries beyond, the Biblical maxim prevailed 'in sorrow shalt thou bring forth children',[29] which was taken very seriously. During the sixteenth century, midwives could actually lose their life for administering analgesic potions during labour. In 1591, midwife Agnes Sampson was burned at the stake in Edinburgh for relieving the pains of childbirth.[30] In spite of the many damning accusations contained in the *Malleus Maleficarum*, there is however little concrete evidence of how many midwives were charged with witchcraft and subsequently executed.

In his *Observations in Midwifery* Percivall Willughby (1596-1685) states the accepted fact that 'it is decreed and pronounced' for women to bring forth children in sorrow. Hence, any pain relief was out of the question during the seventeenth century.[31] Even in 1853, when Queen Victoria (1819-1901) declared herself eager to try the analgesic effects of a new drug, chloroform, during the birth of her eighth child, Prince Leopold, the mindset regarding painful labour had not altered. The Queen encountered serious, publicly voiced reservations and objections, not only from parliamentarians, but especially from ecclesiastic authorities, regarding the use of pain relief in childbirth.[32]

Midwifery training and licensing

As mentioned in the opening paragraphs of this chapter, childbirth was not considered a category of medicine until the early seventeenth century. Rather, childbirth formed a part of everyday life and was strictly 'women's business'. Initially there was no formal training for midwives and no need for them to obtain a licence. Medieval European midwives were reliant on traditional knowledge from their mothers and grandmothers, as well as practical knowledge learned by experience and observation. It is likely that they were mature, married women, who had themselves borne children – 'indeed right up until the end of the seventeenth century, personal experience of childbirth was still generally regarded as an essential qualification'.[33]

Midwifery training and licensing became regulated in different European countries at different times. On the Continent, town authorities began to take an interest in the practices of midwives around the start of the fourteenth century and 'from this period on we find references to midwives in municipal account books', and ordinances, regarding their various duties and activities.[34] Significant progress in the field of midwifery was made during the sixteenth century – a field that had remained almost stagnant for one and a half thousand years. In Germany and the Netherlands, the practices of midwives were government controlled towards the end of the sixteenth century. Aspiring midwives in these and other European countries were mandated to undergo an apprenticeship with an experienced midwife for three years, and were then examined by physicians on their relevant medical knowledge, before being registered.

While midwives were subject to formal examinations in continental Europe during the sixteenth century, no such requirements existed in England, where throughout this century, licensing lay firmly in the hands of the Church[35] and was not accompanied by any stipulation for the midwife's training.[36] Authorities mainly feared that midwives could make use of sorcery and witchcraft in their profession. In order to be licensed, they therefore had to apply to the Bishop's Court, and solemnly swear a long and detailed oath regarding their craft. By the early seventeenth century however, an apprenticeship system for midwives was introduced in England.

Advances in midwifery

During the sixteenth century, several factors combined to significantly advance the field of midwifery. First, the publication of numerous midwifery guides. Notable amongst these was *Der Swangern Frauwen und Hebammen Rosegarten*,[37] published in 1513 by Eucharius Rösslin (died 1526), city physician for the German city of Frankfurt. The book was later translated into English by Thomas Reynalde and became known as the *Byrth of Mankynde*, published in 1545 – the book was so popular that it was still widely read in the eighteenth century. The *Byrth of Mankynde*, discussed not only childbirth and infant care but also sexuality and reproduction, and 'it is reasonable to assume that Thomas Raynalde's decision to include the new Vesalian drawings of the female sexual anatomy […] was a major factor in the book's commercial success'[38] – especially the depiction of female genitalia. Dozens of other important works of the same genre were published during the sixteenth and seventeenth century.[39]

Advances in midwifery were also made through the work of sixteenth century French surgeon Ambroise Paré, contributing to a greater medical understanding of the process of labour and the resulting progress in operative midwifery. In this respect, Paré is especially remembered for re-introducing the podalic version of delivery – the practice of turning the child in cases of mal-presentation and delivering it feet-first – which was already known to the ancients. As word of the involvement in childbirth of prominent men like Paré spread, it encouraged male attendance at childbirth.

Significant progress in the field of midwifery also came about through academic anatomical studies – to which midwives had no access. Hence, credit for improvement in the field was given to men, thereby further promoting their entry into this vocation. The development of male orientated obstetrics started in France and gradually spread throughout Europe. Consequently, in the mid-seventeenth century a new order of medical practitioners was recognised, known in the English language as the man-midwife [40] – basically a contradiction in terms.

An insight into traditional midwifery

Over the centuries traditional midwives would generally call in a surgeon when the manual removal of a dead foetus was not possible – surgeons were licensed to use instruments such as hooks, knives and crotchets. But with the advent of man-midwives, conventional midwives increasingly sought their help in cases of complications, or 'obstetrical disasters'. One such 'man-midwife' in the seventeenth century was Percivall Willughby.

In his book, *Observations in Midwifery*, written around 1670, Willughby meticulously recorded one hundred and fifty case histories of births he had attended. His records give a vivid insight into traditional midwifery practices, which were still extant during the seventeenth century – practices that had remained virtually unchanged for well over a thousand years. Often he was called in to 'clean' up, after grossly botched deliveries and he relates several cases in which the midwife was unable to deliver what was by then a dead child.

Not much is known about the competence and efficiency of traditional midwives over the centuries, and many were accused of being backward and indeed dangerous. Most midwives came from the lower classes and were uneducated. In fact, 'if midwives were literate, it seems to have been coincidental rather than a prerequisite of their work'.[41] Although there were many midwives who were careful, knowledgeable and sympathetic, many were not so inclined and were of the 'meanest sort' who, 'not knowing otherwise to live', had taken up midwifery 'for a shilling or two'.[42]

While their practices remained consistent over hundreds of years, midwives, as may be expected, varied in character and in competence: typically, upon arrival the midwife would check the woman's abdomen to see if the child had 'fallen down' and then carry out an internal examination, after applying fresh butter or other oils to her unwashed hands, to establish the amount of cervical dilatation. If labour was well under way she would encourage the mother to assume her favourite position: kneeling or crouching, or else sitting on the birthing stool that the midwife had brought with her.

Often, midwives dealt with the prolonged terrors of labour by kneading and pressing on the distended abdomen in order to expel the foetus. Midwives were often known to stretch the vulva and neck of the womb[43] in order to 'facilitate' delivery. Not only could this cause swelling and lacerations, but also the onset of deadly childbed fever. Willughby relates that there were those who 'through ignorance or impatience' would tear the woman's delicate membranes with their nails, or cut them with scissors'.[44] In addition, midwives were unable to stem haemorrhage or to resuscitate a baby, while eclampsia or fits were probably viewed as supernatural omens of impending death.

It was believed in ancient times, and through the centuries that the unborn child could be literally 'stuck to the spine'. In this context, Willughby comments that midwives were known to use much force and violence to bring forth the child they were to deliver, often pulling with such strength on the delicate limbs of babies, as to completely wrench them off,[45] thereby killing the child in the process. He relates several cases, attesting to the ignorance of various midwives: 'Anno 1648, I was desired by an eminent midwife, joined with two other midwives, to come to a labouring woman in much distress'.[46] Before he saw the woman the midwives told him that she could not be delivered because a 'great lump of flesh'[47] was blocking the passage. They repeatedly told him to cut the lump out. However, on examining the woman Willughby determined that the 'lump' was in fact the child's head. 'These midwives would not believe me, but told me several strange stories, to induce me to cut it forth'.[48] Several hours later, the woman was delivered of a dead child. Had Willughby done as the midwives entreated him, he would have caused great blood loss and would have cut away part of the womb together with the child's head. In spite of the many negative incidents described, it should perhaps be stated that Willughby was definitely not anti-midwife – two members of his family were highly respected midwives.

Male-midwifery – 'working blind'

The fact that there was initial reluctance to call in man-midwives was largely due to society's unwillingness or taboo, to let men deal with women's 'secret parts' – it was simply considered immodest and inappropriate for a man to be present at childbirth. Although physicians and man-midwives frequently attended women in labour by the late seventeenth and early eighteenth century, they had to work entirely by touch – it was called 'working blind'. For modesty sake they worked with their hands under the sheets, 'feeling' their way around, as they were not allowed to see the patient's perineal region.[49] Unsurprisingly, this practice could lead to serious mistakes.

Many women categorically refused attendance by a man, even if this meant death through birthing complications. There were in fact many cases where the appearance of physicians at a birth 'aroused the most dreadful apprehensions in women'.[50] Therefore, in a difficult delivery, physicians would often advise on a course of action without physically seeing the patient. Various ploys were also initiated to discretely mask male attendance, such as keeping the room in relative darkness. Man midwife Percivall Willughby, described a case where he crept into the lying-in-chamber on all fours, to avoid detection, after being called in by a worried midwife, to attend a Puritan lady.[51]

Even during the mid-nineteenth century the practice of 'working blind', when working on female genitalia and reproductive organs, continued – physicians still firmly stressed the need for 'decorum'. Renowned English surgeon, Sir Astley Cooper (1768-1841), taught that catheters inserted into a woman's urethra to draw urine, should always be inserted 'under the bed clothes'.[52] Students were instructed to examine pregnant women by 'feeling', without seeing the physical part. They were expected to know the relative location of urethra and vagina, and during examinations and subsequent treatments would then orient themselves 'from the position of the clitoris, lest acts performed blind should go horribly wrong'.[53]

In time it became quite fashionable 'for families aspiring to a higher social status to have male practitioners attend births' [54] – male practitioners charged higher fees than traditional midwives, hence affording such a luxury, showed off a family's wealth. Accompanying these changes were enormous advances in the understanding of the anatomy and physiology of childbirth and the nature of obstetric complications.[55]

The growth of male-midwifery led to the development of socalled lying-in-hospitals and outpatient lying-in charities, used mainly by poor, destitute married women. These hospitals, established around Western Europe and England from the early to mid eighteenth century onwards, were typically used for teaching obstetrics and midwifery to mostly male students.[56] By the end of the eighteenth century, almost half of all deliveries in England are estimated to have been attended by medical practitioners.[57] Ironically, the same doctors who attended to 'fashionable' home births, charging high fees, would deliver the babies of poor women, unable to afford a traditional midwife, at the lying-in-hospitals.

An important factor, aiding the development of man-midwifery during the eighteenth century was the widespread use of the forceps. Although the forceps had already been developed by physician William Chamberlen (1540-1596) during the sixteenth century, he kept his invention secret. His useful innovation was passed down to his sons, and not divulged until one hundred and fifty years later. This was in fact not an unusual occurrence at the time, as many patent medicines and devices were kept secret during past centuries in order to boost the reputation and income of select medical practitioners.[58] With the help of forceps, the foetus could now be easily extracted during difficult presentations. To begin with though, the use of the forceps further widened the gap between male-midwives and their traditional counterparts, as women were banned from using forceps and all other instruments. These were for male use only.

A 'dishonerable vocation'

Eventually, policies, controls, and regulations saw the emergence of a new generation of well-trained and competent female and male midwives in Europe. Many elite 'man-midwives' were physicians, while so-called surgeon-apothecaries – the forerunners of our modern general practitioners – had taken up midwifery throughout provincial England, as well as in the cities. By the mid-eighteenth century midwifery was properly regulated, and schools for midwifery had been set up for prospective midwives *and* for doctors.

Initially though 'man-midwives' had no place in the medical system. Neither the Royal College of Physicians nor the Royal College of Surgeons were willing to accept these 'new practitioners into the fold'.[59] The medical profession in general held midwifery in low regard. Man-midwives were derided as 'quasi-practitioners', who were invading a female domain because they were unable to succeed in general medicine. In 1804 the College of Physicians followed the Company of Surgeons in prohibiting men-midwives from election to its Fellowship. The Company of Surgeons, which had been founded with the specific purpose of creating a body of 'pure surgeons', were especially unwilling to practice a branch of medicine that they believed would lower their status – after their long battle in the past to sever connections with barbers. Any member found to be practising obstetrics was instantly expelled.[60] Both medical Colleges regarded the activity of delivering babies as 'contrary to decency and common sense'.[61]

In 1827 the President of of the Royal College of Surgeons derided efforts to regularise this 'dishonerable vocation'.[62] In fact, in the 1830's their leaders still derided obstetrics as an activity 'foreign to the habits of Gentleman of enlarged academical education'.[63] Hence, obstetrics was marginalised, lying outside mainstream medicine. It was not until 1929 that the College of Obstetrics and Gynaecology was established, and even then its foundation was initially opposed on the grounds that it was not a proper medical specialty.[64]

Important reforms in obstetrics

Towards the end of the eighteenth century, reformist English physicians Charles White (1728-1813) and Alexander Gordon (1752-1799) both advocated cleanliness of patients, attendants, and tools, as well as plenty of fresh air. 'This might almost be counted as the first steps towards asepsis, for general cleanliness in the eighteenth century left something to be desired'.[67] In his *Treatise on the Management of Pregnant and Lying-In Women* (1773), White advised on pregnancy, stressing that the rigid 'tightness of stays' and 'petticoat bindings pressing on the enlarged womb'[68] did much harm to mother and child.

White described conditions in 'lying-in rooms' during the late eighteenth century – conditions that had not changed much over hundreds of years, and were not conducive to the mother's or baby's health. According to White, the delivery room was always extremely hot, with a large fire in the room irrespective of the season; in addition, a great number of people would at all times be congregated in the chamber; and all windows, curtains, and every crevice would be tightly shut to avoid the new mother catching cold. To further avoid this she was smothered in blankets, often inducing profuse 'sweating'. Hence the air in the lying-in room was 'rendered foul and unfit for respiration'.[69] He also elaborated on the traditional diet for new mothers – diets that would slow, if not stop normal intestinal function because of the lack of solid food.

To make matters worse, new mothers usually remained in bed in a horizontal position for days, sometimes weeks – thus preventing stools, post-natal bleedings, and discharge from being expelled.[70] Hence, infection could occur from 'decomposition in the uterus of retained products, such as fragments of membrane, clots and lochia'.[71] Lochia or post-natal bleedings, and other matter, such as the partially retained afterbirth, could stagnate in the womb and in the 'folds of the vagina and become quite putrid'.[72] Infection could also enter through the external genitalia if they had been damaged in labour, or from contact with soiled hands, instruments, or dirty linen.[73] White was the first physician to advocate clean linen as soon as a woman was delivered; no fire in the room in summer; nothing that would induce the new mother to sweat; open windows and curtains for fresh air; a not too tightly bound belly; and frequent sitting up and walking by the patient. All these aforementioned prescribed practices would in fact be viewed as common sense in modern times.

As had been the case for centuries, infection following childbirth still killed hundreds of mothers during the nineteenth century – if the birth process did not prove fatal, the next greatest risk was puerperal – or childbed – fever. It was not until the anti-infection work of Hungarian physician Ignaz Philipp Semmelweis (1818-1865), known as 'the saviour of mothers', that mortality rates from childbirth improved. In 1847, Semmelweis discovered that the incidence of puerperal fever, which was still very common and often fatal in nineteenth century hospitals, could be drastically reduced by hand washing with a chlorinated lime solution.[74]

In spite of his groundbreaking discovery, Semmelweis's ideas were rejected, ridiculed, and scorned by the medical community. Many doctors were in fact highly offended at the suggestion that they should wash their hands before examining patients. Semmelweis continued to be harassed by the medical community, and it was only many years after his death, that his findings earned widespread acceptance when Louis Pasteur established the germ theory of disease, and German physician Robert Koch highlighted the role of microscopic pathogens in causing disease.[75]

By the end of the nineteenth century, the foundations of modern obstetric and midwifery had been laid: the Obstetrical Society of London began issuing 'certificates of competence' to midwives in 1872; by 1902 the Central Midwives Board to regulate the profession had been set up; and in 1947, the Midwives Institute (established in 1881), became the Royal College of Midwives.[76]

The last chapter in this book provides a glimpse into a relatively little known and yet so vital part of medical history…

DIAGNOSING DEATH – A DIRE DILEMMA

The fear of being buried alive[1] is ancient and debates about the exact moment of transition between life and death in humans, have been taking place since antiquity. Prior to modern sophisticated methods of determining brain and cardiac death,[2] the fear of premature burial was indeed justified.[3] Medical diagnoses were rudimentary and various conditions – which may render the human body motionless, cold and unresponsive for lengthy periods of time – were not competently and adequately understood.

The historical progression of recognising the specific signs of death stretches back many centuries. Physicians of ancient Greece spoke of imminent 'signs of death'. Hippocrates addressed this issue in his work *Prognostikon*, where he advocated that once certain 'signs of death' had been observed in a patient, the physician's work was done. Such 'signs' designated that it was time for him to collect his fee and withdraw. In other words, it was not the clinical responsibility of physicians to diagnose or certify their patients' death.[4] Hence it was left to family and friends, to make the ultimate decision of pronouncing their loved-one dead. At the time, any concerns and uncertainties regarding the criteria of death were addressed by an Athenian law, which required that no person should be interred before the third day. Some city-states in Greece even waited six to seven days before burying their dead.

Similarly, awareness about the criteria of death existed during Roman times. Galen advocated caution with regard to conditions such as asphyxia and coma, because it had been recognised that in such cases the signs of life could be absent for prolonged periods. Hence, ancient Greeks and Romans made use of potent caustics such as *sal ammoniac* and 'spirit of hartshorn', which were capable of restoring vital functions in cases of syncope. In other words, even if heartbeat and breathing were absent, signs of life could be restored. However, in spite of such measures many classical writers and physicians mention premature burial having taken place: Roman senators awakening on funeral pyres and people walking back home after having been buried.

In his *Natural History*, Pliny the Elder cites numerous examples of people who were buried prematurely and '...who have returned to life when they were about to be laid in the grave'.[5] For example, the case of senator Acilius Aviola, a man of considerable wealth and power, who was assumed dead by his physician and servants and came to life on the funeral pyre. Unfortunately, the ill-fated man could not be rescued from the ferocity of the flames and was burnt alive.[6] The same misfortune befell a Roman praetor named Lucius Lamia.[7] Hence Pliny fittingly declared: 'Such is the condition of humanity, and so uncertain is men's judgement, that they cannot determine even death itself'.[8]

Uncertainties about the signs of death

Although death has never been easy to define, certain historical eras exhibit far greater fear and indecision over the boundaries between life and death than others. Intense almost manic concern about the uncertainties of signs of death began in the 1740's and lasted for more than a century. A thesis by distinguished Danish anatomist Jaques-Bénigne Winslow (1669-1760),[9] professor of anatomy at Jardin du Roi University in Paris, began a movement of burial reform, which was to spread rapidly to most European countries. In his thesis *Morte incertae signa*,[10] published in 1740, he made the assertion that the signs of death used by medical professionals at the time were not dependable. Hence, people were at risk of being buried alive. In his thesis Winslow states that '...nothing is less certain than Life, or more uncertain than the Signs of Death, at least such Symptoms as are commonly taken for Signs of Death'.[11]

In fact, medical practitioners of the past freely admitted to being undecided and doubtful as to whether a patient was indeed dead or still alive. In his book *Buried Alive – The Terrifying History Of Our Most Primal Fear*, Jan Bondeson cites hundreds of cases of individuals buried, dissected, or embalmed while still very much alive. Indeed, there are deplorable speculations that as many as one tenth of all people in eighteenth and nineteenth century Europe, and even later than that, were buried while still clinically alive.[12] In his book *Death and Sudden Death*, Professor Paul Brouardel (1837-1906), Dean of the Faculty of Medicine Paris in 1902, writes: '...we are obliged to acknowledge that we have no sign or group of signs sufficient to determine the moment of death with scientific certainty in all cases'.[13]

Before brain death was understood, life or death was determined solely on the presence or absence of a heartbeat. But, before the invention of the modern stethoscope in the mid-nineteenth century,[14] attending medical practitioners or family members could easily miss a weak heartbeat and a low rate of respiration. Unless someone had died a violent death, it was impossible to establish with certainty that the person had definitely expired.

Accepted signs of death

Accepted signs of death by physicians during the eighteenth and nineteenth centuries included '...livid Spots which appear on the Skin, and the cadaverous Scent of the Subject, which is widely different from all other Smells, even that arising from the Excrements'.[15] It is obvious from this quote by Winslow taken from his thesis *The uncertainty of signs of death*[16] that although contemporary tests for signs of life were better than in ancient times, the only sure way of diagnosing death was to wait for decomposition and the appearance of livid spots to set in. He did not consider the absence of respiratory movement and a pulse to be dependable signs of death.[17] Instead he advocated a series of numerous grim tests to be administered on the presumed corpse to make the dead body flinch or elicit some other kind of response.

Bizarre as they might sound, such tests were indeed routinely carried out by physicians: sharp pencils were inserted up the nose to cause pain; pieces of horseradish, onions and garlic pushed up the nostrils to revive the person; whips and stinging nettles applied to the skin; acrid enemas given; salt and pepper blown up the nose to see if a corpse would sneeze; trumpets blown very close to the ears; vinegar, salt and warm urine poured down the throat; the soles of the feet cut with razors; long needles pushed under the toenails, scalding hot wax dripped on the corpse's forehead and most extreme of all a red hot poker thrust into the rear end of the corpse in an attempt to make it flinch.[18] Furthermore, Winslow recommended the pricking of a corpse's hands and feet with needles and the laceration of shoulders and arms with razor-sharp instruments to '…strip [them] of the epidermis'.[19], [20]

The fear of premature burial

Winslow's thesis on medical practitioners' inadequate recognition of the signs of death soon caused a stir amongst Parisian faculty members and drew the attention of Jean-Jacques Bruhier d'Ablaincourt (died 1756). Bruhier, a physician as well as an author, offered to loosely translate Winslow's thesis from Latin into French. Winslow's agreement to this proposition proved to be a decision with far-reaching consequences in European history. In 1745, Bruhier's book *Dissertation sur l'incertitude des signes de la mort*,[21] became an instant success in France and immediately captured the general public's imagination about the possibility of premature burial. For the rest of his life, Bruhier dedicated himself to burial reforms,[22] publishing his third most impressive book on the subject in 1749. In this volume he again cited countless examples of premature burials, which would have convinced even the most ardent sceptic that the risk of being buried alive in the eighteenth century was *not* negligible. Soon his fame spread, and this once unknown, middle-aged medical practitioner acquired international acclaim.

German, Swedish, Italian and other translations of Bruhier's book appeared, announcing the uncertainties of signs of death across Europe. People were terrified by the physical torment and ghoulishness described in Bruhier's books: scratch marks and other signs of 'life' found in coffins, which had been unearthed; uncovered coffins containing agonisingly contorted corpses with gnawed fingers, bashed broken hands and bodies, from the desperate struggle to break free. He told of 'corpses' sitting up at their funeral, or waking up on the dissection table. In other instances 'corpses' had been found outside their coffins in vaults and tombs, with bloody, broken hands evidencing their desperate effort to escape.

While many alleged Bruhier to be a horror mongerer, spreading panic and fear, most people at the time *were* justifiably terrified of premature burial, with pamphlets and literature circulating that at least one tenth of all people were buried alive. By the early nineteenth century, the danger of premature burial had become one of the most-feared perils of everyday life and a torrent of pamphlets and academic theses were dedicated to this subject by writers all over Europe.[23] It seemed preferable to be dissected, autopsied or even decapitated, just to make doubly sure that death had indeed occurred. Many made provisions in their wills for their physician to ensure that death had taken place before burial: requests for the throat to be cut, all fingers to be cut off, the heart pierced by a metal pin, the head cut off altogether, or the jugular vein cut.

Britain had for some time remained aloof to the continental obsession, viewing the incessant premature burial preoccupation, especially by the Germans and the French, with wry amusement – until two English editions of Bruhier's book appeared in 1746 and 1751. The result was a veritable panic and heightened public anxiety about the subject of premature burial. Almost immediately the English started producing their own horror stories about the topic. We have only to think of the macabre writings of Edgar Allan Poe (1809-1849), tapping into, and fuelling public fear, with short stories such as *The Premature Burial.*

The fear of premature burial in Europe was also greatly exacerbated by the increased use of coffins during the eighteenth and nineteenth centuries. Although wooden coffins were already utilised as early as the thirteenth century, their use was then exclusively for the wealthy – as they were simply too expensive. As the use of coffins became more commonplace for all classes of people in the eighteenth and nineteenth centuries, the perception of being firmly enclosed in a private, securely sealed wooden shell, covered by several meters of heavy ground, 'sank' in and added to the overwhelming panic.

But, nowhere did the abject fear and horror at the prospect of premature interment take a greater hold than in Germany. Here, in an almost frenzied response, the medical profession and general public took on the uncertainty of death, and the best way to prevent people from being buried alive. Consequently, from the mid-seventeen hundreds onwards, a new literary genre was born in Germany. A '…veritable torrent of serious theses, alarmist pamphlets, and amusing anecdotes about swooning ladies rescued from the tomb',[24] people awakening in their premature coffins or tombs and suffering the most abject tortures, before finally being rescued or succumbing to a frightful end.

Waiting mortuaries – 'hospitals for the dead'

In 1787, as the discussion about 'signs of death' raged in several European countries, French physician François Thiérry (1719-1793) made the profound statement that most people actually died much later than '…the onset of traditional signs of death'.[25] He therefore proposed so-called 'waiting mortuaries' in all major French cities for these still conscious, technically alive, individuals. In Germany the idea of waiting mortuaries was immediately and enthusiastically taken up, and implemented in Weimar by the renowned, highly awarded and honoured German physician, Christoph Hufeland (1762-1836).[26]

Few waiting mortuaries were built outside of Germany, with Denmark, Sweden, Belgium, the Netherlands and Austria being the only other countries to house these 'hospitals for the dead'. In France, Italy, Spain and America, the debate for and against the provision of waiting mortuaries raged on for over a century, but ultimately no such mortuaries were ever built in these countries. By far the largest number of these buildings were accommodated in Germany.

German waiting mortuaries, or 'hospitals for the dead', were huge, impressive, ornate, architecturally designed buildings, featuring elaborate columns and facades. Inside were rows upon rows of beds for the presumed deceased, lifeless 'patients'. Male and female corpses were segregated in different halls, as were rich and poor. Every corpse had their lifeless hands and feet attached to a complex system of cords leading to a bell suspended above each bed. The bells were to signal even the slightest movement. Macabrely, as corpses distended with a build-up of gases, they often shifted, causing false alarms.

Generally, all corpses would lie in waiting mortuaries for at least thirty-six hours before burial. The wards were kept well aired in summer – although nothing could obliterate the fetid reek – and were heated during winter. Several watchmen supervised all wards. Attendants monitored the corpses around the clock for signs of life, while a doctor would do his rounds on a daily basis. Waiting mortuaries also housed facilities for the watchmen, as well as a resuscitation room, which was well equipped with surgical instruments and a complete pharmacy. Watchmen lived on the premises, worked in shifts, and were not allowed to smoke or drink alcoholic beverages or receive visitors. Apart from overseeing the corpses, they were kept busy, cleaning the beds of corpses and everything around them, in an attempt at controlling the abominable stench of decomposing flesh.

Hufeland lobbied fervently to have young, educated men employed as attendants in German waiting mortuaries instead of the superstitious, ignorant, 'old crones' employed in the old-fashioned mortuaries of his time. To make his point, Hufeland often recounted a story about one of the 'corpse-women', who, upon seeing a 'corpse' crawl out of bed, thought it was the devil, and repeatedly struck the poor man over the head with a broom, yelling at him to get back to where he had come from.[27]

Support for waiting mortuaries started to diminish in the 1790's. Not only did they cost large amounts of money to build and maintain, but they were also disturbing, distasteful, and objectionable places. Many people simply refused to give up their deceased loved ones to be brought to these foul smelling, grandiose hospitals for the dead. By the mid-nineteenth century many of the smaller waiting mortuaries in Germany had closed or been converted to other uses. However, large *Leichenhäuser*, or mortuaries, were still built in the big German cities at considerable expense, as late as the nineteenth century: 1871 in Hamburg; 1865 in Mainz; 1872 in Ulm; 1875 in Stuttgart.

Surprisingly, Germany experienced a resurgence in the debate about premature burial in the 1880's, probably triggered by the cholera epidemic of that time. Henceforth it became obligatory in Germany for all corpses to be supervised for signs of life, such as in Munich, which had six waiting mortuaries where corpses were placed in separate rooms and kept for forty-eight to seventy-two hours. Macabrely, these and other German mortuaries were open to visitors, who could stroll around at leisure and inspect the pale deathly faces surrounded by flowers, their hands and feet attached to strings and bells. A 1967 article in *Der Spiegel*, confirmed that certain German mortuaries still used signalling devices as late as the 1940's.[28]

The inevitable question arises as to why Germans were so obsessed with hospitals for the dead – more so than any other European nation. The answer is two-fold: Christoph Hufeland, a fervent advocate of waiting mortuaries, was a highly respected and influential physician in the 1790's, and even a century later, no one dared question his legacy. In addition, well past the mid-nineteenth century, German medical practitioners continued to adhere to the idea that putrefaction was the only *sure* sign of death.[29]

In spite of the fact that waiting mortuaries were not built in many European countries, many prominent physicians, in England and on the Continent gave credit to the founding of these specialist buildings. The *Lancet*, dated September 20 1845, comments that '...it is but little use to descant upon an evil without pointing out a remedy. In Frankfort, Munich and in various other towns, houses, properly situated, have been fitted up for the temporary reception of the dead. [...] This plan is evidently much preferable to that which is followed in France'.[30] The article further comments that the German plan, although with some modification, should be followed in Britain.

Similarly, the *British and Foreign Medico-Chirurgical Review* of 1855 stated: 'To Germany belongs the credit of having executed these designs in such wise that they should not prove the positive sources of more danger to the living [...]. Where doubt of the reality of death has existed, Hufeland devised the plan that Frankfort-on-the Main incorporated with its reform in sepulture and establishment of extra-mural cemeteries in 1823'.[31] In 1905 British social reformer William Tebb (1830-1917) commented in his book *Premature Burial And How It May Be Prevented*: 'Of all the various methods that have been suggested or introduced for the prevention of premature interment, none has been attested with such satisfactory results as the erection of [waiting] mortuaries in Germany'.[32]

The safety coffin – saved by the bell

However, by the 1790's an alternative method of safeguarding the dead had emerged. Although support for waiting mortuaries had diminished, this is not to say that fears and anxieties about premature burial were not at a heightened frenzy in Europe. Such fears and anxieties resulted in the timely, reassuring invention of various curious devices, which could be incorporated into coffins, with a means of communication to the outside – such as a cord with a bell attached externally. The presumed deceased, enclosed 'six feet under', could then indeed be 'saved by the bell' – although there is no evidence as to the phrase ever having been used in this connection. Several such devices, known as 'safety coffins' were patented in Germany, England and America.

None other than the ruler of one of the German states, Duke Ferdinand of Brunswick (1721-1792), is thought to have designed the first safety coffin. Having an unnatural fear of premature burial himself, the Duke had a special coffin constructed. The coffin had a window, an airhole and a lid with key mechanism – in other words, the lid was not nailed down. Inside the coffin were pockets where duplicate keys to the lid, as well as the vault, were sequestered. However, such extravagant coffins, as well as vault burials, were certainly not the norm for most people. Therefore, numerous alternative devices, sporting tubes, airholes, ropes, strings and bells – all leading above ground – were designed. Unfortunately, every one of these was financially out of reach for the poor.

The first security coffin with any practical value was designed and personally tested by German physician Dr. Adolph Gutsmuth. A long tube linked the buried coffin to the outside world. When a mechanism was triggered from within, the tube would admit light and air into the coffin, and also afford the opportunity to feed the awakened corpse through it. In order to prove the effectiveness of his invention the good doctor had himself buried alive for several hours, while being sustained from above with soup, sausages and beer, all fed through the tube. Soon improvements on Gutsmuth's model appeared – again in Germany. A superior coffin model sported the tube, as well as a bell and a trumpet, to make oneself heard above ground should the need arise. Critics of this model however pointed out that a weak, sickly, feeble person awakening in a coffin would hardly have the strength or presence of mind to work intricate mechanisms of strings, bells and tubes, which needed to be opened – not to mention blowing enough air out of the tube to sound a trumpet. This criticism immediately prompted other designs to be put forward.

Yet another repository for the dead was an attempt to combine a miniature 'waiting mortuary', with a security coffin. This device became known as the 'portable death chamber'. The model sported a door and a window at the top of the chamber, as well as a bell on the outside. Watchmen would be employed to look through the window at regular intervals and listen out for peels of the bell. If and when putrefaction was definitely noticed, a trapdoor would be operated to let the body fall into a grave underneath the 'portable death chamber'.

During the second half of the nineteenth century, the German fixation on security coffins continued with more than thirty different designs patented. Designs included inbuilt devices, such as drainage systems, security tubes, varying filters or powerful bellows for air circulation, firecrackers instead of bells on the outside, sirens mounted on the inside of the breathing tube, and even a pyrotechnical rocket launched through the security tube.

Not to be outdone by its continental neighbours, the British ensured against premature burial with the Bateson 'Life Revival Device'. In 1852 George Bateson was granted a patent for the device, also known as 'Bateson's Belfry'. The advertising of this apparatus as '...a most economical, ingenious, and trustworthy mechanism, superior to any other method, and promoting peace of mind amongst the bereaved'[33] shows a clear demand for a reasonably priced alarm system to protect the newly interred. Bateson's Belfry consisted of a simple iron bell on a pole, mounted on the lid of the coffin over the deceased's head. The bell was connected to the corpse's hand by a rope or wire through the coffin. Any signs of life from within the casket would sound the alarm on the outside. Instantly popular, hundreds of coffins were fitted with the Bateson's belfry, and its designer became a highly respected, wealthy man. In 1859 Bateson was awarded an O.B.E. by Queen Victoria for his invention.[34]

Later British models sported powerful springs, and, most outrageous of all, an ejection seat for use in vault burials – although it is unknown whether that particular safety coffin was ever manufactured. In the United States no less than twenty-two patents for security coffins were applied for between 1868 and 1925. [35]

In search of reliable signs of death

It was generally felt that premature burial was now largely preventable by the various burial reforms, which had been instituted in European countries. However, longer waiting times before actual interment, waiting mortuaries and safety coffins, were not seen as the ultimate solution. The construction of waiting mortuaries during the eighteenth and nineteenth centuries clearly represented an inability of physicians to positively identify the living from the dead in the absence of putrefaction. Even though support for waiting mortuaries was diminishing by the 1790's, debate about diagnosing the signs of death raged on in Europe, and spread to America.[36] Perhaps this explains the specific instructions the first President of the United States of America, George Washington gave to those in attendance, when he was on his deathbed: 'Have me decently buried and do not let my body be put into the vault, less than three days after I am dead. Do you understand me?'. [37]

Reliable signs of actual death *had* to be found and effectively established by medical science. It was deemed important that the specific signs of death used by medical practitioners were such that all doctors, not only specialists, could use or apply them. In addition, it was agreed that past fierce and often-violent tests for signs of life, as described by Winslow, were of no practical value. After all, what was the point in cutting off someone's fingers in order to revive them, if that person would then spend the rest of their life without these appendages?

Various 'safe' methods of testing for death were now created. French physician Antoine Louis (1723-1792) devised one such 'safe' method. He suggested using powerful bellows to administer enemas of tobacco smoke up the apparently deceased person's rear end! Such enemas were considered practical and were used in the Netherlands, England and Germany, to revive not only those presumed dead, but also those who had drowned or were unconscious. Meanwhile, German medical practitioners and inventors were also experimenting with electricity to revive the dead. A galvanic gadget designed by German physician Johann Caspar Creve (1769-1853), was intended to test 'irritability' of a corpse's arm muscles. But, because of widespread scepticism regarding galvanism, this apparatus did not succeed. Similar electrical gadgets were invented but also failed due to a lack of faith in electrical implements.[38]

By the 1830's Hufeland's doctrine of putrefaction was still widely accepted in continental Europe, as no worthwhile progress regarding reliable signs of death had been made. Since the Germans adhered strictly to Hufeland's ideas, it was left to the French to zealously seek alternative answers and solutions. Their fervour is evidenced clearly by the sheer number of medical theses dealing with acceptable and plausible signs of death – all in all, more than thirty such theses were published between 1800 and 1835. However, no conclusive answers could be agreed upon and premature burial was still a real possibility.

Eventually, in 1839, the French Academy of Sciences in Paris offered a prize of 1500 gold francs, the *Prix Manni*, to be given to anyone submitting reliable proof for signs of death. The prize was offered for the third time in 1846, as no worthy contribution had yet been made. During the third round of the *Prix Manni*, one of the contestants, French physician Eugène Bouchut (1818-1891), suggested that the newly invented stethoscope should be used – applied for at least two minutes – to positively diagnose the cessation of heartbeat. When Bouchut was declared the winner of the *Prix Manni* in 1848 his thesis attracted instant international attention. The century long debate regarding the diagnosing of death seemed to be over at last. However, this was not to be. Bouchut had many critics regarding the unreliability of his postulation, and the French Academy of Sciences received hundreds of objections from medical practitioners citing examples of 'living' people with no audible heartbeat.

'Death-trance' or apparent death

As far back as 1808, German physician Hufeland had already published *Der Scheintod*, or 'apparent death'. His hypothesis was that a state of deep unconsciousness or 'death trance' always excluded real death. He further postulated that such a trance was indistinguishable from real death and that such a state could last for days or even weeks. In other words, although the apparently dead person lacked pulse, muscle reflex, and respiratory movement, this could be a trance from which the person, usually a woman, could be awakened. To strengthen his premise, he cited hundreds of actual examples of this scenario having taken place.

Similarly, some decades later, the American *Dictionary of Medicine* of 1884, described a condition called 'death-trance' in which '…no manifestation of consciousness can be observed or elicited by the most powerful cutaneous stimulation, and on recovery no recollection of the state is preserved; but in some cases volition only is lost, and the patient is aware of all that passes, although unable to give the slightest evidence of consciousness'.[39] Furthermore, the *Dictionary of Medicine* stated emphatically that people had most certainly been buried in this state. Just such a case, of a man 'seized' by a trance during illness, was reported in the *Lancet* in 1889.[40] Aware of everything around him, but unable to move or communicate, the man was about to be covered with the coffin lid, when as a result of his mental anguish, he broke out in a profuse sweat. Fortunately, those around him duly observed this, and he lived to tell of his harrowing ordeal.

The *Lancet* edition of 22 December 1883 [41] cited a remarkable case of 'death trance' reported by William Gairdner (1824-1907), Professor of Medicine at Glasgow University. Apparently, the trance lasted for more than twenty-three weeks and attracted considerable attention and discussion in medical circles. The young lady in question was to all intents and purposes in a condition of suspended consciousness, evidencing no signs of sensation, '...connected to the physical world only through a few insignificant reflexes'.[42]

Similarly, in the January 12, 1884 edition of the *Lancet*, Professor Gairdner quoted the case of a young woman in a state of trance for several weeks. When this particular story was published in one of the local newspapers, it elicited a flurry of similar accounts from dozens of people who had been prematurely buried while in a 'trance', only to be saved at the last moment.[43] Many such stories were cited in various medical books, journals and newspapers of the time, further fuelling public debate and apprehension.[44]

But, the medical establishment was no closer to 'diagnosing death' than it had been a hundred years earlier. On 31 October 1885 the *British Medical Journal*, discussing the difficulties of distinguishing real death from apparent death under the heading 'Death or Coma', stated that '... hardly any sign, short of putrefaction, can be relied upon as infallible'.[45]

Given the recognised inability of physicians in the past to 'diagnose death', it seems astounding, if not incredulous, that textbooks on forensic medicine have little or nothing to say regarding this topic. Furthermore, given the intense, anxious, century-long debate in European countries by the medical establishment and the general public concerning premature burial, it seems shocking that this part of medical history has been swept under the proverbial carpet – comprehensive books on the history of medicine fail to mention the centuries long debate regarding the uncertainty of the signs of death.[46] Perhaps the reluctance by medical historians to explore a history of the signs of death, stems from the fact that if it were known that physicians had repeatedly buried their mistakes alive, this would detract considerably from the real medical breakthroughs of those centuries.

Throughout past decades, concern about premature burial never quite disappeared and as late as 1940, an article in the *Scientific American* asserted that 'frequent' errors in diagnosing death were still resulting in premature burials.[47] With advances in medical technology, several factors have contributed to more accurate diagnoses of death. Progress into the understanding of causes of various diseases and their accompanying prognoses have led to a better perception of what the natural progression of a disease might be in an individual.

Even in modern times the diagnosis of death is still most often made on clinical grounds, such as the absence of a pulse or heartbeat, lack of respiration, the observation of fixed dilated pupils and a lack of any response to external stimuli. However, these are now aided by additional medical investigations employing technological devices such as cardiac monitors. In addition, neurological determination of death criteria, establishing the cessation of neurological activity in the brain - so-called 'brain death'- has become a field of enquiry in its own right in modern medicine.

BIBLIOGRAPHY

Aberth John, *The Black Death – The Great Mortality of 1348-1350 – A Brief History with Documents,* The Bedford Series in History and Culture, Stratford Publishing Services, Boston 2005.

Abbot Elisabeth, *A History of Celibacy*, Scribner, New York 2000.

Adair Mark J, *Plato's View of the 'Wandering Uterus', The Classical Journal* 91:2, 1996.

Adami George, *Charles White of Manchester and the Arrest of Puerperal Fever*, University Press of Liverpool, Hodder and Stroughton, London 1922.

Adams F., *On hysterical suffocation*, In: On the Causes and Symptoms of Acute Diseases, in book II of The Extant Works of Aretaeus, the Cappadocian, New Sydenham Society, London 1856.

Adams Norman, *Dead and Buried: The Horrible History of Body Snatching*, Bell Publishing Company, New York 1972.

Achterberg Jeanne, *Woman as Healer – A panoramic survey of the healing activities of women from prehistoric times to the present*, Shambhala Publications, Boston 1990.

Allen Prudence, *The Concept of Woman: The Aristotelian Revolution 750 BC – AD 1250*, William Eerdmans Publishing 1997.

Archibald Elizabeth, *Did Knights Have Baths? The Absence of Bathing in Middle English Romance*, In: Cultural Encounters in the Romance of Medieval England, Edited by Corinne Saunders, DS Brewer Publishing 2005.

Aretaeus, ed. Karl Hude, *Collection of Greek Medical Authors*, In: Aedibus Academiae Scientiarum, Berlin 1958, Book 4:13, pp. 85-90.

Aristotle's Masterpiece, Illustrated Edition, New York 1846

Original manuscript viewed on: https://archive.org/details/8709661.nlm.nih.gov Accessed April 2014

Armstrong John W., *The Water of Life*, Health Research Books, 2000.

Arrizabalaga Jon, Henderson John and French Roger, *The Great Pox: The French Disease in Renaissance Europe,* Yale University Press 1997.

Auf der Heide Arthur, *The Scientific Study of Mummies*, Cambridge University Press, Cambridge 2003.

Bächtold-Stäubli Hans, *Handwörterbuch des Deutschen Aberglaubens*, Vols. I – X, de Gruyter Publishers, Berlin 1987, Vols. 1-10.

Bacon Francis, *Sylva Sylvarum: Or a Natural History in Ten Centuries*, reprint of 1627 edition, Kessinger Publishing 1996, p134. Original manuscript viewed on: http://books.google.com.au/books?id=IXyOUr9kylUC&q=moss#v=snippet&q=moss&f=false Accessed January 2014

Bailey James Blake, *The Diary of a Resurrectionist 1811-1812*, Swan Sonnenschein & Co., London 1896. Original manuscript viewed on: http://archive.org/stream/

diaryofresurrect/ Accessed May 2013

Baldwin John W., *The Language of Sex: Five Voices from Northern France around 1200*, Chicago University Press, Chicago 1994.

Ball Philip, *The Devil's Doctor – Paracelsus and the World of Renaissance, Magic and Science*, Farrar, Straus and Giroux, New York 2006.

Blackmore Richard Sir, *A Treatise of the Spleen and Vapours: Or Hypocondriacal and Hysterical Affections*, Printed for J. Pemberton, London 1726.

Bondeson Jan, *Buried Alive – The Terrifying History Of Our Most Primal Fear*, Barnes and Noble Books, New York 2006.

Bourke John G., *Scatalogic Rites of all Nations*, Kessinger Publishing, Montana USA 2003. (Originally published as *Notes and Memoranda Bearing upon the Use of Human Ordure and Human Urine*, 1888.)

Bowie Fiona, *Hildegard of Bingen and medieval women's sexuality*, In: Diskus 2:1, pp. 1-14, 1994.

Bradis Henning, *Diarium*, published by Hänselmann, Hildesheim 1896.

Brain Peter, *Galen on Bloodletting: A Study of the Origins, Development, and Validity of His Opinions, with a Translation of the Three Works*, Cambridge University Press, 1986.

Brown Elisabeth A. R., *Death and the Human Body in the Later Middle Ages: The Legislation of Boniface VIII on the Division of the Corpse*, University of California Press 2003.

Brown Kevin, *The Pox – The life and death of a very social disease*, Sutton Publishing Limited, Gloucestershire 2006.

Brody Nathaniel Samuel, *The Disease of the Soul – Leprosy in Medieval Literature*, Cornell University Press, London 1974.

Brouardel P. and Benham Lucas, *Death and Sudden Death*, Baillière, Tindall & Co., London 1902. Original manuscript viewed on: http://archive.org/stream/ deathsuddendeath00brouuoft#page/n3/mode/2up Accessed July 2014

Brugis Thomas, *The marrow of physick or: A learned discourse of the several parts of mans body*, 1669. British Library, Original manuscript viewed on: http:// eebo.chadwyck.com.rp.nla.gov.au/search/full_rec?SOURCE=pgimages. cfg&ACTION=ByID&ID=V58925 Accessed July 2013

Budge, Sir Ernest A. Wallis, *The Mummy: A Handbook of Egyptian Funerary Archaeology*, Cambridge University Press; Reissue edition, July 2010.

Bullough Vern L., *The Subordinate Sex*, University of Illinois Press, 1974.

Burland Margaret, *Meaning and its Objects: Material Culture in Medieval and Renaissance France*, Yale University Press 2006.

Cadden Joan, *The Meanings of Sex Difference in the Middle Ages: Medicine, Science and Culture*, In: Cambridge Studies in the History of Medicine, Cambridge University Press 1995.

Cameron M. L., *Anglo-Saxon Medicine*, Cambridge University Press, Cambridge 1993.

Cawthorne Nigel, *The Curious Cures of Old England*, Piatkus Books Ltd., London 2005.

Celsus C., *De Medicina*, edited by W. G. Spencer, Loeb Classical Library, London 1935.

Chaucer Geoffrey, *The Canterbury Tales*, A Complete Translation into Modern English by Ronald Ecker and Eugene Crook, Hodge & Braddock Publishers 1993.

Chauliac Guy de, *Inventarium Sive Chirurgica Magna*, edited by Michael McVaugh, In: Studies in Ancient Medicine, Brill Publishing 1997.

Clark Andrew Sir, *Anaemia or Chlorosis of Girls, Occurring More Commonly between the advent of Menstruation and the Consummation of Womanhood*, In: Lancet 1887, Vol. 2, p 1003-1004.

Clark George Sir, *History of the Royal College of Physicians of London*, In: British Medical Journal, January 1965, pp. 79-82.

Clark Stuart, *Thinking with Demons: The Idea of Witchcraft in Early Modern Europe*, Oxford University Press, 1999.

Cockayne Oswald, *Leechdoms, Wortcunning, and Starcraft of Early England*, 3 vols. (London, 1865; reprint, 1961), vol. II: 110-13.

Cohn Samuel K., *The Black Death and the Transformation of the West*, European History Series, Harvard University Press, 1997.

Crawfurd Raymond, *The Last Days of Charles II*, Claredon Press, Oxford 1909.

Crawfurd Raymond, *The King's Evil*, Claredon Press, Oxford 1911.

Culpeper Nicholas, *Pharmacopoeia Londinensis* or *The London Dispensatory*, Royal College of Physicians of London, originally published 1649. Original manuscript viewed on: https://archive.org/details/2548018R.nlm.nih.gov Accessed February 2013

Cunningham Andrew and Grell Ole Peter, *The Four Horsemen of the Apocalypse*, Cambridge University Press, Cambridge 2000.

Dannenfeldt Karl, *Egyptian Mumia: The Sixteenth Century Experience and Debate*, In: Sixteenth Century Journal 16:2, 1985.

Darwin F. (ed.), *Charles Darwin; His Life Told in an Autobiographical Chapter, And in a Selected Series of His Published Letters*, London 1892.

Demaitre Luke, *Leprosy in Premodern Medicine: A Malady of the Whole Body*, JHU Press 2007.

Donnison Jean, *Midwives and Medical Men – A History of the Struggle for the Control of Childbirth*, Historical Publications, London 1999.

Douglas Mary, *Witchcraft and Leprosy: Two Strategies of Exclusion*, Cultural Studies Project, Massachusetts Institute of Technology, 1991, 25 pages.

Drife J., *The start of life: a history of obstetrics*, In: Postgraduate Medical Journal, 2002, Volume 78:919, pp. 311-315.

Duff Charles, *A Handbook on Hanging*, EP Publishing, Rowman & Littlefield, 1974.

Dunant, Sarah, *Syphilis, sex and fear: How the French disease conquered the world*, In: The Guardian, Saturday 18 May 2013.

Dunn-Hensley Susan Michele, *Powerful Purity: The Sacred Virgin in Early Modern Literature*, Proquest Publishing, Kansas 2007.

Ehrenreich Barbara and English Deirdre, *Witches, Midwives and Nurses*, Feminist Press, New York 2010.

Ellul Max, *The Sword and the Green Cross: The Saga of the Knights of Saint Lazarus from the Crusades to the 21st Century*, Authorhouse Publishing UK 2011.

Evans Richard J., *Rituals of Retribution: Capital Punishment in Germany 1600 – 1987*,

Oxford 1996.

Evenden D., *The Midwives of seventeenth century London*, Cambridge University Press, 2000.

Fabricius Johannes, *Syphilis in Shakespeare's England*, Kingsley Press, Michigan 1994.

Ferrari Giovanna, *Public Anatomy Lessons and the Carnival: The Anatomy Theatre of Bologna*, In: Past and Present 117, 1987, pages 50-106.

Ficino Marsilio, *De Vita II* (1489), 11: 196-199. Translated by Sergius Kodera.

Foucault Michel, *Discipline and Punish*, translated from the French by Alan Sheridan, Harmondsworth, 1977.

Frith John, *Syphilis – Its early History and Treatment until Penicillin and the Debate on its Origins*, In: Journal of Military and Veterans' Health, Volume 20:4 2012.

Furdell Elizabeth Lane, *The Royal Doctors: 1485-1714 – Medical Personnel at the Tudor and Stuart Courts*, University of Rochester Press 2001.

Gatrell V.A.C., *The Hanging Tree – Execution and the English people 1770-1868*, Oxford University Press, Oxford 1994.

Getz Faye. *Medicine in the English Middle Ages*. Princeton University Press, 1998.

Gilman Sander L., King Helen, Porter Roy, Rousseau G. S., Showalter Elaine, *Hysteria Beyond Freud*, University of California Press 1993.

Gordon Alexander, *Treatise on the Epidemic Puerperal Fever of Aberdeen*, C.G.Robinson, Paternoster Row, London 1795.

Gordon-Grube Karen, 'Anthropophagy in Post-Renaissance Europe: The Tradition of Medicinal Cannibalism', In: American Anthropologist, 90 (1988) p. 405-409.

Gottfried Robert S., *The Black Death – Natural and Human Disaster in Medieval Europe*, The Free Press, New York 1983.

Gray Earnest, *The Diary of a Surgeon in the Year 1751- 1752*, Apple Century Company, New York 1937.

Green Monica, *The Transmission of Ancient Theories of Female Physiology and Diseases Through the Early Middle Ages* (PhD thesis), Princeton University, New York 1985.

Green Monica, *Making Women's Medicine Masculine: The Rise of male Authority in Pre-Modern Gynaecology*, Oxford University Press, 2008.

Greilsammer Myriam, *The midwife, the priest, and the physician: the subjugation of midwives in the Low Countries at the end of the Middle Ages*, In: Journal of Medieval and Renaissance Studies, 21:2, 1991 p. 285-329.

Grigsby Bryon Lee, *Pestilence in Medieval and Early Modern English Literature*, In: Studies in Medieval History and Culture, Routledge University Press 2004.

Hæger Knut, *The Illustrated History of Surgery*, revised by Sir Roy Calne, AB Nordbok, Gothenburg Sweden 2000.

Hall Marshall, *The Morbid and Curative Effects of Loss of Blood*, E.L. Carey & A. Hart, Philadelphia, 1830.

Harper K.N., Zuckerman M.K., Harper M.L., Kingston J.D., Armelagos G.J.. *The origin and antiquity of syphilis revisited: an appraisal of old world pre-Columbian evidence for treponeal infection.* In: Yearbook Phys Anthropol 2011: 54: 99-133. Viewed on: http://www.ncbi.nlm.nih.gov/pubmed/22101689 Accessed May 2013

Hatcher John, *The Black Death – A Personal History*, Da Capo Press, Philadelphia USA 2008.

Hayden Deborah, *Pox: Genius, Madness and the Mysteries of Syphilis*, Basic Books 2003.

Heer F., *The Medieval World*, New American Library, New York 1961.

Helmont, Jean Baptiste van, *A ternary of paradoxes the magnetick cure of wounds, nativity of tartar in wine, image of God in man*, translated, illustrated and amplified by Walter Charleton, University of Michigan, Digital Library Production Service 2005.

Original manuscript viewed on: http://name.umdl.umich.edu/A43289.0001.001 Accessed October 2012

Henryson Robert, Heaney Seamus, *The Testament of Cresseid and Seven Fables*, Translated by Seamus Heany, Faber Press, Mitchigan 2009.

Herodotus, *The Persian Wars*, transl. by George Rawlinson, The Modern Library, New York 1942.

Hindson Bethan, *Attitudes towards menstruation and menstrual blood in Elizabethan England*, In: Journal of Social History, Cengage Learning, University of Sheffield 2009.

Hippocrates, *Aphorisms*, From the Latin Version of Verhoofd, by Elias Marks, M.D., Collins &Co. New York 1817.

Hobbes Thomas, Curley Edwin M., *Leviathan: With Selected Variant from the Latin Edition of 1868*, Editor: Edwin M. Curley, Hackett Publishing, London 1994.

Homes Urban Tigner, *Daily living in the twelfth century, based on observations of Alexander Neckam in London and Paris*, University of Wisconsin Press, 1952.

Horrox Rosemary, *The Black Death*, Manchester University Press, Manchester 1994.

Huntsinger Wolf Elizabeth, *Georgetown Mysteries and Legends*, John F. Blair Publishing, 2007.

Jager Eric, *The Book of the Heart*, University of Chicago Press, 2000.

Jarald Edwin, Sheeja Edwin, Vaibhav Tiwari, 2008, *Antioxidant and Antimicrobial Activities of Cow Urine*, In: Global Journal of Pharmacology 2 (2): 20-22, 2008.

Jevons F. R., *Paracelsus's Two-Way Astrology – What Paracelsus meant by 'Stars'*, In: The British Journal for the History of Science 2:2, December 1964, pp.139-147. Viewed on:

http://www.jstor.org/stable/4025012 Accessed September 2012

Jorden Edward, *A briefe discourse of a disease called the suffocation of the mother*, Publisher John Windet, London 1603, Digitised 24 Aug 2011 by University of California.

Kanner Leo, *The Folklore and Cultural History of Epilepsy*, In: *Medical Life*, 34.4, 1930.

Karlen A., *Man and Microbes*, GP Putnam's Sons, New York 1995.

Kassell Lauren, *Medicine and Magic in Elizabethan London: Simon Forman: Astrologer, Alchemist and Physician*, Oxford University Press, 2005.

Katzenberg Anne and Saunders Shelley, *Biological Anthropology of the Human Skeleton*, John Wiley & Sons, 2011.

Kelly John, *An Intimate History of the Black Death, the Most Devastating Plague of all Time*, Harper Perennial, Harper Collins, London 2006.

Kerridge IH, Lowe M., *Bloodletting: The story of a therapeutic technique*, In: Medical Journal of Australasia 1995, No. 163, pp. 631-633.

King Helen, *Once upon a text: Hysteria from Hippocrates*, In: Hysteria beyond Freud, University of California Press 1998, pp. 3-90.

King Helen, *Hippocrates' Woman: Reading the Female Body in Ancient Greece*, Routledge University Press, 2002.

King Helen, *The Disease of Virgins: Green Sickness, Chlorosis, and the Problems of Puberty*, Psychology Press, 2004.

Kingston Jeremy, *Healing without Medicine*, Aldus Books, London 1976.

Kontoyannis Maria, Katsetos Christos, *Midwives in early modern Europe (1400-1800)*, In: Health Science Journal, Volume 5:1, 2011, pp: 31-36.

Krieger Heinz-Bruno, *Elmsagen – Ein Beitrag zur Volkskunde des Elmgebietes*, Braunschweig-Schöppenstedt Verlag, Oeding 1967.

Krieger Heinz-Bruno, *Von Pflichten und Künsten der alten Scharfrichter im Lande Braunschweig*, Braunschweig-Schöppenstedt Verlag, Oeding 1967. Original manuscript viewed on: http://www.elmsagen.de/erzaehl.asp Accessed September 2013

Kudlein Fridolf, *The Seven Cells of the Uterus: the doctrine and its roots*, In: Bulletin of the History of Medicine 39 (1965): pp. 415-423.

Lacey Andrew, *The Cult of King Charles the Martyr*, Boydell & Brewer 2003.

Laqueur Thomas, *Making Sex: Body and Gender from the Greeks to Freud*, Harvard University Press 1990.

Lassek A. M., *Human Dissection – Its Drama and Struggle*, Charles Thomas Publishing, Illinois USA 1958.

Leonetti Georges, *et al.*, '*Evidence of Pin Implantation as a Means of Verifying Death During the Great Plague of Marseilles (1722)*'. In: *Journal of Forensic Science* 42:4 (1997).

Leroux Gaston, *The Phantom of the Opera*, translated by Alexander Teixeira de Mattos, Harper Perennial, USA 1991.

Lewin Ralph A., *Merde: Excursions in Scientific Cultural and Socio-Historical Coprology*, Random House, London 1999.

Lindemann Mary, *Medicine and Society in Early Modern Europe*, Cambridge University Press 1999.

Lindemann Mary, *Health and Healing in Eighteenth Century Germany*, John Hopkins University Press 2001, p.223-6, 346)

Linebaugh Peter, *The Tyburn Riot Against Surgeons*, In: Albion's Fatal Tree: Crime and Society in Eighteenth Century England, Pantheon Books, New York 1975.

Lobis Seth, *The Virtue of Sympathy: Magic, Philosophy and Literature in Seventeenth Century England*, Yale University Press, 2015.

Loudon Irvine, *Death in Childbirth*, Clarendon Press, Oxford 1992.

Loudon Irvine, *The Making of Man-Midwifery*, In: Bulletin of the History of Medicine, 1996, Volume 70:3, pp. 507-515.

Loudon Irvine, *General practitioners and obstetrics: a brief history*, In: Journal of the Royal Society of Medicine Nov. 2008, 101:11, pp. 531-535.

Lowe K.J.P., *Church and Politics in Renaissance Italy: The Life and Career of Cardinal Francesco Soderini*, Cambridge University Press 2002.

Macaulay Thomas Babington, *The History of England from the Accession of James II*,

Volume 3, Chapter XIV, Porter & Coates Philadelphia 2008 (EBook #2612). Viewed on: http://www.gutenberg.org/files/2612/2612-h/2612-h.htm Accessed June 2014

McCord Sheri, *Healing by Proxy: The Early Modern Weapon-Salve*, English Language Notes, 2009, Vol. 47 Issue 2, p13.

MacDonald Helen, *Human Remains – Dissection and its Histories*, Yale University Press, London 2006.

MacLean Ian, *The Renaissance Notion of Women: A Study in the Fortunes of Scholasticism and Medical Science in European Intellectual Life*, Cambridge University Press, 1983.

Mafart B., Pelletier J., Fixot M., *Post-mortem Ablation of the Heart: A Medieval Funerary Practice*, In: International Journal of Osteo-Archaeology Vol. 14, 2004, pp. 67-73.

Magner Lois N., *A History of Medicine*, CRC Press, Florida USA, 1992.

Major R.H., *Classic Descriptions of Disease*, Springfield, USA: Charles C Thomas, 1932.

Manchester K., *Tuberculosis and Leprosy in Antiquity*, In: Medical History, Volume 28, Issue 2, April 1984, pp. 162-173.

Marks Elias, *The Aphorisms of Hippocrtaes*, Translated from the Latin Version of Verhoofd, by Elias Marks, M.D., Collins &Co. New York, 1817.

McClive Cathy, *Menstrual Knowledge and Medical Practice in Early Modern France c.1555-1761*, In: Menstruation: A Cultural History, eds. Andrew Shail and Gillian Howie, Hampshire 2005.

McNeill William Hardy, *Plagues and Peoples*, Anchor Books 1998.

Meaney A. L., *Variant Versions of Old English Medical Remedies and the Compilation of Bald's Leechbook, Anglo-Saxon England* 13 (1984) pp. 235-68.

Meek Heather, *Of Wandering Wombs and Wrongs of Women: Evolving Conceptions of Hysteria in the Age of Reason*, In: English Studies in Canada, Volume 35, No 2-3, June/September 2009, p. 105-128.

Merians Linda Evi, *The Secret Malady: Venereal disease in eighteenth-century Britain and France*, University Press of Kentucky 1996.

Merskey Harold, Merskey Susan, *Hysteria or 'suffocation of the mother'*, In: Canadian Medical Association Journal, 1993, 148 (3), pp. 399- 405.

Miller Timothy S., Smith-Savage Rachel, *Medieval Leprosy Reconsidered*, In: International Social Science Review, Vol. 81, No. 1-2, 2006.

Mitchinson W., *Hysteria and Insanity in Women: A nineteenth century Canadian perspective*, In: Journal of Canadian Studies, 1986, 21 (3) 87-105.

Moog Ferdinand P., *Between Horror and Hope: Gladiators Blood as a Cure for Epileptics in Ancient Medicine*, In: Journal of the History of Neuroscience, 12.2, 2003, 137-43.

Moore R. I., *The Formation of a Persecuting Society: Authority and Deviance in Western Europe 950-1250*, John Wiley & Sons, 2008.

Moore Wendy, *The Knife Man – Blood, Body-Snatching and the Birth of Modern Surgery*, Bantam Press, London 2005.

Morabia A. P.C.A. Louis, *The birth of clinical epidemiology*, In: Journal of Clinical Epidemiology 1996, No. 49, pp. 1327-1333.

Mortimer Ian, *The Time Traveller's Guide to Medieval England*, Vintage Books, London 2009.

Morton R.S., *Some early Aspects of Syphilis in Scotland*, In: British Journal of Venereal Diseases, 38 (1962), p. 175-180.

Mukherjee Siddhartha, *The Emperor of all Maladies*, Fourth Estate, London 2011.

Musacchio Jacqueline, *The Art and Ritual of Childbirth in Renaissance Italy*, Yale University Press, New Haven 1999.

Najemy John M., *Italy in the Age of the Renaissance: 1300-1550*, Oxford University Press 2004.

Neaman Judith S., *Suggestion of the Devil – The Origins of Madness*, Anchor Books, New York 1975.

Newman Paul B., *Daily Life in the Middle Ages*, Google eBook, McFarland Press 2001.

Numbers Ronald & Amundsen D.W. eds., *Caring and Curing: Health and Medicine in the Western Religious Tradition*, Macmillan, New York 1986.

Nutton Vivian, *Logic, Learning, and Experimental Medicine*, In: Science, Vol. 295, No 5556, 2002.

Opie Iona and Tatem Moira, *A Dictionary of Superstitions*, Oxford Press, New York 1989.

Oppelt Wolfgang, *Über die Unehrlichkeit des Scharfrichters*, Lengfeld 1976.

Ordinary's Account, *Proceedings from the Old Bailey, London Criminal Court,* Original manuscript viewed on: http://www.oldbaileyonline.org/browse.jsp?path=ordinarysAccounts%2FOA17360726.xml and http://www.oldbaileyonline.org/browse.jsp?path=ordinarysAccounts%2FOA17440217.xml Accessed July 2012

Pachter Henry, *Paracelsus: Magic into Science*, Henry Schuman Publishing, New York 1951.

Padilla Mark William, *Rites of Passage in Ancient Greece: Literature, Religion, Society*, Bucknell University Press, 1999.

Pagel Walter, *Paracelsus: An Introduction to Philosophical Medicine in the Era of the Renaissance*, Karger Medical and Scientific Publishers, 1982.

Park Katherine, *The Criminal and the Saintly Body: Autopsy and Dissection in Renaissance Italy*, In: Renaissance Quarterly, Vol. 47, No. 1.

Payne, J.F. *English Medicine in the Anglo-Saxon Times.* Oxford: Clarendon Press, 1904.

Peris Teresa Fuentes, *Visions of Filth: Deviancy and Social Control in the Novels of Galdós*, Liverpool University Press, Liverpool 2003.

Persels Jeff, Ganim Russell, *Fecal Matters in Early Modern Literature and Art: Studies in Scatology*, Ashgate Publishing, London 2004.

Pettigrew Thomas Joseph, *On Superstitions connected with the History and Practice of Medicine and Surgery*, Barrinton & Haswell, Philadelphia 1844.

Pettit Edward, *Anglo-Saxon Remedies, Charms, and Prayers From British Library Ms Harley 585: the Lacnunga*, 2 vols., Lewiston, New York 2001, vol. II: 77.

Phillips Kate, *Capturing the Wandering Womb Childbirth in Medieval Art*, In: The Haverford Journal, 3, 2007, pp. 40-55.

Pliny the Elder, *Natural History – A Selection*, translated by J.F. Healy, Penguin Books, London 1991.

Pliny, *Natural History*, Translated by H. Rackham, W.H.S. Jones, D.E. Eichholz, 10 volume edition, BOOK XXVIII, Harvard University Press, Massachusetts 1949. Original manuscript viewed on: http://www.masseiana.org/pliny.htm Accessed

September 2013

Pollington Stephen, *Leechcraft – Early English Charms, Plantlore and Healing*, Anglo-Saxon Books, London 2008.

Porter Roy, *The Greatest Benefit to Mankind – A Medical History of Humanity from Antiquity to the Present*, Harper Collins Publishing, London 1999.

Porter Roy, *Blood and Guts – A Short History of Medicine*, Penguin Books, London 2002.

Porter Roy (editor), *The Cambridge History of Medicine*, Cambridge University Press, Cambridge 2006.

Pouchelle Marie-Christine, *The Body and Surgery in the Middle Ages*, Rutgers University Press, New York 1990.

Prioreschi Plinio, A History of Medicine: Medieval Medicine, Volume 5, Horatius Press, Omaha USA 2003.

Probst Christian, *Fahrende Heiler und Heilmittel Händler – Medizin von Marktplatz und Landstraße*, Rosenheimer Verlagshaus, Zwickau 1992.

Quain Richard (editor), *A Dictionary of Medicine*, Appleton & Company, New York 1884. Original manuscript viewed on: http://archive.org/stream/cu31924000286280#page/n13/mode/2up Accessed April 2012

Quétel Claude, *History of Syphilis*, John Hopkins University Press, Baltimore 1990.

Quincy John, *Complete English Dispensatory* or *Pharmacopoia Offininalis and Extemporanea*, London 1730. Original manuscript viewed on: http://catalogue.nla.gov.au/Record/3171660 Accessed February 2013

Radcliffe Walter, *Milestones in Midwifery*, Wright Publishing, London 1967.

Rawcliffe Carole, *Medicine and Society in Later Medieval England*, Sandpiper Publishers, New York 1999.

Rawcliffe Carole, *Leprosy in Medieval England*, Boydell and Brewer Incorporated 2009.

Raynalde Thomas, *The Birth of Mankind: Otherwise named the Woman's Book*, Editor Elaine Hobby, Translated by Richard Jonas, Ashgate Publishing 2009.

Reed C.S., *The codpiece: Social fashion or medical need?*, Occasional Medical History Series, In: Internal Medicine Journal 34:684-686, 2004, Sydney Australia.

Renaud Lauren, *Even Royal Molars Decay*, In: Medicine, Health and Society (Vanderbilt University). Original manuscript viewed on: http://www.wondersandmarvels.com/2011/12/even-royal-molars-decay.html Accessed January 2013

Rhodes Philip, *An Outline History of Medicine*, Cambridge University Press 1986.

Richardson Ruth, *Death, Dissection and the Destitute*, University of Chicago Press, Chicago 2000.

Richardson Samuel, *Familiar Letters on Important Occasions*, R. West Publishing, Philadelphia 1978.

Risse Guenter B., *Mending Bodies, Saving Souls: A History of Hospitals*, Oxford University Press 1999.

Roach Mary, *Stiff: The Curious Lives of Human Cadavers*, W.W. Norton & Company, New York 2003.

Roach Mary, *Bonk : the curious coupling of science and sex*, W.W. Norton & Co., New York 2009.

Root-Bernstein Robert and Michèle, *Honey, Mud, Maggots and Other Medicinal*

Marvels, Macmillan Publishers, London 1999.

Rosen Barbara, *Witchcraft in England 1558-1618*, University of Massachusetts Press 1969.

Rosen William, *Justinian's Flea – Plague, Empire and the Birth of Europe*, Viking Press 2007.

Rosenstrauch Hazel, *Karl Huß, der empfindsame Henker – Eine böhmische Miniatur*, Matthes und Seitz Verlag, Berlin 2012.

Sabine Ernest L., *Latrines and Cesspools of Mediaeval London*, In: *Speculum*, In: The Medieval Academy of America, Volume 9, Issue 03, July 1934, pp. 303-321.

Salisbury Joyce E., editor, *Sex in the Middle Ages: A Book of Essays*, Garland Publishing, New York 1991.

Salzman L. F., *English Life in the Middle Ages*, Oxford University Press, London 1926.

Sathansivam Arunkumar et al 2010, *Antimicrobial Activities of Cow Urine Distillate against some Clinical Pathogens*, In: Global Journal of Pharmacology 4 (1): 41-44, 2010.

Saunders J. B. and O'Malley D., *The Illustrations from the Works of Andreas Vesalius of Brussels*, Dover Publications, New York 1950.

Sawday Jonathan, *The Body Emblazoned*, Routledge Publishing 2013.

Schmidt Franz, *A Hangman's Diary: Being the Authentic Journal of Master Franz Schmidt, Public Executioner of Nuremberg 1573–1617*, translated by C. Calvert and A.W. Gruner, edited by Albrecht Keller, published by Patterson Smith, 1973.

Schmidt Joseph, *Holy and Unholy Shit*, In: *Fecal Matters in Early Modern Literature and Art: Studies in Scatology*, Jeff Persels and Russell Ganim (editors), Ashgate Publishing, Michigan 2004.

Schütte Otto, *Der Scharfrichter in Braunschweig*, In: Festschrift für Paul Zimmermann, Wolfenbüttel, 1914, 204-211.

Shakespeare William, *The Tragedy of Macbeth*, Editor: Nicholas Brooke, Oxford World's Classics Series, Oxford University Press, Oxford 1998.

Shakespeare William, *Hamlet*, Editor Robert Hapgood, Cambridge University Press, Cambridge 1999.

Sharp Jane, *The Midwives Book or The Whole Art of Midwifery* Discovered, published in 1671. Original manuscript viewed on: http://books.google.com.au/books/about/The_Midwives_Book_Or_the_Whole_Art_of_Mi.html?id=VizP6wtqtQIC&redir_esc=y Accessed August 2014

Sharp Jane, *The Midwives Book or The Whole Art of Midwifery Discovered*, editor Elaine Hobby, Women Writers in English 1350-1850 Series, Oxford University Press 1999.

Sheldon D.C., *Man-midwifery history: 1730-1930*, In: Journal for Obstetrics and Gynaecology, 2012 Nov;32(8):718-23.

Shelton Herbert M., *Syphilis: Is it a Mischievous Myth or a Malignant Monster*, published by Health Research Centre, Mokehumne California 1962.

Siena Kevin Patrick, *Sins of the Flesh: Responding to sexual Disease in Early modern Europe*, Centre for Reformation and Renaissance Studies, Victoria University, Toronto Canada 2005.

Siraisi Nancy G., *History, Medicine, and the Traditions of Renaissance Learning*, University of Mitchigan Press, 2007.

Siraisi Nancy G., *Medieval and Early Renaissance Medicine: An Introduction to Knowledge and Practice*, University of Chicago Press, 2009.

Smith Virginia, *Clean: A History of Personal Hygiene and Purity*, Oxford University Press, 2007.

Spierenburg Pieter, *The Spectacle of Suffering – Executions and the Evolution of Repression: From a pre-industrial metropolis to the European experience*, Cambridge University Press, Cambridge 1984.

Stapelberg Monica-Maria, *Old Wives' Tales? A select background to the origins of popular beliefs, traditions and superstitions*, Zeus Publishing, Australia 2005.

Stapelberg Monica-Maria, *Curious and Curiouser – A background to some fascinating beliefs and traditions*, Multi-Media Publications, Canada 2011.

Stapelberg Monica-Maria, *Strange But True – a historical background to popular beliefs and traditions*, Crux Publishing, London 2014.

Steele Robert (editor), *Three Prose Versions of the Secreta Secretorum*, Volume 1, published by Kegan Paul, Trench, Trübner & co., London 1898.

Stein Claudia, *Negotiating the French Pox in Early Modern Germany*, Ashgate Publishing 2009.

Steinacker Karl, *Vom Galgen, Pranger und Nachrichter Braunschweigs im 18. Jahrhundert*, In: Braunschweig Heimat Jahrgang 24, 1933, 51-54.

Stengel Alfred (1896), *Diseases of the Spleen*, In: Thomas Stedman (ed.) Twentieth Century Practice, Vol.7, London, Sampson Low, Marsten and Co., pp 231-525.

Stockman Ralph, *Observations on the Causes and Treatment of Chlorosis*, In: British Medical Journal, Dec 14, 1895, 2: 1473-1476. Original text viewed on: http://www.ncbi.nlm.nih.gov/pmc/articles/PMC2509359/ Accessed August 2014

Storl Wolf L., *Healing Lyme Disease Naturally*, North Atlantic Books, California 2010.

Stuart Kathy, *Defiled Trades and Social Outcasts: Honor and Ritual Pollution in Early Modern Germany*, Cambridge University Press, Cambridge 1999.

Sugg Richard, *Good Physic but Bad Food: Early Modern Attitudes to Medicinal Cannibalism and its Suppliers* In: Social History of Medicine, 19:2 (2006), p. 227.

Sugg Richard, *Mummies Cannibals and Vampires – The History of Corpse Medicine from the Renaissance to the Victorians*, Routledge Group, London 2011.

Suskind Patrick, *Perfume: The Story of a Murderer*, Penguin, London 2007.

Taylor Joseph, *The Danger Of Premature Interment – Proved From Many Remarkable Instances*, Simkin and Marshall, London 1816.

Original manuscript viewed on: http://publicdomainreview.org/2011/08/15/the-danger-of-premature-interment-1816/ Accessed January 2014

Tebb William, *Premature burial, and how it may be prevented, with special reference to trance catalepsy, and other forms of suspended animation*, Second Edition by Walter R. Hadwen M.D., Swan Sonnenschein & Co.Limited, London 1905.

Original manuscript viewed on: http://archive.org/details/prematureburialhootebbuoft Accessed November 2013

Temkin Owsei, *The Falling Sickness – A History of Epilepsy from the Greeks to the Beginnings of Modern Neurology*, John Hopkins University Press, Baltimore 1994.

Thomas Jane Resh, *Behind the Mask: The Life of Queen Elizabeth I*, Clarion Books, UK 1998.

Thompson Lloyd, *Syphilis*, Lea & Febiger, 1920.

Thorndike Lynn, *A History of Magic and Experimental Science During the First Thirteen Centuries of our Era*, Volume II, Columbia University Press, New York 1923.

Thorwald Jürgen, *Science and Secrets of Early Medicine*, Thames & Hudson, London 1962.

Tikhomirov E. *Epidemiology and Distribution of Plague*. In : WHO. Plague Manual: Epidemiology, Distribution, Surveillance and Control. 2011. Viewed on: http://www.who.int/csr/resources/publications/plague/whocdscsredc992a.p Accessed November 2011

Turner Cecil Howard, The *Inhumanists*, A Ouseley Publishing, London 1932.

Twain Mark. *The Innocents Abroad,* Signet Classics, New York 1997.

Vanneste Sarah, *The Black Death and the Future of Medicine: The Effects of the Second Plague Pandemic on the Practice and Development of Medicine*, Lambert Academic Publishing, 2010.

Vicary Thomas, *The English Man's Treasure*, Imprinted at London By Thomas Creed, 1599. Original manuscript viewed on: http://archive.org/stream/englishmanstreas00vica#page/n9/mode/2up Accessed March 2013

Vadakan Vibul, *The Asphyxiating and Exsanguinating Death of President George Washington*, In: The Permanente Journal, Spring 2004, Volume 8, No. 2.

Vigarello Georges, *Concepts of Cleanliness: Changing Attitudes in France since the Middle Ages*, translated from French by Jean Birell, In: Cambridge Studies in Medieval Literature Past and Present Publications, Cambridge University Press 1988.

Von Hutten Ulrich, *Of the Wood Called Guaiacum*, trans. Paynel Tom, Berthelet, London 1540.

Von Klein Carl H., *The Medical Features of the Papyrus Ebers*, American Medical Association Press, Chicago 1905.

Von Staden Heinrich, *The Discovery of the Body: Human Dissection and Its Cultural Contexts in Ancient Greece*, In: The Yale Journal of Biology and Medicine 65 (1992), pp. 223-241.

Wagner Christiane, Failing Jutta, *Vielmals auf den Kopf gehacket – Galgen und Scharfrichter in Hessen,* Verlag M. Naumann, Hanau 2008.

Warner John Harley, Edmonson James, *Dissection: Photographs of a rite of passage in American medicine, 1880-1930*, Blast Books 2009.

Watts Sheldon J., *Epidemics and History: Disease, Power and Imperialism*, Yale University Press 1999.

Wallis Patrick, On: 'Bullein, William', In: *Oxford Dictionary of National Biography*, first published 2004.

Weeks A., *Paracelsus: Speculative Theory and the Crisis of the Early Reformation*, State University of New York Press, New York 1997.

Weiss-Krejci Estelle, *Restless Corpses – Secondary Burial in the Babenberg and Habsburg Dynasties*, In: Antiquity 75, 769-780, 2001.

White Charles, *Treatise on the Management of Pregnant and Lying-In Women*, Edward and Charles Dilly Printers, London 1773.

Wilson Adrian, *The Making of Man-Midwifery: Childbirth in England, 1660-1770*, Harvard University Press, 1995.

Wilson F. P., *The Plague in Shakespeare's London*, Oxford University Press, Oxford 1927.

Willughby Percivall, *Observations in Midwifery*, edited by Henry Blenkinsop, H.T. Crooke & Son, Warwick 1863.

Winslow Jacques-Bénigne, *The Uncertainty of the Signs of Death, and the Danger of Precipitate Interments and Dissections*, London 1746. Original manuscript viewed on: http://catalogue.nla.gov.au/Record/3207095 Accessed January 2014

Winslow, Charles-Edward Amory, *The Conquest of Epidemic Disease – A Chapter in the History of Ideas*, Wisconsin University Press, 1980.

Withington John, *A Disasterous History of the World: Chronicles of War, Earthquakes, Plague and Flood*, Hachette, London 2008.

Wittlin Alma, Stephanie, *Museums: in search of a usable future*, MIT Press, Virginia 1970.

Woolley Benjamin, *The Herbalist – Nicholas Culpeper and the fight for medical freedom*, Harper Perennial, London 2005.

Wright Thomas, *Homes of Other Days – A history of domestic manners and sentiments in England*, Trübner & Co., Paternoster Row, London 1871.

Young Sidney, *Annals of the Barber-Surgeons of London*, East and Blades Publishing, London, 1890. Original manuscript accessed March 2013 on: https://archive.org/details/annalsofbarbersuooyoun.

Zaner Richard M., *Death: Beyond Whole-Brain Criteria*, Kluwer Academic Publishers, Netherlands 1988.

Ziegler Philip, *The Black Death*, Harper Perennial Modern Classics, Harper Collins, London 2009.

ENDNOTES

Introduction

1. Crawfurd Raymond, *The Last Days of Charles II*, Claredon Press, Oxford 1909, p. 28-30.
2. Porter Roy, *The Greatest Benefit to Mankind – A Medical History of Humanity from Antiquity to the Present*, Harper Collins Publishing, London 1999, p. 12.

Chapter 1
Medical practitioners of the past

1. The thirteenth century English word 'physic', meaning 'medicine' or 'remedy', became *physician* from Latin *physica* meaning 'natural science' and *physicum* or *physicus*, denoting 'remedy'. The word 'doctor' is a Latin word meaning anyone who is a teacher, including those who have mastered theology, law, philosophy and medicine.
2. Marcus Aurelius (121-180) and his son Commodotus.
3. Ball Philip, *The Devil's Doctor – Paracelsus and the World of Renaissance, Magic and Science*, Farrar, Straus and Giroux, New York 2006, p. 54.
4. Quoted by Woolley Benjamin, *The Herbalist – Nicholas Culpeper and the fight for medical freedom*, Harper Perennial, London 2005, p. 46.
5. Rhodes Philip, *An Outline History of Medicine*, Cambridge University Press 1986, p. 20-21.
6. Woolley 2005, p. 39.
7. Chaucer Geoffrey, *The Canterbury Tales, A Complete Translation into Modern English* by Ronald Ecker and Eugene Crook, Hodge & Braddock Publishers 1993, General Prologue lines 413-46.
8. Woolley 2005, p. 40.
9. The word 'university' is derived from the Latin *universitas magistrorum et scholarium*, meaning 'community of teachers and scholars'. The term was coined by the University of Oxford 1096 – the oldest university in the English-speaking world. The origin of many medieval unversities is traceable to Christian monastic and cathedral schools, some of which appeared as early as the sixth century.
10. Leading medical schools were the Italian Universities of Bologna (founded in 1088 and considered the first university) and Padua, which began training physicians in 1219 and 1222 respectively; the Universities of Montpellier (formally founded in 1289) and Paris (founded in 1160); the University of Oxford (founded in 1096), the world's second oldest university, where medicine was taught since the thirteenth century, and the University of Cambridge 1209.
11. Modelled after the educational system advocated by the Parisian philosopher and theologian Peter Abelard around the year 1100 CE.
12. Abd Allāh ibn Sīnā commonly known by his Latinized name Avicenna, was a Persian

polymath. He wrote almost 450 treatises on a wide range of subjects, 40 of them on medicine. His most famous works are *The Book of Healing*, and *The Canon of Medicine*, which were standard medical texts at many medieval universities as late as 1650, providing a complete system of medicine according to the principles of Galen and Hippocrates.

13. Ball 2006, page 56.
14. Brody Nathaniel Samuel, *The Disease of the Soul – Leprosy in Medieval Literature*, Cornell University Press, London 1974, p. 43.
15. Ibid.
16. Rhodes 1985, p. 36.
17. Quoted in Ball 2006, p.57.
18. In *Astronomia Magna*, his major work on the subject of astrology.
19. Ball 2006, p. 238.
20. The practice of visual analysis of a patient's urine was based on the ancient 'catarrh theory' of disease. The name 'catarrh' derives from Hippocrates' use of *katarrhoos*, which refers to a 'flowing down' of humors from the head. Illness was thought to stem from 'vapours' ascending through the body from the stomach to the brain, where they condensed to mucous. From the brain this harmful, poisonous fluid was thought to flow down to the lungs and the joints, manifesting in a range of rheumatic symptoms, as well as coughing and fevers. Up to the seventeenth century, the Latin term *catarrhus* was used to define a 'cold' of the brain, producing large quantities of an unbalanced humor, that passed from the brain, through the palate to the lungs. In modern terminology 'catarrh' is regarded as an inflammation of the mucous membranes, especially of the air passages.
21. Hæger Knut, *The Illustrated History of Surgery*, revised by Sir Roy Calne, AB Nordbok, Gothenburg Sweden 2000, p. 79.
22. Quoted in Ball 2006, p.58.
23. Rhodes 1985, p. 36.
24. Online *Etymological Dictionary*.
25. Porter Roy, *The Greatest Benefit to Mankind – A Medical History of Humanity from Antiquity to the Present*, Harper Collins Publishing, London 1999, p. 116.
26. Furdell Elizabeth Lane, *The Royal Doctors: 1485-1714 – Medical Personnel at the Tudor and Stuart Courts*, University of Rochester Press 2001, p. 7.
27. Pagel Walter, *Paracelsus: An Introduction to Philosophical Medicine in the Era of the Renaissance*, Karger Medical and Scientific Publishers, 1982, p. 15.
28. Porter 1999, p. 187.
29. Ibid.
30. Giving rise to so-called 'laudable pus', which was erroneously thought to be a good sign of healing – a premise stemming from Hippocrates' theory on the treatment of wounds – a theory which remained influential for centuries.
31. He also introduced dressing wounds with clean bandages and ointments, and designed functional artificial hands, which looked perfectly natural under gloves. The artificial hands had two pairs of fingers , which could be moved for simple grabbing and releasing tasks.
32. Rhodes 1985, p. 51.
33. Membranes surrounding the brain.
34. Rawcliffe Carole, *Medicine and Society in Later Medieval England*, Sandpiper Publishers, New York 1999, p. 125.
35. Rhodes 1985, p. 36.
36. Moore Wendy, *The Knife Man – Blood, Body-Snatching and the Birth of Modern Surgery*, Bantam Press, London 2005, p. 103.

37. Ibid., p. 107-108.
38. Mukherjee Siddhartha, *The Emperor of all Maladies*, Fourth Estate, London 2011 p. 61-62.
39. Originally the pole featured a small brass basin – representing the vessel in which leeches were kept – at the top. Another basin at the bottom of the pole depicted the vessel, which received the patient's blood.
40. Merians Linda Evi, *The Secret Malady: Venereal disease in eighteenth-century Britain and France*, University Press of Kentucky 1996, p.23.
41. Porter 1999, p. 119.
42. Ibid.
43. Inside the anus are a number of small glands, which may become blocked, forming an abscess. An anal abscess is usually treated by surgical drainage. About fifty percent of these abscesses may develop into a fistula, in which a small tunnel connects the infected gland inside the anus to an opening on the skin around the anus. http://my.clevelandclinic.org/health/diseases_conditions/hic_anal_fistula
44. Richardson Ruth, *Death, Dissection and the Destitute*, University of Chicago Press, Chicago 2000, p. 35.
45. Under the patronage of King Henry VIII.
46. Its first master was Thomas Vicary (1490-1561), while William Clowes (1544-1603) was one of its most active members.
47. After surgery had been defined as a separate craft, an act was passed by Henry VIII in 1543, attacking surgeons for their 'small cunning', branding them as money-grabbers who tended to hurt and injure rather than cure their patients (Woolley 2005, p. 38). As an advocate for herbal medicine, the monarch, proceeded to protect the rights of herbalists to practice under an act, known as the 'Quack's Charter'. This meant that anyone with 'experience and knowledge' could perform the function of a surgeon, as long as the use of a scalpel was not required. Exactly who would determine the level of 'experience and knowledge' was left undetermined.
48. Woolley 2005, p. 36.
49. Ibid., p. 35.
50. Clark George Sir, *History of the Royal College of Physicians of London*, In: British Medical Journal, January 1965, p. 79.
51. Woolley 2005, p 36.
52. Clark 1965, p. 79.
53. Porter 1999, p. 288.
54. Clark 1965, p. 80.
55. Altogether the College published ten editions up until 1851.
56. Rawcliffe 1999, p. 148.
57. Porter 1999, p. 289.
58. In 1421, English physician Gilbert Kymer petitioned Parliament to ban women from practising medicine (Porter 1999, p. 129). Women were completely excluded from entry to the Royal College of Physicians of London until 1909, when a bylaw was passed allowing them to take examinations.
59. Woolley 2005, p. 9.
60. Porter 1999, p. 288.

Chapter 2
Humoral bodies – a healthy balance

1. Porter Roy, *The Greatest Benefit to Mankind – A Medical History of Humanity from Antiquity to the Present*, Harper Collins Publishing, London 1999, p.9.
2. Rhodes Philip, *An Outline History of Medicine*, Cambridge University Press 1986, p. 12.
3. Cameron M. L., *Anglo-Saxon Medicine*, Cambridge University Press, Cambridge 1993, p.159.
4. At the time he named them 'roots', the term 'element', having been ascribed to Plato.
5. Mukherjee Siddhartha, *The Emperor of all Maladies*, Fourth Estate, London 2011, p. 48.
6. Ibid.
7. Phlegm was a broad term for any colorless or whitish discharge, except semen and milk.
8. Yellow bile was thought to be the fluid found in the gallbladder.
9. Blood was linked to the liver, to spring and to a sanguine state of mind. The sanguineous personality was thought of as amorous, outgoing, and prone to optimism, a cheerful temperament and a wildness of spirit. Sanguine people were thought to have florid complexions from an excess of blood. Phlegm was linked to the spleen, to winter and to a phlegmatic state of mind. Phlegmatic personalities were calm, slow, and prone to apathy. As they were thought to be dominated by the phlegm humor, they were prone to watery swellings in the body. Yellow bile was linked to the gall bladder, to summer and a choleric state of mind, quick-witted, bold, energetic, querulous, and prone to anger. Quick of temper, cholerics tended to have red hair.
10. Porter 1999, p. 58.
11. Ibid.
12. King Helen, *The Disease of Virgins: Green Sickness, Chlorosis, and the Problems of Puberty*, Psychology Press, 2004, p. 58.
13. Chyle refers to a white milky body fluid formed from pancreatic juice and bile.
14. King 2004, p. 58-59.
15. Before Harvey's theory of circulation, the Galenic body was thought to contain veins, carrying food to nourish the body; and arteries originating from the heart that carried pneuma, although they were also thought to contain some blood. 'In addition to chyle, blood and pneuma, there are additional fluid components of the normal Galenic body which may appear in excessive quantities, making it necessary to intervene medically to remove them: normally the gall bladder purges the blood of yellow bile, the spleen removes black bile, and the kidneys remove water. Yellow bile and black bile are by-products of the process by which the liver converts chyle into blood' (King 2004, p. 58-59).
16. Meaning 'toxic'.
17. Humoral theory could not explain epidemics such as malaria, cholera and the Black Death. These were ascribed to poisonous vapours or *miasma* a noxious form of 'bad air'. Miasmic theory, the substantial change in air quality, was first advocated by Hippocratic writers and further advanced by Galen.
18. Porter 1999, p. 57.
19. Ibid., p. 117.
20. As opposed to this practice, renowned French surgeon Henri de Mondeville (1260-1316) recommended the gentle bathing of wounds, followed by dry dressings. He encouraged healing without pus formation, an approach which met with much opposition from supporters of conventional wound salves: plasters and powders designed to promote suppuration.
21. Mukherjee Siddhartha, *The Emperor of all Maladies*, Fourth Estate, London 2011, p. 53.
22. Ibid.

Chapter 3
Phlebotomy, purges and other medical marvels

1. Numerous and varied are the beliefs surrounding this vital body fluid. Believed to contain the life force and essence of humans and animals, as well as the soul, blood has for thousands of years been used in all major religious rites for sacrificial purposes. It has also been employed in magic, witchcraft and folk medicine. Bloodshed in sacrifice symbolises human or animal life being given back to God its creator. In ancient times the offering of sacrificial blood was the most holy covenant between man and God, which is why Moses ritually purified his people by sprinkling them with the blood of sacrificed animals. The tradition of pouring sacrificial blood directly onto the ground, so that the Earth Mother could reabsorb the life force, or of sprinkling blood on an altar, was once common to all cultures. Over millennia the concept of blood has become incorporated in our social attitudes, our language and especially in common phrases. Hence, we speak of 'cold-blooded' murder, 'bad blood' being the result of quarrels and feuds, anger making a man's 'blood boil', a particularly amorous person being 'hot-blooded', aristocracy as 'blue-blooded' and inherited characteristics as 'running in the blood' (Stapelberg Monica-Maria, *Strange But True – a historical background to popular beliefs and traditions*, Crux Publishing, London 2014, p. 212).

2. Porter Roy, *The Greatest Benefit to Mankind – A Medical History of Humanity from Antiquity to the Present*, Harper Collins Publishing, London 1999, p. 57.

3. Ibid., p. 77.

4. The definition of phlebotomy is 'bloodletting as a medical operation' (*The Concise Oxford Dictionary*). Venesection is the practice of 'cutting a vein'. In modern times the term 'phlebotomy' defines the practice of drawing or 'collecting' blood, with a syringe, for diagnostic rather than therapeutic reasons.

5. Porter 1999, p. 77.

6. Ibid.

7. Brain Peter, *Galen on Bloodletting: A Study of the Origins, Development, and Validity of His Opinions, with a Translation of the Three Works*, Cambridge University Press, 1986, p. 86.

8. Ibid.

9. Rhodes Philip, *An Outline History of Medicine*, Cambridge University Press 1986, p. 37.

10. Hall Marshall, *The Morbid and Curative Effects of Loss of Blood*, E.L. Carey & A. Hart, Philadelphia, 1830, p. 166.

11. Cameron M. L., *Anglo-Saxon Medicine*, Cambridge University Press, Cambridge 1993, p.165.

12. Porter 1999, p. 133.

13. Saunders J. B. and O'Malley D., *The Illustrations from the Works of Andreas Vesalius of Brussels*, Dover Publications, New York 1950, p. 15.

14. Vesalius, a budding humanist, accepted the Greek view, which led him into a fiery and intemperate dispute with Thriverius Brachelius (1504-1554)' (Saunders 1950, p. 15), who had written two comprehensive works on bloodletting, which supported Arabic practice.

15. The first to speak out on what was termed the true Hippocratic and Galenical technique of bloodletting was Paris physician Pierre Brissot. He based his standpoint on the successful treatment of pleurisy patients during an epidemic of 1514. He contended that since pleurisy existed in a part of the body drained by the vena cava, it did not matter whether blood was let from the right or the left side. Moreover, opening a vein of the arm on the affected side of the body, would still preserve sufficient remoteness in the Hippocratic sense. As a result, Brissot was bitterly attacked by the conservative element, and eventually two camps

were formed, engaging in a violent polemic over the question (Saunders 1950, p. 17-18).

16. One UK pint equals 0.568 litres.

17. Crawfurd Raymond, *The Last Days of Charles II*, Claredon Press, Oxford 1909, p. 28.

18. The amount of 8 ounces of blood equals 236.6 ml.

19. Crawfurd 1909, p. 28.

20. Hæger Knut, *The Illustrated History of Surgery*, revised by Sir Roy Calne, AB Nordbok, Gothenburg Sweden 2000, p. 123.

21. Ibid., p. 130.

22. Quoted in: Magner Lois N., *A History of Medicine*, CRC Press, Florida USA, 1992, *p. 218.*

23. Vadakan Vibul, *The Asphyxiating and Exsanguinating Death of President George Washington*, In: The Permanente Journal, Spring 2004, Volume 8, No. 2, p. 76.

24. Cantharidin (from Greek *kantharis*, meaning beetle) is a powerful irritant and blister-inducing substance obtained from blister beetles. Various blister beetles, including 'Spanish Fly', were popularly used in the past by apothecaries. The main irritant in Spanish Fly is cantharidin, which was first isolated in 1810 by French chemist Pierre Robiquet. He found that cantharidin had poisenous properties comparable to those of stychnine.

25. Vadakan 2004, p.76.

26. Ibid., p. 79.

27. Ibid.

28. Hall 1830, p. 153.

29. Ibid., p. 145.

30. Ibid., p. 147.

31. Ibid., p. 153.

32. Ibid., p. 160.

33. Ibid., p. 154.

34. Ibid., p. 152.

35. Mukherjee Siddhartha, *The Emperor of all Maladies*, Fourth Estate, London 2011, p. 61-62.

36. Ibid.

37. Bloodletting through leeching meant the attachment of annelid worms, of the species *Hirudo medicinalis*, to the patient. Leeches remove old blood and at the same time inject anticoagulating, vasodilating substances. Hirudin, the potent thrombin inhibitor of leech saliva, has been cloned and is used in modern times in the treatment of cardiological and hematological disorders.

38. In Egypt, the tomb of the scribe Userhat (1567-1308 BCE) depicts the application of leeches to a patient. The oldest known written account describing the application of leeches, is by a Greek named Nicander (died 135 BCE). In this account he explains how blood-sucking 'worms' were applied to specific body-parts containing excess blood.

39. 'Leechcraft' became synonymous with Anglo-Saxon medicine and denoted the art of healing in general. Several works of leechcraft survive from Anglo-Saxon times (512-1154 CE) in England, among them the *Herbarium Apuleius* (480-1050 CE), one of the most copied herbal manuscripts, containing recipes and uses of over 100 herbs. The *Herbarium Apuleius* is available in modern English. Also available in modern English is the *Leechbook of Bald* (925 CE).

40. Hæger 2000, p. 128.

41. After his death, his portrait was hung in the National Gallery and a proposal was put forward to erect a statue of Morison in front of the British College of Health. The idea was however 'nipped in the bud' by the magazine *Punch*, with the suggestion that a large brass plaque should instead be installed in the English graveyard filled with the largest number of patients killed by Morison's pills.

42. Woolley Benjamin, *The Herbalist – Nicholas Culpeper and the fight for medical freedom*, Harper Perennial, London 2005, p. 64.
43. Ibid., p. 67.
44. Kerridge IH, Lowe M., *Bloodletting: The story of a therapeutic technique*, Medical Journal of Australasia 1995, No. 163, pp. 631-633.
45. Ibid.
46. Morabia A. P.C.A. Louis, *The birth of clinical epidemiology*, In: Journal of Clinical Epidemiology 1996, No. 49, pp. 1327-1333.

Chapter 4
Opening up the dead – a dismembered history

1. From Latin *dissecare*, 'to cut to pieces'.
2. Von Staden Heinrich, *The Discovery of the Body: Human Dissection and Its Cultural Contexts in Ancient Greece*, In: The Yale Journal of Biology and Medicine 65 (1992), p. 241)
3. The belief in the power of the corpse as a source of contamination was deeply ingrained in ancient Greece. According to their sacred laws, the human corpse was seen as a major source of pollution for all who came into contact with it. Therefore, all people and objects, thought to have been contaminated by the corpse, had to undergo extensive purification rites, following the burial of a corpse.
4. Specific cultural perceptions of human skin and cutting through the skin were extant at the time. The skin was seen as symbolising the wholeness and integrity of an individual, who might otherwise be at risk of dissolution or fragmentation. ' It is significant that, with a few notable exceptions, the skin is the only part of the sacrificial victim that is neither burnt as a gift to the gods nor eaten by the human participants in the sacrifice. After sacrifice, the skin remains behind, either on display in a temple or other public space, or in the hands of a priest' (Von Staden 1992, p. 228). The skin was seen as a sacred reflection of the body held within. In other words, both internal physical disorder and moral pollution was thought to be physically apparent on the skin. This is why for centuries, skin diseases were seen as manifestations of moral or religious pollution that could be symbolically 'washed' away through purification. Hippocratic writers pointed to healthy skin as a sign of a well-ordered body. Hence, to forcibly violate the skin, by cutting into it was to 'interfere with the surface version both of the physical and of the moral condition of a person' (Von Staden 1992, p. 228). But what were the reasons provoking Herophilus and Erasistratus to breach such deeply entrenched beliefs and cultural mores? At the time of Herophilus and Erasistratus two schools of philosophy were extant in Athens: Stoicism and Epicureanism. Although representing opposing traditions on most issues, both schools of thought agreed that all creatures, animate and inanimate, were nothing but matter or 'void'. Even the soul, which Aristotle had still identified as 'the form that is always joined to matter, now is constructed as being nothing but matter of a certain kind or in a certain state. According to both Stoics and Epicureans, neither death nor the corpse is to be feared: death is simply either a change in the state of matter or a rearrangement of matter' (Von Staden 1992, p 233). Hence so-called Rationalists justified human dissection by claiming that the causes of diseases of the internal organs should be investigated.
5. Von Staden 1992, p. 223.
6. From around 1250, autopsies had become customary in Italian, French and German towns, with surgeons called in to investigate homicide and to establish cause of death

(Porter p. 132) – the step from post-mortem to dissection was small.

7. The first Crusade proclaimed by Pope Urban II took place in 1095. After two centuries of conflict for control of the Holy Land, the mission ended in failure with the last crusade taking place in 1291.

8. Mafart B., Pelletier J., Fixot M., *Post-mortem Ablation of the Heart: A Medieval Funerary Practice*, In: International Journal of Osteo-Archaeology Vol. 14, 2004, pp. 67-73.

9. He decreed that death on Christian soil was to be followed by burial – remains were not to be exhumed until the flesh had naturally disappeared into the earth.

10. The practice however continued amongst royalty and nobles. The kings of France starting with Philip the Fair (1268-1314) obtained special consideration for themselves and all family members, for this practice, from each newly elected Pope. English kings similarly continued the custom. For example, when King Henry V of England died at Vincennes near Paris in 1422, his corpse was cut up and boiled before being returned to England. Another example is Louis IX of France. After his death during the crusades in 1216, his entrails were entombed in a church in Sicily, while his skeleton – obtained by boiling the dismembered body, and his ablated heart, were returned home to France. Edward I (1239-1307), wished for his heart to be embalmed after death and taken to the Holy Land, whereas his body was to be dismembered, then boiled, and the bones carried into Scotland on his last campaign. Similarly, when Robert the Bruce, King of Scotland, died in 1329, his body was buried in Dunfermline after excision of the heart. In keeping with the king's last request, James Douglas, his comrade-in-arms, took the heart on crusade to the Holy Land. Although Douglas was killed in battle in 1330, Robert's heart was returned and buried at Melrose Abbey in Scotland. (Stapelberg Monica-Maria, *Strange But True – a historical background to popular beliefs and traditions*, Crux Publishing, London 2014, p. 205)

11. Rhodes Philip, *An Outline History of Medicine*, Cambridge University Press 1986, p. 34.

12. Nutton Vivian, Logic, *Learning, and Experimental Medicine*, In: Science, Vol. 295, No 5556, 2002, pp. 800-801.

13. Bologna clearly led the way with the first public dissection taking place around 1315; in Spain, the first public dissection occurred in 1404; in Germany anatomy teaching using human corpses did not become customary before the 1550's (Porter Roy, *The Greatest Benefit to Mankind – A Medical History of Humanity from Antiquity to the Present*, Harper Collins Publishing, London 1999, p. 133). In England, public dissections were performed at the University of Oxford from 1549 onwards, and at Cambridge, Caius College, since 1565.

14. One of the main historical rooms of the Bologna medical school – a grand anatomical theatre – was housed in the Archiginnasio of Bologna. This was once the main building of the University completed around 1563. In 1638 it was replaced by a bigger theatre, completely made of spruce wood. This theate underwent several modification and reached its final shape between 1733 and 1736, decorated with the carved wooden statues of renowned physicians.

15. Ferrari Giovanna, *Public Anatomy Lessons and the Carnival: The Anatomy Theatre of Bologna*, In: Past and Present 117, 1987, p. 12.

16. It had to be completely rebuilt following bombings during WW2 in 1943.

17. Public anatomy lessons were held at carnival time: In Pisa from 1544 onwards until the early eighteenth century; in Rome until the late seventeenth century, and thereafter during Lent; in Ferrara at least from 1600 onwards; in Turin at least from 1729 onwards; in Padua public anatomy lessons were held either at Christmas or during the carnival during the sixteenth and seventeenth centuries (Ferrari 1997, p. 168).

18. Porter 1999, p. 133.
19. Quoted in Ferrari 1987, p. 199.
20. Ferrari 1987, p. 51.
21. Moore Wendy, *The Knife Man – Blood, Body-Snatching and the Birth of Modern Surgery*, Bantam Press, London 2005, p. 76.
22. The Renaissance began in Italy and is estimated to lie between 1400 and 1700.
23. Ferrari 1987, p. 98.
24. Ball Philip, *The Devil's Doctor – Paracelsus and the World of Renaissance, Magic and Science*, Farrar, Straus and Giroux, New York 2006, p. 67.
25. Gatrell V.A.C., *The Hanging Tree – Execution and the English people 1770-1868*, Oxford University Press, Oxford 1994.
26. Sawday Jonathan, *The Body Emblazoned*, Routledge Publishing 2013.
27. At public executions it was not so much the physical elimination of the convict that counted, as the excessive dimension of the punishment inflicted. Chronicles describe executions, which included horrific tortures, additional forms of bodily mutilation such as amputations and other operations – analogous to those carried out during anatomical dissection – performed on the convict prior to his death as an integral part of the punishment.
28. Woolley Benjamin, *The Herbalist – Nicholas Culpeper and the fight for medical freedom*, Harper Perennial, London 2005, p. 46.
29. Ibid., p. 47.
30. Ferrari 1987, p. 88.
31. Ibid.
32. Ibid., p. 90.
33. Lassek A. M., *Human Dissection – Its Drama and Struggle*, Charles Thomas Publishing, Illinois USA 1958, p. 75.
34. Ibid.
35. Porter 1999, p. 133.
36. Lassek 1958, p. 75.
37. Ibid.
38. Ibid.
39. Porter 1999, p. 133.
40. Ibid.
41. Saunders J. B. and O'Malley D., *The Illustrations from the Works of Andreas Vesalius of Brussels*, Dover Publications, New York 1950, p. 22-23.
42. First in the Ambrosian Library in Milan and later in the Royal Library in Windsor.
43. Saunders 1950, p. 22-23.
44. Ibid., p. 14.
45. Ibid.
46. Ibid., p.12
47. A vault or building in which human skeletal remains were housed.
48. Mukherjee Siddhartha, *The Emperor of all Maladies*, Fourth Estate, London 2011, p. 53.
49. Saunders 1950, p.13.
50. Ibid.
51. Hæger Knut, *The Illustrated History of Surgery*, revised by Sir Roy Calne, AB Nordbok, Gothenburg Sweden 2000, p. 117.
52. Moore 2005, p. 118
53. The first sterilised medical gloves were used in 1890 by William Halsted, while disposable latex medical gloves were initially manufactured in 1964.

54. Warner John Harley, Edmonson James, Dissection: *Photographs of a rite of passage in American medicine, 1880-1930*, Blast Books 2009.
55. Moore 2005, p. 118.
56. Ibid., p. 119.
57. Richardson Ruth, *Death, Dissection and the Destitute*, University of Chicago Press, Chicago 2000, p. 31.
58. Ibid.

Chapter 5
Surgeons and the gallows – a spectacle of suffering

1. MacDonald Helen, *Human Remains – Dissection and its Histories*, Yale University Press, London 2006, p. 2.
2. Linebaugh Peter, *The Tyburn Riot Against Surgeons*, In: Albion's Fatal Tree: Crime and Society in Eighteenth Century England, Pantheon Books, New York 1975, p. 69.
3. Whilst executions for murder and robbery were common, and death sentences could be passed for picking pockets or stealing food, these sentences for minor offenders were often not carried out. During that time 35,000 death sentences were handed down in England and Wales. Of these 'only' 7000 executions (Gatrell V.A.C., *The Hanging Tree – Execution and the English people 1770-1868*, Oxford University Press, Oxford 1994, p.7) took place – men and women hanged amongst jeering crowds on public scaffolds. At the end of the eighteenth century the number of people hung for petty crimes was causing public unrest and in 1823, Sir Robert Peel reduced the number of offences resulting in capital punishment by over 100.
4. Death sentences for minor offenders were often not carried out. Statistics for the rate of executions over the centuries in England are difficult to determine with any degree of accuracy. Nevertheless, according to some estimates an alarmingly high number of people died on the scaffold right through to the 1820's (Gatrell 1994, p.8).
5. Moore Wendy, *The Knife Man – Blood, Body-Snatching and the Birth of Modern Surgery*, Bantam Press, London 2005, p. 79.
6. Hobbes Thomas, Curley Edwin M., *Leviathan: With Selected Variant from the Latin Edition of 1868*, Editor: Edwin M. Curley, Hackett Publishing, London 1994, p. 76.
7. Adams Norman, *Dead and Buried: The Horrible History of Body Snatching*, Bell Publishing Company, New York 1972, p. 12.
8. Richardson Ruth, *Death, Dissection and the Destitute*, University of Chicago Press, Chicago 2000, p. 53.
9. *Barber Surgeon's Company Records* in *Annals of the Barber-Surgeons of London* 1890, S. Young 1890.
10. Moore 2005, p. 77.
11. Linebaugh 1975, p. 68.
12. Gatrell V.A.C., 1994.
13. Richardson 2000, p. 37.
14. Ibid., p. 109.
15. Anatomisation, from Greek *anatomia*, 'to cut up'.
16. The bodies of murderers were either gibbeted – hung in chains until all flesh had rotted away – or anatomised. Some criminals however preferred the latter option to the indignity of rotting in chains. In larger towns the place of execution differed from where bodies were gibbeted i.e. exposed after death – the public excution serving as a deterrent to a

towns inhabitants, while bodies hung in chains outside the towns were seen as a warning to all who entered. In modern times it is difficult to imagine such conditions, but in the past a familiarity with decaying bodies desensitised towns' inhabitants with regard to the horrific site, as well as smell and hygiene.

17. *Political Anecdotist* of 1831, No 3, 2.7.1831.
18. Linebaugh 1975, p. 79-80.
19. Mass executions at Tyburn were common, and sometimes up to twenty-three convicts were 'turned-off' the carts all at once (Moore 2005, p. 78).
20. Richardson 1978, p. 127.
21. Ferrari Giovanna, *Public Anatomy Lessons and the Carnival: The Anatomy Theatre of Bologna*, In: Past and Present 117, 1987, p. 60.
22. Spierenburg Pieter, *The Spectacle of Suffering – Executions and the Evolution of Repression: From a pre-industrial metropolis to the European experience*, Cambridge University Press, Cambridge 1984, p. 90.
23. Stapelberg Monica-Maria, *Strange But True – a historical background to popular beliefs and traditions*, Crux Publishing, London 2014, p. 196.
24. Linebaugh 1978, p. 102.
25. *Proceedings from the Old Bailey, London Criminal Court: Ordinary's Account*, 26th July 1736, *Ordinary's Account*, 26th July 1736.
26. In the early part of the nineteenth century the 'New Drop Gallows' was standardised, making certain that the condemned felon fell at least one foot. This ensured a somewhat 'quicker' death – that is if struggling for several agonising minutes after the drop fell, could be defined as such. After falling only one foot, death was still typically by strangulation, with the executioner often having to hang onto the prisoner's legs for some time.
27. Sawday Jonathan, *The Body Emblazoned*, Routledge Publishing 2013, p. 61.
28. Taylor Joseph, *The Danger of Premature Interment*, London 1816, p. 62-63.
29. Adams 1972, p. 20-25.
30. Moore 2005, p. 81.
31. *Lancet* 261, 1951, pp. 1222-1224.

Chapter 6
Resurrectionists and anatomists – a 'grave' alliance

1. See Chapter 1 – Medical practitioners of the past
2. MacDonald Helen, *Human Remains – Dissection and its Histories*, Yale University Press, London 2006, p. 28.
3. Moore Wendy, *The Knife Man – Blood, Body-Snatching and the Birth of Modern Surgery*, Bantam Press, London 2005, p. 73.
4. Moore 2005, p. 72.
5. Ibid., p. 25.
6. MacDonald 2006, p. 11.
7. Body snatching for anatomy purposes was however not new. As early as the fourteenth century, Pope Boniface VIII excommunicated body-snatchers and condemned anatomy as a practice abominable to both God and humankind.
8. Adams Norman, *Dead and Buried: The Horrible History of Body Snatching*, Bell Publishing Company, New York 1972, p. 1.
9. Ferrari Giovanna, *Public Anatomy Lessons and the Carnival: The Anatomy Theatre of Bologna*, In: Past and Present 117, 1987, p. 60.

10.   Gray Earnest, *The Diary of a Surgeon in the Year 1751- 1752*, Apple Century Company, New York 1937, p. 35.

11.   Bailey James Blake, *The Diary of a Resurrectionist 1811-1812*, Swan Sonnenschein & Co., London 1896, p.61-62.

12.   Moore 2005, p. 89.

13.   Shelton Don, *The Real Mr. Frankenstein – Sir Anthony Carlisle, Medical Murders and the Social Genesis of Frankenstein,* available as ebook only, *p. 128.*

14.   Moore 2005, p. 90.

15.   Ibid., p. 90.

16.   Lassek A. M., *Human Dissection – Its Drama and Struggle*, Charles Thomas Publishing, Illinois USA 1958, p. 119.

17.   *Moore 2005, p. 74.*

18.   Moore 2005, p. 118.

19.   Bailey 1896, p.59.

20.   In the past it was a customary sign of mourning to toll the 'passing or soul bell'. This bell announced someone's demise, thus ensuring the prayers of all Christian people. The sounds of the 'soul bell' were also thought to frighten away all those evil spirits ever on the ready to molest and terrify the soul in its passage to the hereafter. Because the ringing of this specific bell protected the soul of the deceased it was called the 'soul bell' (Stapelberg Monica-Maria, *Curious and Curiouser – A background to some fascinating beliefs and traditions,* Multi-Media Publications, Canada 2011, p.66).

21.   Bailey 1896, p. 40.

22.   Ibid., p.65-68.

23.   Adams 1972, p. 82.

24.   Ibid, p. 84.

25.   Darwin F. (ed.), *Charles Darwin; His Life Told in an Autobiographical Chapter, And in a Selected Series of His Published Letters*, London 1892, p. 22.

26.   Lassek 1958, p. 182.

27.   Richardson Ruth, *Death, Dissection and the Destitute*, University of Chicago Press, Chicago 2000, p. 102.

28.   Moore 2005, p. 94.

29.   Ibid., p. 92.

30.   Ibid., p. 95.

31.   Bailey 1896, p. 48.

32.   The serious concern for grave robbing was not new and is evident from the 1615 epithet on William Shakespeare's tombstone: *Good friend, for Iesus sake forebeare To digge the dust enclosed heare. Bleste be ye man spares these stones, And curste be he moves my bones.*

33.   *Richardson 2000, p. 7.*

34.   Traditional post-mortem observances embodied the belief that customs practiced or enacted by survivors of the departed could affect the dead person's soul in their passage to the afterlife – this being a vague notion of intermediate purgatory or limbo between death and judgement. In accordance with such beliefs, the closing of the eyes and the mouth was done soon after death – often a Bible was propped under the chin until *rigor mortis* had set in. Then the body was washed, symbolising a baptism for the next life and dressed in grave-clothes or a shroud. In England the custom of corpse dressing with sprigs of rosemary, to signify love, was observed for hundreds of years. Another custom to be observed was the practice of orientation: The arms were placed cross-wise over the chest; the legs straightened and ankles often tied together to prevent the dead from 'walking'. Usually the corpse was positioned feet facing the door – hence the saying 'they carried

him out feet first'. (Stapelberg Monica-Maria, *Strange But True – a historical background to popular beliefs and traditions*, Crux Publishing, London 2014, p. 193-194).

35. Adams 1972, p.

36. Bailey 1896, p. ix.

37. Adams 1972, p. 88.

38. It should be pointed out that Dr. Knox was not only a brilliant anatomist but also extremely popular amongst his students. A highly controversial man on the Edinburgh medical scene, he would sneer and jibe at rival teachers during lectures. But, he expected his students to have the best and once unflinchingly paid £800 out of his own pocket to ensure a steady supply of cadavers. As a result, attendance rate for his classes was between 300 and 400 students – and when the number reached 500 it was the 'largest anatomical class ever to gather in Britain' (Adams 1972, p. 103).

39. Adams 1972, p. 94.

40. MacDonald 2006, p. 33.

41. Ibid., p. 33.

42. *Political Anecdotist* No 3, 2.7.1831.

43. Richardson 2000, p. 95.

44. Jeremy Bentham was an English author, jurist, philosopher as well as a legal and social reformer. He is best known for his advocacy of utilitarianism. He argued for individual and economic freedom, the separation of church and state, freedom of expression, equal rights for women, the decriminalising of homosexual acts, the abolition of slavery, and was also an early advocate of animal rights.

45. Adams 1972, p. 3.

46. Richardson 2000, p. 64.

47. It took John Hunter some thirty years to amass his collection of 65,000 anatomical, embryological and pathological preparations – most of which were destroyed during WW II. The restored preparations are on public display in the Royal College of Surgeons.

48. Moore 2005, p. 26.

49. Hæger Knut, *The Illustrated History of Surgery*, revised by Sir Roy Calne, AB Nordbok, Gothenburg Sweden 2000, p. 155.

Chapter 7
Sewer pharmacology – filthy medicine

1. In addition, many superstitious beliefs connected to animal dung still abound worldwide: smeared on various body parts it is believed to promote bodily hair in puberty, used to treat skin lesions and burns or applied as a remedy against baldness.

2. Proverbs 5:15.

3. Urine, was known as: the 'soma' beverage, the 'mother of medicine', the 'water of life', the 'living water' within, 'life's elixir', the 'water of Shiva', and the 'water of a thousand flowers'.

4. In sympathetic magic the effective principle is that 'like cures like' or 'like influences like'. Therefore, anything regarded as evil may be used to repel evil. For instance, during the Middle Ages, in times of plague, it was firmly believed that any poisonous substance such as arsenic, carried on one's person, would draw unto it the contagious air thought responsible for the spread of the plague. Another more current example can be found in a CNN report of 9 June 2014 titled: 'Albino activist fights witchcraft murders'. The news item relates that in Tanzania and other African countries, where little is known about the

genetic disorder affecting albinos, atrocities committed against them are still prevalent. In Tanzania alone, dozens of albinos have been mutilated and slaughtered in recent years, their limbs hacked off and used in potions or magic rituals to bring 'good luck'. The news item further states that traditionally, albinos in African societies are viewed with great superstition, regarded as demons, ghostlike evil beings, or spirits. It is most likely that because albinos are regarded as fundamentally 'evil' by these societies, witchdoctors use their body parts to repel evil – hence inviting good fortune or 'luck'. Similarly, vile excretions may have been used by the ancients to drive away evil forces responsible for illness and disease (Stapelberg Monica-Maria, *Strange But True – a historical background to popular beliefs and traditions*, Crux Publishing, London 2014, p. 3).

5. From the Papyrus Ebers, c. 1500 BC.
6. Magical properties have always been ascribed to human urine, worldwide. During the Middle Ages the urine of those claiming to have been bewitched was used to try witches. So-called 'witch-cakes' were baked with the urine of someone believed to be bewitched and this would cause the evil to be reverted back to the witch. Human urine was supposed to be imbued with hidden virtues. Spitting into one's urine or washing the hands in urine was regarded as a sure way of keeping evil forces at bay. In Scotland it was customary to sprinkle cattle and livestock once yearly with urine for protection against evil forces. On New Year's Day it was customary in some parts of Britain during the early nineteenth century, to sprinkle the whole family with urine for good luck! (Stapelberg Monica-Maria, *Old Wives' Tales? A select background to the origins of popular beliefs, traditions and superstitions*, Zeus Publishing, Australia 2005, p. 302).
7. Armstrong John W., *The Water of Life*, Health Research Books, 2000. p.14.
8. Bourke John G., *Scatalogic Rites of all Nations*, Kessinger Publishing, Montana USA 2003, p. 279. (Originally published as *Notes and Memoranda Bearing upon the Use of Human Ordure and Human Urine*, 1888.)
9. Galen writes that Xenocrates lived in the second generation before himself. Xenocrates is quoted several times by Galen, and also by Clement of Alexandria, Pliny, Aëtius and Alexander of Tralles.
10. Bourke 2003, p. 290.
11. Ibid., p 293-294.
12. Ibid., p. 286-290.
13. Pliny, *Natural History*, Translated by H. Rackham, W.H.S. Jones, D.E. Eichholz, 10 volume edition, Harvard University Press, Massachusetts 1949, Book XXVIII, section LI.
14. Ibid., Book XXVIII, section XVIII..
15. Ibid., Book XXII, section LVIII.
16. Ibid., Book XXVIII, section XVIII.
17. Ibid., Book XXVIII, section XVIII.
18. Suskind Patrick, *Perfume: The Story of a Murderer*, Penguin, London 2007, p.3.
19. Culpeper Nicholas, *Pharmacopoeia Londinensis* or *The London Dispensatory*, Royal College of Physicians of London, originally published 1649, p. 209.
20. Ibid., p. 76-77.
21. Ibid.
22. Ibid., p. 77.
23. Ibid., p. 206.
24. Ibid., p. 77.
25. Ibid.
26. Ibid., p. 209.
27. Bourke 2003, p. 303.

28. Quincy John, *Complete English Dispensatory* or *Pharmacopoia Offininalis and Extemporanea*, London 1730, p.307.
29. Ibid., p.111.
30. Ibid., p.249.
31. Also referred to as *Pharmacopoia Offininalis and Extemporanea.*
32. Schmidt Joseph, *Holy and Unholy Shit*, In: *Fecal Matters in Early Modern Literature and Art: Studies in Scatology*, Jeff Persels and Russell Ganim (editors), Ashgate Publishing, Michigan 2004, p. 109.
33. Bourke 2003, p. 298-299.
34. Ibid.
35. Ibid.
36. Also known as the *Therapeutic Faecal Pharmacy.*
37. Schmidt 2004, p. 113.
38. Another interesting discovery regarding this subject matter was made at 'Pusan National University' in South Korea and reported in the *New Scientist Magazine* in November 2008. Researchers found that the excrement of the musk-rat contains a potent antibiotic that can kill *salmonella* bacteria, as well as the *vibrio* bacteria, which are a common cause of food poisoning.
39. According to clinical studies documented in the medical research report *Immuno-Stimulation by Bacillus Subtilis Preparations*, by micro-biologist J. Harmann, cell wall components of ingested *bacillus subtilis* activate nearly all systems of the human immune defense.
40. 'British officers serving in the Sahara during World War II observed Arabs urinating on the open wounds of British soldiers. At first the British officers were shocked and interpreted the action as gross insubordination and an offence to flag and country. But these actions were actually a way of cleaning and sterilising wounds, developed by people who rarely have access to plentiful water. And it is still used today' (Root-Bernstein Robert and Michèle, *Honey, Mud, Maggots and Other Medicinal Marvels*, Macmillan Publishers, London 1999, p. 122.). Amongst the Aztecs the use of urine to clean wounds was widely advocated in their medical texts. Similarly, Meriwether Lewis and William Clark wrote in 1806, when on their expedition to map the North-West Territories that various American Indian tribes washed themselves in urine every morning although they also bathed in springs and rivers (Root-Bernstein Robert and Michèle, *Honey, Mud, Maggots and Other Medicinal Marvels*, Macmillan Publishers, London 1999, p. 122.) As is widely known, Indian culture confers a special place to the cow, and regards it as a veritable medical dispensary. Cow dung is still used in modern times as manure to produce the best quality grains, fruits, and vegetables, while cow urine is regarded as 'divine medicine', also used as a natural pesticide for crops. Although this seems bizarre in a modern age, some studies, such as *Antioxidant and Antimicrobial Activities of Cow Urine* (Jarald Edwin, Sheeja Edwin, Vaibhav Tiwari, 2008, *Antioxidant and Antimicrobial Activities of Cow Urine*, In: Global Journal of Pharmacology 2 (2): 20-22, 2008) and *Antimicrobial Activities of Cow Urine Distillate against some Clinical Pathogens* (Sathansivam Arunkumar et al 2010, *Antimicrobial Activities of Cow Urine Distillate against some Clinical Pathogens*, In: Global Journal of Pharmacology 4 (1): 41-44, 2010) published in the Global Journal of Pharmacology have shown that cow urine does in fact have anti-bacterial, anti-fungal and antioxidant properties, as well as immune-modulator characteristics. In modern times forms of urea are commonly used as humectants in cosmetics, and also as preservatives in hypoallergenic products. Urea is also the principal source of nitrogen for fertilisers. Urea is a chemical component found in urine, although it is also made artificially. 'Urea

is officially described as a buffering agent, humectant, and skin-conditioning agent-humectant for use in cosmetic products, there is a report stating that Urea also is used in cosmetics for its desquamating and antimicrobial action. In 2001, the Food and Drug Administration (FDA) reported that Urea was used in 239 formulations.' (*Final Report of the Safety Assessment of Urea*, In: PubMed, 2005;24, Suppl 3:1-56).

41. It seems that not only were physicians of the past on the right track with their disgusting medications, but the practice is finding a modern resurgence. A recent newspaper headline in the London *Daily Mail* confirms and expounds on the latest research into this yucky matter: 'Doctors treat patients' super bug infections with transplant of feces from a healthy relative'. This fecal transplant procedure involves taking a stool sample from a healthy person, mixing it with saline and transferring it into the colon of someone infected with the superbug *Clostridium difficile*. "The technique helps restore the natural balance of bacteria in the gut, U.S scientists told a meeting at the American College of Gastroenterology in Washington"' (London *Daily Mail*, 2 November 2011). *Clostridium difficile* is a very nasty bacterium, which has become more virulent over the last decade and is speedily developing resistance to antibiotics. The bacterium poses a significant problem in hospitals and nursing homes.

Chapter 8
Corpse medicine – medical cannibalism

1. Sugg Richard, *Mummies Cannibals and Vampires – The History of Corpse Medicine from the Renaissance to the Victorians*, Routledge Group, London 2011, p. 1.

2. Gordon-Grube Karen, *Anthropophagy in Post-Renaissance Europe: The Tradition of Medicinal Cannibalism*, American Anthropologist 90, 1988, p. 406.

3. Quincy John, *Complete English Dispensatory or Pharmacopoia Offininalis and Extemporanea*, London 1730, p. 232.

4. Ibid., p. 43.

5. Ibid., p. 476.

6. Ibid., p. 482.

7. Ibid., pp. 485, 593.

8. Ibid., p. 623.

9. Ferrari Giovanna, *Public Anatomy Lessons and the Carnival: The Anatomy Theatre of Bologna*, In: Past and Present 117, 1987, p. 102.

10. Wagner Christiane, Failing Jutta, *Vielmals auf den Kopf gehacket – Galgen und Scharfrichter in Hessen*. Verlag M. Naumann, Hanau 2008, p. 130.

11. Macbeth, Act 4, Scene 1.

12. Early editions of the *Pharmacopoeia Londinensis* issued in 1621, 1632, 1639 and 1677 prescribed compounds which were varied and complex. Some contained as many as seventy different ingredients ground-up: crab's eyes, blind puppies, earthworms, shells, precious stones, coral, human or animal excrement as well as human skull and the moss growing upon it. Apothecary Nicholas Culpeper translated the *Pharmacopoeia Londinensis* from Latin into English in 1653 an act which outraged physicians countrywide. Up until this time medical texts were exclusively published in Latin, making all medical knowledge elitist and closed to the uneducated. Culpeper however demystified medicine for the common people. The *Pharmacopoeia Londinensis* or *London Dispensatory* was sold at an affordable price and incorporated instructions on how to use the various cures contained therein.

13. *Pharmacopoeia Londinensis* 1947, p. 241, 246, 252.
14. Ibid., p. 47.
15. Ibid., p. 77.
16. Ibid., p. 47.
17. Ibid., p. 77.
18. Stuart Kathy, *Defiled Trades and Social Outcasts: Honor and Ritual Pollution in Early Modern Germany*, Cambridge University Press, Cambridge 1999, p 157.
19. Ibid., p 158.
20. Gordon-Grube 1988, p. 406.
21. In 1609 Oswald Crollius's *Treatise of Signatures*, describing methods of preparing chemical medicine, was published.
22. Gordon-Grube 1988, p. 406.
23. Ferrari 1987, p. 189.
24. The notion of 'sensitivity' retained by a corpse, also provided the basis for a legal norm, the *jus feretri*, according to which the 'reaction' of a dead body in the presence of its presumed assassin constituted valid proof.
25. Stuart 1999, p. 158.
26. Helmont, Jean Baptiste van, *A ternary of paradoxes the magnetick cure of wounds, nativity of tartar in wine, image of God in man*, translated, illustrated and amplified by Walter Charleton, University of Michigan, Digital Library Production Service 2005.
27. The horrific practice of gibbeting was already used in Britain and other parts of Europe in the thirteenth century, but legalised in Britain by the Murder Act of 1752. The additional punishment of gibbeting, or hanging in chains, was used when the courts wished to make an example of a particular criminal. It meant that after the hanging the felon was stripped, the body dipped in molten tar, re-dressed and placed into an iron cage, suspended either from the original gallows or a gibbet. These were usually positioned at highly visible locations such as crossroads or hilltops as a grim reminder that crime did not pay. Although protected by the tar covering, the corpse would eventually rot and decompose – exposed to the elements and pecked at by birds. This, fate worse than death from a prisoner's point of view – because no burial took place – was regularly implemented up to 1834.
28. Quincy 1730, p. 230.
29. Wagner Christiane, Failing Jutta, *Vielmals auf den Kopf gehacket – Galgen und Scharfrichter in Hessen*, Verlag M. Naumann, Hanau 2008 p. 96.
30. Gordon-Grube 1988, p. 407.
31. Ficino Marsilio, *De Vita II* (1489), 11: 196-199. Translated by Sergius Kodera.
32. Sugg 2011, p. 17.
33. Temkin Owsei, *The Falling Sickness – A History of Epilepsy from the Greeks to the Beginnings of Modern Neurology*, John Hopkins University Press, Baltimore 1994, p. 12.
34. Kanner Leo, *The Folklore and Cultural History of Epilepsy*, in: Medical Life, 34.4, 1930, p 198.
35. Grimm Jacob, *Teutonic Mythology*, Vol.1, 2, 3 & 4, George Bell and Sons, London 1883, Vol. IV, p. 1824.
36. Evans Richard J., *Rituals of Retribution: Capital Punishment in Germany 1600–1987*, Oxford 1996, p. 90-98.
37. Wagner Christiane, Failing Jutta, *Vielmals auf den Kopf gehacket – Galgen und Scharfrichter in Hessen*, Verlag M. Naumann, Hanau 2008, p. 62.
38. Ibid., p. 63.
39. Ibid., p. 100.
40. Moog Ferdinand P., *Between Horror and Hope: Gladiators Blood as a Cure for Epileptics in*

Ancient Medicine, In: Journal of the History of Neuroscience, 12.2, 2003, 137-43, p. 138.

41. Wagner 2008, p. 125.

42. The implicit belief in the supernatural healing powers of sovereigns is a relic of the ancient doctrine of the divinity of kingship. See Chapter 12 – Medical magic – healing by touch and sympathy.

43. Stapelberg Monica-Maria, *Strange But True – a historical background to popular beliefs and traditions*, Crux Publishing, London 2014, p. 9.

44. Sugg 2011, p. 85.

45. Crawfurd Raymond, *The King's Evil*, Claredon Press, Oxford 1911, p. 101.

46. Moog 2003, p. 138-143.

47. *Peter Moosleitner's Interessantes Magazin*, 1. August 1993, p. 30.

48. Sugg 2011, p. 81.

49. Stapelberg 2014, p. 10.

50. Wagner Christiane, Failing Jutta, *Vielmals auf den Kopf gehacket – Galgen und Scharfrichter in Hessen*, Verlag M. Naumann, Hanau 2008, p. 130.

51. Culpeper Nicholas, *Pharmacopoeia Londinensis or The London Dispensatory*, Royal College of Physicians of London, originally published 1649, p. 77.

52. Ibid., p. 47

53. Ibid., p. 77.

54. Ibid., p. 47.

55. Opie Iona and Tatem Moira, *A Dictionary of Superstitions*, Oxford Press, New York 1989, p.359.

56. Phillipus Aureolus Theophrastus Bombastus von Hohenheim, known simply as Paracelsus, held that illness was the result of external agents attacking the body rather than humoral imbalances. Hence he advocated the use of chemicals against disease-causing agents. He was renowned for his medical ability and his unorthodox views at the time. For instance, he was known to have publicly burned established medical texts. In modern times he is recognised as the first medical scientist. He wrote the first complete work on the causes, symptoms and treatment of syphilis; he recommended that epileptics should be treated as sick persons and not as lunatics possessed by demons. Despite his rigorous scientific studies, his work was closely connected to the mystical alchemical tradition. Aware that invisible forces were always at work in a fourth dimension, he employed various types of divination, astrology, amulets and incantations. The system of medicine he espoused was built primarily on chemistry, with a '…liberal dose of cosmology and astrology' (Hæger 2000, p. 103) thrown in.

57. Gordon-Grube 1988, p. 408.

58. In medieval times sphagnum moss was used as a spur-of-the-moment bandage during jousting and a dressing for wounds in battle, because of its naturally antiseptic properties and absorbency to soak up blood – it was similarly applied during both World Wars. As sphagnum moss inhibits the growth of bacteria and fungi, it is used in refined form in modern times as an environmentally-friendly alternative to chlorine in swimming pools and as a hospital grade herbal disinfectant and cleaner concentrate.

59. Bacon Francis, *Sylva Sylvarum: Or a Natural History in Ten Centuries*, reprint of 1627 edition, Kessinger Publishing 1996, p 134.

60. Helmont, Jean Baptiste van 2005, p. 4.

61. *Irish Examiner Newspaper*, 25 May 2011.

62. Sugg 2011, p. 24.

63. Brugis Thomas, *The marrow of physick or: A learned discourse of the several parts of mans body*, 1669, p. 65. British Library.

64. Woolley Benjamin, *The Herbalist – Nicholas Culpeper and the fight for medical freedom*, Harper Perennial, London 2005, p. 344.

65. Furdell Elizabeth Lane, *The Royal Doctors: 1485-1714 – Medical Personnel at the Tudor and Stuart Courts*, University of Rochester Press 2001, p. 160.

66. Crawfurd Raymond, *The Last Days of Charles II*, Claredon Press, Oxford 1909, p. 29.

67. Ibid., p. 29.

68. West Kennet Long Barrow, in which humans were buried from between 3700 BCE to 2000 BCE, is one of the largest and best-preserved monuments of its kind in Britain.

69. Sugg 2011, p. 94.

70. Ibid., p.98.

71. Ibid., p.98.

72. Wagner 2008, p. 128.

73. Quoted in Wagner Christiane, Failing Jutta, *Vielmals auf den Kopf gehacket – Galgen und Scharfrichter in Hessen*, Verlag M. Naumann, Hanau 2008, p. 128.

74. Culpeper, *Pharmacopoeia Londinensis*, p. 47. See also: Brockbank William, *Sovereign Remedies: A Critical depreciation of the 17th Century London Pharmacopoeia*, In; Medical History Volume 8, 1964. And: Linebaugh Peter, *The Tyburn Riot Against Surgeons*, In: Albion's Fatal Tree: Crime and Society in Eighteenth Century England, ed. Douglas Hey, New York 1975.

75. Wagner 2008, p. 116.

76. Are cannibalistic tendencies in medicine still prevalent even in modern times? In March 2011 the *Journal of Science-Based Medicine* published an article titled *Eating Placentas: Cannibalism, Recycling, or Health Food?* under the category 'Nutrition, Obstetrics and Gynaecology'. The article discusses placentophagy, its evolutionary survival value and possible benefits for modern women. After giving birth, most mammals eat the afterbirth or placenta, but most humans do not. However, in modern times eating the placenta is promoted by various New Age, holistic, and 'back-to-nature' pundits. Does this constitute cannibalism? Given, that the assertion of the placenta being part of a woman's body is inaccurate, the answer is 'yes'. Although a maternal component is present, placental tissue is mainly derived from the fertilized egg and carries the fetus' genome. So technically, eating the placenta does fit the definition of cannibalism: eating the flesh of your own species. Dried human placenta, ingested, is still used in traditional Chinese medicine to treat infertility, impotence and other conditions.

Chapter 9
Yummy mummy

1. Budge, Sir Ernest A. Wallis, *The Mummy: A Handbook of Egyptian Funerary Archaeology*, Cambridge University Press; Reissue edition, July 2010, p. 202.

2. Gordon-Grube Karen, '*Anthropophagy in Post-Renaissance Europe: The Tradition of Medicinal Cannibalism*', American Anthropologist, 90 (1988) pp. 405-409, p. 406.

3. Intentional mummification in Egypt dates to 3500 BCE. However, deliberate mummification was also a feature of other ancient cultures: In China, more than 1000 mummies dating back to 1500 BCE, were found in 1989 in a remote corner of the Taklamakan desert in Xinjiang, China's westernmost province. Ancient mummies discovered in Peru and other parts of South America date back to 4000 BCE, the oldest ever found.

4. Pouchelle Marie-Christine, *The body and Surgery in the Middle Ages*, Rutgers University

Press, New York 1990, pp. 74, 166.

5. In ancient times, bitumen was found in abundance throughout the Middle East, but especially in Mesopotamia. From north to south along the Tigris and Euphrates rivers, the country was littered with bitumen seepages and crude oil springs. The description of bitumen as 'mankind's oldest engineering material' can be supported by a considerable amount of evidence. The ancient Sumerians (3000 years BCE) attached ivory or mother-of-pearl eyes into the eye sockets of their statues with this sticky black substance, also using it to insulate their houses against flooding and to waterproof their boats.

6. Sanskrit for asphaltum.

7. Pedanius Dioscorides who lived circa 40 – 90 CE was a Greek physician and pharmacologist. He is renowned for his work *De Materia Medica*, a five volume encyclopedia about herbal medicine and related medicinal substances, that was widely read for more than 1,500 years.

8. Ibn Sīnā or commonly known by his Latin name Avicenna (980-1037 CE).

9. Siraisi Nancy, *History, Medicine, and the Traditions of Renaissance Learning*, University of Mitchigan Press, 2007, p. 232.

10. Ball Philip, *The Devil's Doctor – Paracelsus and the World of Renaissance, Magic and Science*, Farrar, Straus and Giroux, New York 2006, p. 274.

11. Culpeper Nicholas, *Pharmacopoeia Londinensis* or *The London Dispensatory*, Royal College of Physicians of London, originally published 1649, pp. 241, 246, 252.

12. Quincy John, *Complete English Dispensatory* or *Pharmacopoia Offininalis and Extemporanea*, London 1730, p. 484.

13. Ibid., p. 527.

14. Shakespeare William, *Hamlet*, Editor: Robert Hapgood, Cambridge University Press, Cambridge, 1999, Act 4, Scene 3:32-33, p. 225.

15. 'In Northern Europe amongst royalty, aristocrats, and ecclesiastics, post-mortem ablation of the heart was a widespread, common funerary practice. This process involved separate, independent burial not only of the body but also the entrails, as well as the excised heart in locations of sacred worship. For example, when King Heinrich III died in October 1056 in Bodfeld, Germany, his heart was buried separately from his body. When Henry I of England died in France in 1135 his entrails, as well as his brain and eyes were buried in Rouen and his body was returned to England for interment in Reading Abbey. The crusading English King Richard I, known as Richard Lionheart, decreed before his death in 1199 that his brain and entrails be buried in Charroux, France, his body in the Abbey of Fontevreau, and his heart in the Cathedral of Rouen. The heart of Frederick Wilhelm IV (1795–1861), King of Prussia, and member of the House of Habsburg, is buried at his parents' feet in the Mausoleum of Charlottenburg, Berlin. Since the seventeenth century, the hearts of all members of the House of Habsburg have been buried separately from their bodies in the Augustiner Church in Vienna. The desire to apportion one's remains to various favoured locations was to solicit prayers from the living for salvation of one's soul in more than one place of religious foundation' (Stapelberg Monica-Maria, *Strange But True – a historical background to popular beliefs and traditions*, Crux Publishing, London 2014, p. 205).

16. Mafart B., Pelletier J., Fixot M., *Post-mortem Ablation of the Heart: A Medieval Funerary Practice*, In: International Journal of Osteo-Archaeology Vol. 14, 2004, pp. 67-73, p. 72.

17. Auf der Heide Arthur, *The Scientific Study of Mummies*, Cambridge University Press, Cambridge 2003, p. 523.

18. Ibid., p. 523.

19. Twain, Mark. *The Innocents Abroad*, Signet Classics, New York 1997, p. 642.

20. Gordon-Grube 1988, p. 406.

21. Venice treacle was popular throughout the ancient world including China and India and was known as a cure-all. Pharmacists throughout Europe sold it as late as 1884.

22. Wittlin Alma, Stephanie, *Museums: in search of a usable future*, MIT Press, Virginia 1970, p. 30.

23. Wallis Patrick, On: 'Bullein, William', In: *Oxford Dictionary of National Biography*, first published 2004.

24. Meaning 'treacle' during the Middle Ages.

25. Shakespeare William, *The Tragedy of Macbeth*, Editor: Nicholas Brooke, Oxford World's Classics Series, Oxford University Press, Oxford 1998, pp. 168-169, 4.1.23. Maw and gulf stand for stomach and throat.

26. Sugg 2011. p. 21.

27. Occasionally one hears references about the fashionable Victorian trend of mummy 'unwrapping' parties. Supposedly, these little *soirees* were quite in vogue amongst the upper class British during the 1830's. Victorian gentlemen would bring back a mummy or two from their travels to Egypt, or buy an actual mummy at auction and subsequently invite friends to witness the 'unwrapping of the mummy', followed by refreshments. Purportedly, the charms and amulets found within the wrappings were given out as gifts and it was similarly fashionable to keep the hand or foot of a mummy as a display piece. The facts are however quite different and not a single report is in existence of a mummy being unwrapped at a social function just for sheer entertainment. Consequently, how did the myth come about? A specific 'party' invitation was probably to blame. It announced a gathering at Lord Londesborough's home with 'a mummy from Thebes to be unrolled at half-past two'. But, surviving accounts from that specific 10th day of June 1850 prove that this was not a social gathering, but an academic lecture for members of the Society of Antiquaries. It seems that this occasion was an exception and that mummy unwrappings were generally only held in lecture halls and at universities, not in private homes.

28. Budge 2010, p.202.

29. Ibid., p. 202.

30. Gordon-Grube 1988, p. 407.

31. Ibid., p. 407.

32. Sugg 2011, p. 205.

33. Ibid., p.205.

34. Dannenfeldt Karl, *Egyptian Mumia: The Sixteenth Century Experience and Debate*, In: *Sixteenth Century Journal* 16:2, 1985, pp. 163-80, 176.

35. Quincy 1730, pp. 86, 221.

36. Budge 2010, p. 203.

Chapter 10
The Executioner's Healing Touch

1. Spierenburg Pieter, The Spectacle of Suffering – Executions and the Evolution of Repression: From a pre-industrial metropolis to the European experience, Cambridge University Press, Cambridge 1984, p. 16.

2. Ibid, p. 16.

3. Ibid, p. 17.
4. See Klemettilä Hannele, Epitomes of Evil – Representations of Executioners in Northern France and the Low Countries in the Late Middle Ages, , In: Studies in European History 1100-1800.
5. Wagner Christiane, Failing Jutta, Vielmals auf den Kopf gehacket – Galgen und Scharfrichter in Hessen, Verlag M. Naumann, Hanau 2008, pp. 66, 89.
6. Stuart Kathy, Defiled Trades and Social Outcasts: Honor and Ritual Pollution in Early Modern Germany, Cambridge University Press, Cambridge 1999, p. 27.
7. Stuart 1999, p. 154.
8. Krieger Heinz-Bruno, Elmsagen – Ein Beitrag zur Volkskunde des Elmgebietes, Braunschweig-Schöppenstedt Verlag, Oeding 1967.
9. Bradis Henning ' Diarium', published by Hänselmann, Hildesheim 1896, p. 2.
10. Hildesheim Urkundenbuch VII. Nr. 871, quoted in Krieger Heinz-Bruno, Von Pflichten und Künsten der alten Scharfrichter im Lande Braunschweig, http://www.elmsagen.de/erzaehl.asp?Kap=E21
11. Probst Christian, Fahrende Heiler und Heilmittel Händler – Medizin von Marktplatz und Landstraße, Rosenheimer Verlagshaus, Zwickau 1992, p. 146.
12. Spierenburg 1984, p. 31.
13. Ibid., p. 31.
14. Being an avid collector, he also ammassed an assortment of selected minerals, as well as documents on the town's history, and a large collection of antiquities. Very soon word of the 'educated' executioner and his significant collection spread. The little spa town became a 'noteworthy' attraction and various distinguished scholars started to correspond with Huß. The viewing of his extensive collection by spa guests, rapidly became part of the town's social program – even Germany's most reputable writer, politician and philosopher, Johann Wolfgang von Goethe, visited Huß on many occasions. After the death of his wife in 1824, the retired Huß approached Prince Metternich regarding his museum collection. The prince agreed to take over the collection, granting Huß free housing, a life-time annuity until his death in 1838, as well as the position of custodian to the collection, which is still housed at the Eger chateau.
15. Stuart 1999, p. 159.
16. Sawday Jonathan, The Body Emblazoned, Routledge Publishing 2013, p. 82.
17. Stuart 1999, p. 154.
18. Wagner 2008, p. 25.
19. Stader Jahrbuch 1975 p. 71.
20. Stuart 1999, p 160.
21. Krieger Heinz-Bruno, Von Pflichten und Künsten der alten Scharfrichter im Lande Braunschweig, http://www.elmsagen.de/erzaehl.asp?Kap=E21
22. Ibid.
23. Ibid., p.61
24. Hæger Knut, The Illustrated History of Surgery, revised by Sir Roy Calne, AB Nordbok, Gothenburg Sweden 2000, p. 157.
25. Ibid., p. 157.
26. Krieger Heinz-Bruno, Von Pflichten und Künsten der alten Scharfrichter im Lande Braunschweig, http://www.elmsagen.de/erzaehl.asp?Kap=E21
27. Probst 1992, p. 152.
28. Ibid.

29. Wagner 2008, p. 131.
30. Ibid., p. 116.
31. Ibid.
32. Wagner 2008, p. 116, p. 128-129.
33. Stuart 1999, p 157.
34. Ferrari Giovanna, Public Anatomy Lessons and the Carnival: The Anatomy Theatre of Bologna, In: Past and Present 117, 1987, pages 50-106, p. 102.
35. Oppelt Wolfgang, Über die Unehrlichkeit des Scharfrichters, Lengfeld 1976, p.376.
36. Franz Schmidt resigned from his post in 1617. His diary is a unique source of social and legal history in his years as executioner. The diary contains information about the 361 executions he carried out by rope, sword, burning and drowning, as well as various forms of punishment he implemented, and details of the crimes on which the sentences were based.
37. Stuart 1999, p. 157.

Chapter 11
Medical magic – healing by touch and sympathy

1. Porter Roy, *The Greatest Benefit to Mankind – A Medical History of Humanity from Antiquity to the Present*, Harper Collins Publishing, London 1999, p. 41.
2. Ibid., p. 40
3. A Member of Parliament, and Chief Secretary to the Admiralty under King Charles II, Samuel Pepys is best known for the diary he kept for almost a decade between 1660 and 1669. The diary relates his every day activities, his business dealings, his personal life, as well as national events and political wranglings during his lifetime. But most importantly the diary gives a graphic account of life during the Plague of London and the Great Fire of London, during the Restoration period. Suffering from bladder stones and resulting infections, Pepys was never without pain in his early adult years. Even after surgical removal of his stones, the lasting effects of the operation continued to plague him in later life.
4. Porter 1999, p. 40.
5. The ancient Sumerians were first to develop this concept of divinely ordained kings, descended from heaven as primary intermediaries between God and humankind. It was believed in ancient cultures that kings and rulers were sons of the Holy Sun. Accordingly, in line with priestly tradition, the first king of Egypt, Menes meaning 'the sole light', and all subsequent ruling sovereigns were seen as the living image of the sun-god Ra. Similarly, the early monarchs of Babylon and Mesopotamia were worshipped as gods in their lifetime. The Roman emperors Constantine, Vespasian and Hadrian, were all regarded as divine. The Emperor of China was regarded as the 'Son of Heaven' and the chief priest of his people. The same notions also existed about Mayan, Aztec and Inca rulers. Even in modern times vestiges of this ancient belief remain in many cultures. For example, the word 'king' in Thai means 'god of the land'. In the same context, the Japanese Emperor has been viewed as a god throughout history and in the twenty-first century Emperor Akihito continues the practice of blessing land and crops (Stapelberg Monica-Maria, *Strange But True – a historical background to popular beliefs and traditions*, Crux Publishing, London 2014, p. 8).
6. Clark Stuart, *Thinking with Demons: The Idea of Witchcraft in Early Modern Europe*, Oxford University Press, 1999, p. 660.
7. Furdell Elizabeth Lane, *The Royal Doctors: 1485-1714 – Medical Personnel at the Tudor and*

Stuart Courts, University of Rochester Press 2001, p. 53.

8. Stapelberg Monica-Maria, *Strange But True – a historical background to popular beliefs and traditions*, Crux Publishing, London 2014, p. 8.

9. Pettigrew Thomas Joseph, *On Superstitions connected with the History and Practice of Medicine and Surgery*, Barrinton & Haswell, Philadelphia 1844, p. 166.

10. Ibid.

11. Furdell 2001, p. 53.

12. Clark 1999, p. 661.

13. Dunn-Hensley Susan Michele, *Powerful Purity: The Sacred Virgin in Early Modern Literature*, Proquest Publishing, Kansas 2007, p. 77.

14. Ibid.

15. Ibid., p. 78.

16. The medical name for the King's Evil at the time.

17. Dunn-Hensley 2007, p. 75.

18. Ibid.

19. Furdell p. 89.

20. Dunn-Hensley 2007, p. 76.

21. Crawfurd 1911, p. 100.

22. Ibid.

23. Lacey Andrew, *The Cult of King Charles the Martyr*, Boydell & Brewer 2003, p. 60.

24. Crawfurd 1911, p. 101.

25. Lacey 2003, p. 60.

26. Furdell p. 126.

27. Macaulay Thomas Babington, *The History of England from the Accession of James II*, Volume 3, Chapter XIV, Porter & Coates Philadelphia 2008 (EBook #2612).

28. Furdell p. 126.

29. Crawford 1911, p. 111.

30. Pettigrew 1844, p. 170.

31. Crawfurd 1911, p. 121.

32. It could of course be argued that during the reign of any monarch, but especially so under Charles II, it would have been dangerous to express disbelief in the 'royal touch', since it evidenced the King's right to the throne by the Grace of God – a fact, which after his long exile in France would have been hailed by his supporters.

33. Crawfurd 1911, p. 102.

34. Ibid., p. 128.

35. Ibid., p. 126.

36. Macaulay 2008.

37. In accordance with the vast majority of seventeenth century European society, this work confirms physician Brown's belief in the existence of angels, witches and witchcraft. During the 1662 Bury St. Edmund's witch trials, Browne's citation of a similar trial in Denmark so influenced the jury that two accused women, were subsequently found guilty and executed for witchcraft.

38. Macaulay 2008.

39. Ibid.

40. Ibid.

41. Quoted by Crawfurd 1911, p. 140.

42. Macaulay 2008.

43. In France the popular custom continued until the coronation of King Charles X on 29 May 1825. After that date the royal touch was never again employed. French kings had

zealously fulfilled this duty for centuries and the royal touch had been an integral part of the coronation ceremony of French monarchs at Reims Cathedral since the late Middle Ages. During the coronation rite the king's hands would be anointed, in the belief that this specifically conferred the ability to heal. Immediately after this ceremonial, the king and his entourage would pilgrimage to the shrine of Saint Marcouf, the patron saint of scrofula sufferers, after which the newly crowned king was thought to possess the gift of healing this disease. It is documented that King Henry IV of France (1553 -1610) on Easter Sunday 1594, touched around nine hundred scrofula suffers and thousands more during his lifetime. Similarly French King Louis XIII touched over eight hundred persons at his coronation in 1610 and his physicians attested to him having touched more than a thousand people in July 1616 (Crawfurd 1911, p. 102). These numbers were exceeded by King Louis XIV of France, who touched no less than 2600 scrofula sufferers at his coronation in 1643, while King Charles XV touched two thousand victims at his coronation in 1722 (Porter 1999, p. 282). During the reign of French King Louis XV (1710-1774) the sentence spoken by the king upon touching sufferers changed to: 'The King touches you, may God heal you', implying that a cure was not guaranteed. In all instances royal physicians and others who witnessed these ceremonies insisted that at least half of all the diseased people touched were healed within days.

44. Paracelsus (1493-1541), which means 'equal or greater than Celsus' was a German-Swiss alchemist and occultist. He named himself after Aulus Cornelius Celsus, a Roman encyclopedist of the first century CE, but his real name was Philippus Aureolus Theophrastus Bombastus von Hohenheim. Paracelsianism was based on the principle of maintaining harmony between the microcosm, represented by man and the macrocosm, represented by nature. Paracelsus' most important legacy is probably his evaluation of scholastic methods in medicine, science and theology – all of which did however not exist as separate from each other during his time. Without disputing their teachings, he was however opposed to the unquestioning acceptance of the old masters Hippocrates, Galen and Avicenna.

45. Jevons F. R., *Paracelsus's Two-Way Astrology – What Paracelsus meant by 'Stars'*, The British Journal for the History of Science 2:2, December 1964, pp.139-147.

46. Ibid., pp.148-155.

47. German theologian, alchemist, occult writer and astrologer.

48. See Agrippa's *Three Books of Occult Philosophy*, Book I, XV.

49. Resh Thomas Jane, *Behind the Mask: The Life of Queen Elizabeth I*, Clarion Books, UK 1998, p. 113.

50. Pettigrew Thomas Joseph, *On Superstitions connected with the History and Practice of Medicine and Surgery*, Barrinton & Haswell, Philadelphia 1844, p. 18.

51. A mixture of red ochre and clay.

52. Ball Philip, *The Devil's Doctor – Paracelsus and the World of Renaissance, Magic and Science*, Farrar, Straus and Giroux, New York 2006, p. 79.

53. Lobis Seth, *The Virtue of Sympathy: Magic, Philosophy and Literature in Seventeenth Century England*, Yale University Press, 2015, p. 40.

54. Pettigrew 1844, p. 207.

55. McCord Sheri, *Healing by Proxy: The Early Modern Weapon-Salve*, English Language Notes, 2009, Vol. 47 Issue 2, p. 9.

56. Croll's books strongly advocated the use of alchemy and chemistry in medicine, as well as promoting botany, the medicinal value of herbs and other sciences put forward by Paracelsus.

57. Or *Medicina Magnetica*, Edinburgh: C. Higgins, Printed in the year 1656.

58. English courtier, diplomat, natural philosopher and founding member of the Royal Society, also noted as the first person to recognise the importance of oxygen or 'vital air' for the sustenance of plants.

59. The world's oldest medical faculty, founded in 1137, and still in operation.

60. Digby, regarded himself as a man of science and firmly disavowed any adherence to demonology. The various ingredients of his concoction had to be prepared according to a specific alchemical and astrological formula. He claimed that the formula had originated in Persia and was given to him by a Carmalite monk. What he failed to mention though, was that a similar cure had been advocated by Paracelsus a century earlier.

61. Quincy John, *Complete English Dispensatory or Pharmacopoia Offininalis and Extemporanea,* London 1730, p. 649.

62. Ibid.

63. Ball 2006, page 79.

Chapter 12
The Great Mortality – the Black Death

1. Aberth John, *The Black Death – The Great Mortality of 1348-1350 – A Brief History with Documnts,* The Bedford Series in History and Culture, Stratford Publishing Services, Boston 2005, p. 3.

2. Tikhomirov E., *Epidemiology and Distribution of Plague.* In : WHO. Plague Manual: Epidemiology, Distribution, Surveillance and Control. 2011. Viewed on: http://www.who.int/csr/resources/publications/plague/whocdscsredc992a.p.

3. The first attested case of 'true' plague was in Constantinople in 542 CE.

4. Tikhomirov E., 2011.

5. In this way the bacterial strains called *Yersinia pestis* are kept moving between hosts. Generally these bacterial strains live in the digestive tract of fleas particularly rat and gerbil fleas, although they can also live in human fleas. When the *bacilli* multiply in the flea's stomach in very large numbers, they cause the flea to 'block up', thus threatening the flea with starvation. The 'blocked up' flea then regurgitates large numbers of *Y pestis* into its victim. Hence the flea's bite is crucial to the dissemination of the plague. Although the toxicity of *Y pestis* varies, all three principal varieties of the plague, namely bubonic, pneumonic and septicemia, are highly lethal. Bubonic is the most common, with blackish gangrenous pustules appearing first at the site of the initial fleabite. Then an enlargement of the lymph nodes follows, after which subcutaneous hemorrhaging occurs causing terrible purple blotches. The hemorrhaging causes cell necrosis and intoxication of the nervous system, leading to neurological and psychological disorders – hence the famous *danse macabre*, which accompanied so many victims of the Black Death.

6. Quoted in Withington John, *A Disasterous History of the World: Chronicles of War, Earthquakes, Plague and Flood,* Hachette, London 2008, p. 63.

7. From *Historia de Morbe*, quoted in Hatcher John, *The Black Death – A Personal History,* Da Capo Press, Philadelphia USA 2008, p. 149.

8. Horrox Rosemary, *The Black Death*, Manchester University Press, Manchester 1994, p.250.

9. Hatcher John, *The Black Death – A Personal History*, Da Capo Press, Philadelphia USA 2008, p. 59.

10. Gottfried Robert S., *The Black Death – Natural and Human Disaster in Medieval Europe,* The Free Press, New York 1983, p. 81.

11. Hatcher 2008, p. 130.

12. Kelly John, *An Intimate History of the Black Death, the Most Devastating Plague of all Time*, Harper Perennial, Harper Collins, London 2006, p. 267.

13. Dressed in white robes emblazoned with a red cross, Flagellants travelled through towns and villages in groups led by a 'master' or 'father' (Gottfried 1983, p. 70). The 'master heard their confessions and '…to the horror of the clergy imposed penance and granted absolution' (Gottfried 1983, p. 70). Flagellants were forbidden to speak, to bathe, shave or change their clothing. Flagellants were seen as martyrs atoning for the sins of the world and most town and village people regarded their visit as an honour. Increasingly however, Flagellants were dominated by marginal elements, including criminals and vagabonds.

14. Ziegler Philip, *The Black Death*, Harper Perennial Modern Classics, Harper Collins, London 2009, p. 70.

15. Before even attempting to treat a patient doctors were obliged to ensure that confession had taken place – in other words, medicine waited its turn and took a secondary position in the sickroom.

16. Kelly 2006, p. 232.

17. Aberth 2005, p. 41.

18. Ibid.

19. However, the well-known French chronicler Jean de Venette (c. 1307 – c. 1370) whose work covers many important events of the fourteenth century including, the Black Death and the Hundred Year War, put the causes of the plague down to a different astrological phenomena: 'In A.D. 1348 the people of France and of almost the whole world were struck by a blow other than war. For, in addition to famine […] and to the wars […] pestilence and its attendant tribulations appeared again in various parts of the world. In the month of August 1348, after Vespers, when the sun was beginning to set, a big and very bright star appeared above Paris, towards the west. It did not seem as stars usually do, to be very high above our hemisphere, but rather very near. As the sun set and night came on, this star did not seem to me or any other friars who were watching it, to move out of place. […] this big star, to the amazement to all of us who were watching, broke into many different rays, and as it shed these rays over Paris towards the east, totally disappeared and was annihilated. It is […] possible that it was a presage of the amazing pestilence to come […]. All this year and the next, the mortality of men and women, of the young even more than the old, in Paris and the kingdom of France, and also in other parts of the world, was so great that it was almost impossible to bury the dead…' (Jean de Venette, *The Chronicle* p. 48).

20. Typically, in line with the trend of ideas at the time, Lutheran pastor Andreas Osiander in 1533 sermonised on the outbreak of the plague in Nürnberg: '…such a scourge comes perchance from the influence of the stars, from the effects of comets, from extraordinary weather conditions and changes of the air, from southerly winds, stinking waters or from rotten vapours of the air' (Gottfried 1983, p. 53).

21. Gottfried, 1983, p. 111.

22. The Greek word for 'pollution'. In historical usage the term 'miasma', representing disease-specific characteristics, is a nineteenth century term. In previous centuries the term 'corrupt air' was used instead.

23. Ziegler 2009, p. 20.

24. Newman Paul B., *Daily Life in the Middle Ages*, McFarland Press 2001, p. 137.

25. Peris Teresa Fuentes, *Visions of Filth: Deviancy and Social Control in the Novels of Galdós*, Liverpool University Press, Liverpool 2003, p. 51.

26. Sabine Ernest L., *Latrines and Cesspools of Mediaeval London*, In: *Speculum*, The Medieval Academy of America, Volume 9, Issue 03, July 1934, pp. 303-321, p. 309.

27. Castles and palaces usually had garderobes on every floor and sometimes also in

individual rooms, with separate flues passing down through the stonework into a moat of running water below (Sabine 1934, p. 304), or into cesspools. In London many wealthy establishments also housed 'privies', which usually jutted out over the Thames so that excrement fell directly into the river. Authorities did however make efforts to clean the build-up of noxious filth by declaring that although latrines could still be built over the stream, the dumping of all other filth and rubbish into the same, was unlawful.

28. The construction of aqueducts and vast cisterns, providing fresh water, as well as the building of public sewers were amongst the many great accomplishment of the Romans – achievements, which long outlasted their reign. Hence, some of these facilities were still in use during the Middle Ages. Apart from those areas which the Romans had not conquered, or where they had established only scattered settlements, or areas on the periphery of the once great Empire, Roman conduits continued to flow. In the major cities, many public Roman baths and waterworks continued to function. In addition, European kings, Charlemagne in the ninth century for instance, built cold bathing facilities in imitation of those found in the larger Roman villas (Newman 2001, p. 139). During the early Middle Ages, monasteries, 'the great preservers of classical knowledge' (Newman 2001, p. 139), were built containing water and sewer systems. Latrines emptied into shafts, through which waste was dumped into cesspits. Ideally monasteries would be built on coastlines, where sewage waste could then be washed away by the tides twice a day and by the twelfth century, several monasteries in England '…had water piped in from several miles away using gravity- powered systems' (Newman 2001, p. 139). This was water collected in reservoirs or from springs on high ground and distributed through pipes made of wood, earthenware, or lead (Salzman 1926, p. 86). The first water main or 'conduit' in London was laid down in the thirteenth century. It brought water from the springs at Tyburn to a fountain in West Cheap and was intended to provide drinking water only, for the poor to drink, and '…for the wealthier classes (who did not drink water, regarding it as the last resource of thirsty poverty), to cook their food with […]. Other conduits were laid down during the fifteenth and sixteenth centuries, and at the end of the sixteenth century something in the nature of water-towers supplied by pumping appears to have been introduced' (Salzman 1926, p. 86).

29. Sabine 1934, p. 307.
30. Ibid.
31. Kelly 2006, p. 17.
32. Salzman L. F., *English Life in the Middle Ages*, Oxford University Press, London 1926, p. 87.
33. Ibid.
34. Ziegler 2009, p. 154.
35. Salzman 1926, p. 87
36. Ibid.
37. Kelly 2006, p. 17.
38. Cawthorne Nigel, *The Curious Cures of Old England*, Piatkus Books Ltd., London 2005, p. 98.
39. Stapelberg Monica-Maria, *Strange But True – a historical background to popular beliefs and traditions*, Crux Publishing, London 2014, p. 66.
40. Ziegler 2009, p. 75.
41. Gottfried 1983, p. 117.
42. Ziegler 2009, p. 73.
43. Winslow, Charles-Edward Amory, *The Conquest of Epidemic Disease – A Chapter in the History of Ideas*, Wisconsin University Press, 1980, p. 95.

44. Aberth 2005, p. 59.
45. Archibald Elizabeth, *Did Knights Have Baths? The Absence of Bathing in Middle English Romance*, In: *Cultural Encounters in the Romance of Medieval England*, Edited by Corinne Saunders, DS Brewer Publishing 2005, p. 101.
46. Archibald 2005, p. 101, quoting French historian J. Michelet.
47. Wright Thomas, *Homes of Other Days – A history of domestic manners and sentiments in England*, Trübner & Co., Paternoster Row, London 1871, p. 271.
48. Official accounts record at least twenty-six public baths in mid-thirteenth century Paris and eighteen in metropolitan London (Newman 2001, p. 153). Considering that the population in Paris numbered about 160,000 at that time, twenty-six public baths is not a great number and indicates that a large proportion of the population probably remained 'unwashed'. The same is applicable to London with eighteen public baths in the mid-thirteenth century and a population of around 60,000. In *Concepts of Cleanliness: Changing Attitudes in France since the Middle Ages*, Cambridge University Press 1988, Professor Georges Vigarello states that bathing during the Middle Ages was '…dominated by notions of play and that when town criers summoned townsfolk to bath, as the water was hot, he was in fact inviting people to a "feast of pleasure"'. Vigarello describes bathhouses as places for eating drinking and sensual delights, where carnal pleasures could be pandered to under the auspices of respectability. In other words, washing was not the purpose of medieval bathing.
49. Achterberg 1990, p. 42.
50. Salzman 1926, p. 26.
51. Archibald p. 113.
52. By the mid-sixteenth century '…grander European palaces were installing plumbed water supplies with full drainage, in the neo-classical style. The built-in bath or grooming suite was a luxury many princes and nobility were eager to acquire' (Smith Virginia, *Clean: A History of Personal Hygiene and Purity*, Oxford University Press, 2007) Emulating the French king Francis II who had a full suite of baths installed at Fontainbleau, Henry III of England had a bath, cold-water cistern and drop-latrine installed at Hampton Court Palace. Another innovation at Hampton Court Palace was the twenty-eight seater communal latrine, known as the 'Great House of Easement' (Smith 2007) His daughter Elizabeth I always travelled with her hip-bath and had bathing facilities in all her palaces and '…there is no reason to think that Elizabeth I did not enjoy her monthly bath "whether she needed it or not" – probably at the time of her menses' (Smith 2007).
53. Smith, 2007
54. Salzman 1926, p. 106.
55. Wright Thomas, *Homes of Other Days – A history of domestic manners and sentiments in England*, Trübner & Co., Paternoster Row, London 1871, p. 166.
56. Salzman 1926, p. 106.
57. Kelly 2006, p. 17.
58. Smith 2007.
59. Vigarello Georges, *Concepts of Cleanliness: Changing Attitudes in France since the Middle Ages*, translated from French by Jean Birell, In: Cambridge Studies in Medieval Literature Past and Present Publications, Cambridge University Press 1988, p. 138.
60. Kelly 2006, p. 17.
61. Although folklorists generally reject this hypothesis, the following well-known nursery rhyme may in fact be a reminder of 'plague times': *Ring around the rosie, A pocketful of posie, Ashes, ashes, all fall down!* The 'ring' mentioned represents the circular *danse macabre*, as the plague was often represented, in which a half-decomposed corpse was

shown pulling apparently healthy young men or woman into a circle of dancers. The 'rosie' is thought to represent the blood-suffused face of the plague-victim; the 'posie' is the presumed prophylactic bag of herbs and flowers; 'ashes, ashes' refers to the sound of sneezing, regarded as a symptom of the plague; and 'all fall down' re-enacts the sure death of the victim.

62. Vigarello 1988, p. 138.
63. From Alfonso de Córdoba, *Letter and Regimen concerning the Pestilence*, In: Aberth 2005, p. 46.
64. He was also chief surgeon to Edward VI, Queen Mary and to Queen Elisabeth I.
65. Vicary Thomas, *The English Man's Treasure: With the true Anatomie of Man's bodie*, Imprinted at London By Thomas Creed, 1599, p. 82.
66. Ibid., p. 64.
67. Ibid., p. 81-82.
68. Most *memento mori* works are the products of Christian art – the prospect of death serving to highlight the emptiness and transience of earthly pleasures and accomplishments. Hence, the outcry *memento mori* focuses one's thoughts on the inevitable prospect of the afterlife.
69. These so-called 'double-decker' tombs featured an ornate carved stone effigy of the person as they were in life on the top level, and as a rotting, naked cadaver on the bottom level. The skeletal or rotting cadaver was often depicted shrouded and sometimes shown with worms devouring the decomposing corpse. These sculptures were intended as a sharp reminder of how transient all earthly glory really is, as we all end up in the same state. Cadaver tombs, with their exacting sculptural program, were made only for high-ranking nobles, usually royalty, bishops or abbots, because one had to be suitably rich to meet the expense of having such a tomb made, as well as powerful enough to be allotted space for one in a church. The term cadaver tomb can also be used for a monument that represents only the cadaver without a likeness of the living person. Some royal tombs were double tombs, for both king and queen.
70. The famous *danse macabre*, the depiction of a dancing Grim Reaper carrying off rich and poor alike, is another well-known example of the *memento mori* theme. Similar depictions of Death decorate many old European churches.
71. Aberth 2005, p. 37.
72. From Matteo Villani, *Cronica*, In: Aberth 2005, p. 37).
73. The chief physicians of the King of France, the German Emperor and the Duke of Burgundy all succumbed to the Black Death. Similarly, several of Pope Clement VI's physicians and surgeons died.
74. The term 'quarantine' comes from the Latin word meaning 'forty'.
75. Aberth 2005, p. 39.

Chapter 13
Leprosy – disease of the soul

1. True leprosy has existed for thousands of years and is referred to and described in numerous ancient sources: Egyptian papyrus scrolls detailing treatments for leprosy date back to 1500 BCE. Amongst the ancient Greeks, Aristotle describes the disease, while

Hippocrates called it the 'Phoenician disease' and also denoted the name *lepra* or 'scaly' disease, to what was probably not leprosy at all, but either psoriasis or another skin disease emitting a disgusting scaly, discharge.

2. Miller Timothy S., Smith-Savage Rachel, *Medieval Leprosy Reconsidered*, In: International Social Science Review, Vol. 81, No. 1-2, 2006.
3. The First Crusade took place in 1099.
4. Several theories have been put forward as to why the incidence of leprosy declined in Europe after the 1300's: One of the prime reasons was most likely the plague, which disseminated a third to half of Europe's population during the fourteenth century and probably killed a higher proportion of already physically weakened lepers. Another factor, similarly affecting those physically compromised by leprosy, must have been the syphilis epidemic, which struck Europe in the fifteenth century, killing thousands of people.
5. Miller Timothy S., Smith-Savage Rachel, 2006.
6. Watts Sheldon J., *Epidemics and History: Disease, Power and Imperialism*, Yale University Press 1999, p. 47.
7. II Kings, 5:20-27; Numbers 12:11; II Chronicles 26:16-23; II Kings 15:1-6.
8. Leviticus 13: 44-46.
9. Leviticus 13:3
10. Brody Nathaniel Samuel, *The Disease of the Soul – Leprosy in Medieval Literature*, Cornell University Press, London 1974, p. 114.
11. Watts 1997, 47-48.
12. Porter Roy Porter, *The Greatest Benefit to Mankind: A Medical History of Humanity*, New York: W.W. Norton & Company, Inc., 1998, pp. 121-22).
13. Watts 1997, pp. 41, 64; and Douglas Mary, *Witchcraft and Leprosy: Two Strategies of Exclusion*, Cultural Studies Project, Massachusetts Institute of Technology, 1991.
14. Manchester K., *Tuberculosis and Leprosy in Antiquity*, In: Medical History, Volume 28, Issue 2, April 1984, pp. 167-68.
15. Ibid., p. 171.
16. Miller, Smith-Savage 2006.
17. Demaitre Luke, *Leprosy in Premodern Medicine: A Malady of the Whole Body*, JHU Press 2007, p. 84.
18. Luke 17: 12-19.
19. Rawcliffe Carole, *Leprosy in Medieval England*, Boydell and Brewer Incorporated 2009, p. 49.
20. This has been highlighted in various monographs through intensive research into Greek sources of the patristic age (300 to 500 CE) as well as sources from Latin Europe during the time of the leprosy epidemic.
21. Risse Guenter B., *Mending Bodies, Saving Souls: A History of Hospitals*, Oxford University Press 1999, p. 174.
22. Brody 1974, pp. 101- 103.
23. Grigsby Bryon Lee, *Pestilence in Medieval and Early Modern English Literature*, In: *Studies in Medieval History and Culture*, Routledge University Press 2004, p. 39.
24. Aretaeus, ed. Karl Hude, *Collection of Greek Medical Authors*, In: Aedibus Academiae Scientiarum, Berlin 1958, Book 4:13, pp. 85-90.
25. Miller, Smith-Savage 2006.
26. Ibid.
27. Ibid.
28. Ibid.
29. By Roy Porter, Sheldon Watts, Guenter Risse, Nathaniel Brody, Carole Rawcliffe.

30. Ellul Max, *The Sword and the Green Cross: The Saga of the Knights of Saint Lazarus from the Crusades to the 21st Century*, Authorhouse Publishing UK 2011, p. 111.
31. Risse 1999, p. 177.
32. Demaitre 2007, p. 80.
33. Watts 1999, p. 48.
34. Risse 1999, p. 170.
35. Ibid.
36. Ibid., p. 171.
37. Brody 1974, p. 35.
38. Risse 1999, p. 170.
39. Brody 1974, p. 58.
40. Moore R. I., *The Formation of a Persecuting Society: Authority and Deviance in Western Europe 950-1250*, John Wiley & Sons, 2008, p. 73.
41. Brody 1974, p. 60.
42. Grigsby 2004, p. 38
43. Ellul 2011, p. 108.
44. Risse 1999, p176.
45. Ibid., p176.
46. Watts 1999, p. 50.
47. Achterberg Jeanne, *Woman as Healer – A panoramic survey of the healing activities of women from prehistoric times to the present*, Shambhala Publications, Boston 1990, p. 47.
48. Risse1999, p. 185.
49. Community regulations for medieval French leprosaria were collected and published by Le Grand, in *Statuts d'hotels-Dieu et de leproseries*. p. 181-83. Quoted in Miller, Timothy S.; Smith-Savage, Rachel, *Medieval Leprosy Reconsidered*, Academic journal article from *International Social Science Review*, Vol. 81, No. 1-2 , 2006.
50. Miller, Smith-Savage 2006.
51. Risse 1999, p. 175.
52. Rawcliffe 2006, pp. 65-71.
53. Baldwin John W., *The Language of Sex: Five Voices from Northern France around 1200*, Chicago University Press, Chicago 1994, p. 214.
54. According to this doctrine, the particular shape and colour of plants' leaves and flowers clearly indicated for which disease they could hopefully be used as a cure. For example, a heart-shaped leaf was meant to cure heart disease; seeds containing a dot resembling the pupil of the eye, such as the herb 'eye-bright' were deemed good for the eyes; foot-shaped roots would ease gout; hard, stony seeds such as those of the gromwell plant were believed to cure 'gravel', a disease due to an aggregation of urinary crystals; the knotty tubers of the *scrophularia*, or figwort plant, were believed to heal any ailment of scrofula, a tubercular disease of the lymphatic glands; the spotted leaves of *pulmonaria officinalis*, or lungwort plant, would aptly soothe tuberculous lungs; nettle tea was recommended for nettle rash; and all yellow flowers, seeds or roots such as the East Indian turmeric, were believed to heal jaundice. The doctrine of signatures existed for a considerable period as a medical reference, and gave rise to the names of many plants based on the resemblance of their roots, seeds and leaves to certain parts of the human body (Stapelberg Monica-Maria, *Old Wives' Tales? A select background to the origins of popular beliefs, traditions and superstitions*, Zeus Publishing, Australia 2005, p. 214).
55. Pettigrew Thomas Joseph, *On Superstitions connected with the History and Practice of Medicine and Surgery*, Barrinton & Haswell, Philadelphia 1844, p. 18.
56. Thomas Jane Resh, *Behind the Mask: The Life of Queen Elizabeth I*, Clarion Books, UK

1998, p. 113.

57. Pettigrew 1844, p. 19.
58. Pliny, *Natural History*, Translated by H. Rackham, W.H.S. Jones, D.E. Eichholz, 10 volume edition, Harvard University Press, Massachusetts 1949, BOOK XXVIII p. 181.
59. The use of snakes for healing purposes was so popular, that snakes were imported to European cities in their thousands, tied together in bundles of twelve. When the 'French Academy of Sciences' tried to ban the import of poisonous snakes in 1820, physicians requested that an exception be made with vipers, as they were thought vital to effect certain cures (Bächtold-Stäubli Hans, *Handwörterbuch des Deutschen Aberglaubens*, Vols. I – X, de Gruyter Publishers, Berlin 1987, Vol. 7, p. 1165.) Generally snakes were dried and pulverised or boiled. The fat gleaned from this process was made into a salve or oil. Snake powder ingested or salve used as a cream, was believed efficacious in curing countless ailments and diseases ranging from arthritis, eye problems, cancer, epilepsy, stomach, kidney and intestinal problems, to boils, skin lesions, toothache and nerve complaints. In addition, the eating of snake flesh, which was only affordable to very wealthy ladies, was even thought to have anti-aging effects. Such examples of the varying pseudo-medicinal uses of snake-products once widely used, serve to explain the popular phrase of 'selling snake-oil', a derogatory term for bogus, fraudulent and ineffective medication, sold as a cure-all (Stapelberg Monica-Maria, *Strange But True – a historical background to popular beliefs and traditions*, Crux Publishing, London 2014, p. 241).
60. Bächtold-Stäubli Hans, *Handwörterbuch des Deutschen Aberglaubens*, Vols. I – X, de Gruyter Publishers, Berlin 1987, Vol. I, p. 1437.
61. Ibid.
62. Pliny, *Natural History*, Translated by H. Rackham, W.H.S. Jones, D.E. Eichholz, 10 volume edition, Harvard University Press, Massachusetts 1949, BOOK XXVI. p. 271.
63. During the Middle Ages the blood from a virgin was regarded as a certain cure for leprosy. This theme is central to the Middle-High-German epic *Der arme Heinrich* (written circa 1195) – 'Poor Henry' – as well as the idea that leprosy was a symbol for sin. The central character of this romance is Heinrich, portrayed as the perfect knight. Blessed with wealth and good looks, he was also courageous, brave and strong in battle. However, his God-given gifts had filled him with personal pride, which is why God struck him down with leprosy. Desperately seeking a cure he consulted the best doctors in Christendom, even visiting the most famous medical school in Salerno. Here, learned physicians told him that his only cure would be the blood from a virgin's heart, willingly given. Although Heinrich eventually found the love of a pure peasant girl, willing to offer her life to restore his health, Heinrich did not accept her offer, valuing her life more than his own health – this selfless act of goodness brought him God's cure (Brody Nathaniel Samuel, *The Disease of the Soul – Leprosy in Medieval Literature*, Cornell University Press, London 1974. 147-57).
64. Risse 1999, p. 179.

Chapter 14
The French Pox – not just French

1. A Caribbean island, comprising the sovereign nations of the Dominican Republic in the

east and Haiti in the west of the island. Hispaniola is located between Puerto Rico in the east and Cuba in the west.

2. Such as osteomyelitis and osteoarthropathy.

3. On 31 July 2001 the British television station Channel 4 presented a documentary titled 'The Syphilis Enigma'. The program gave details about several mid-fourteenth century skeletons from Hull in the UK, showing bone deformation as evidence of syphilis. According to this archaeological research, England seems to have been struck by a mystery epidemic of syphilis one hundred and fifty years before the disease actually became widespread in Europe. Radiocarbon dating tests carried out at Oxford University suggest that there was a severe syphilis epidemic in the town of Hull, as well as in other English towns as early as the 1340's. However, evidence of the disease being prevalent in medieval Europe may be regarded as inconclusive, given the fact that indications of syphilis in skeletons are difficult to distinguish from the damage done by leprosy, which was prevalent at that time. The research on the Hull skeletons was thought to suggests that an intermittent series of smaller syphilis epidemics struck the British Isles. The reason for such outbreaks may lie in voyages of discovery by Norwegian Vikings between 1000-1400 CE, when they first landed on the shores of what is now eastern Canada. Archaeological evidence from numerous locations in North America shows that syphilis was endemic in the New World and because England was one of the main destinations for Norwegian sailors and merchants in this period, such close contact could account for a syphilis outbreak erupting in England. Perhaps this syphilis bacterium had achieved equilibrium with its human hosts, hence becoming less virulent over time.

4. Researchers George Armelagos, a bio-archaeologist at Emory University in Atlanta, Molly Zuckerman, from Mississippi State University and Columbia University's Kristin Harper, claim that evidence as to the excistence of syphilis in Europe before Cloumbus' voyages, is flawed. In 2011 Harper et al evaluated all published reports of pre-Columbian Old World treponeal disease, using a systematic approach involving diagnostic criteria, certainty of diagnosis, and the accuracy and reliability of palaeo-pathological dating and radiocarbon dating. The authors concluded that among the 54 reports they evaluated, using their criteria, they did not find a single case of Old World treponeal disease that had both a certain diagnosis and a secure pre-Columbian date. They came to the overall conclusion that evidence for an Old World origin for syphilis remains absent, and that this further supported the hypothesis that syphilis, or its progenitor, came from the New World. (Harper KN, Zuckerman MK, Harper ML, Kingston JD, Armelagos GJ. *The origin and antiquity of syphilis revisited: an appraisal of old world pre-Columbian evidence for treponeal infection. Yearbook Phys Anthropol* 2011: 54: 99-133.)

5. A contention reinforced by comparative genetic information from numerous scattered strains of the syphilis bacterium, establishing that today's syphilis *is* related to the South American strain – where syphilis dates back at least 7,000 years (George Armelagos, In: American Journal of Physical Anthropology, 49 (4): pp 511-516).

6. Explorers returned to Europe with maize, potatoes, and tomatoes and in turn introduced manioc and the peanut to the Americas. This exchange of plants and animals transformed the European and American way of life. Before 1000 CE, potatoes were not known outside of South America. But, by the mid 1800s, Ireland was so dependent on the potato that a diseased harvest led to the devastating Irish Potato Famine. Similarly, the horse, one of the first European exports to the New World changed the lives of Native American tribes on the Great Plains, as they adopted a nomadic lifestyle based on hunting bison on horseback. Tomato sauce, made from New World tomatoes, became an Italian trademark and tomatoes were widely used in France. The Columbian Exchange has often been

described as the single most important event in modern world history, ultimately affecting almost every society on earth.

7. Porter Roy, *The Greatest Benefit to Mankind – A Medical History of Humanity from Antiquity to the Present*, Harper Collins Publishing, London 1999, p. 165.

8. Salzman L. F., *English Life in the Middle Ages*, Oxford University Press, London 1926, p. 87.

9. In medieval Paris for instance, a number of street names were inspired by *merde*, the French word for 'shit'. Paris street names inspired by *merde*, to name but a few, are: the Rue Merdeux, Rue Merdelet, Rue Merdusson Rue des Merdons and many others. Kelly John, *An Intimate History of the Black Death, the Most Devastating Plague of all Time*, Harper Perennial, Harper Collins, London 2006, p. 17.

10. Salzman 1926, p. 26.

11. Achterberg Jeanne, *Woman as Healer – A panoramic survey of the healing activities of women from prehistoric times to the present*, Shambhala Publications, Boston 1990, p. 77.

12. Venereal syphilis may have mutated from one of the non-venereal forms such as 'yaws', which could suggest Columbus did bring it with him. Yaws is a common chronic infectious disease that occurs mainly in warm humid regions such as the tropical areas of Africa, Asia, South and Central America and the Pacific Islands. It is transmitted mainly through direct skin contact with an infected person. The disease affects mainly the bone, cartilage and skin, featuring lesions that appear as bumps on the face, hands, feet and genital area. The organism causing yaws is considered a subspecies of the organism that causes syphilis.

13. The first stage of syphilis tends to disappear after ten to ninety days, only to reappear much later in the secondary phase of the disease.

14. Hayden Deborah, *Pox: Genius, Madness and the Mysteries of Syphilis*, Basic Books 2003, p.7.

15. Ibid., p.7.

16. Ibid., p.7.

17. Ibid., p.7-11.

18. Although the pox was first recorded in 1495, three years after Columbus returned from his first voyage, the name 'syphilis' to describe this malady was only coined much later. In 1530, physician Girolamo Fracastoro, published the poem *Syphilis sive morbus gallicus* 'Syphilis or the French Disease'. The central character in the story is a swineherd who suffers from a dreadfully disfiguring, debilitating disease – his name is Syphilus. But the term 'syphilis' to denote this disease only came to be popularly used in the late eighteenth century.

19. When Columbus arrived back on the island of Hispaniola, on his third voyage in August 1498, he found one hundred and sixty of his men, which amounted to thirty percent (Hayden 2003, p. 8) sick with the French pox as this disease was by then already known.

20. Frith John, *Syphilis – Its early History and Treatment until Penicillin and the Debate on its Origins*, In: Journal of Military and Veterans' Health, Volume 20:4 2012.

21. Ibid.

22. Najemy John M., *Italy in the Age of the Renaissance: 1300-1550*, Oxford University Press 2004, p. 105.

23. Karlen A., *Man and Microbes*, GP Putnam's Sons, New York: 1995.

24. Shelton Herbert M., *Syphilis: Is it a Mischievous Myth or a Malignant Monster*, published by Health Research Centre, Mokehumne California 1962.

25. Thorwald Jürgen, *Science and Secrets of Early Medicine*, Thames & Hudson, London 1962, p.89, 142, 166, 264.

26. Leviticus 15:2-33.

27. Frith 2012.

28. Arrizabalaga Jon, Henderson John and French Roger, *The Great Pox: The French Disease in Renaissance Europe,* Yale University Press 1997, p.12.

29. Stein Claudia, *Negotiating the French Pox in Early Modern Germany*, Ashgate Publishing 2009, p. 44.

30. Arrizabalaga 1997, p. 26.

31. Ibid.

32. Dunant Sarah, *Syphilis, sex and fear: How the French disease conquered the world,* In: *The Guardian*, Saturday 18 May 2013.

33. Ibid.

34. Ibid.

35. Hayden 2003, p. 17.

36. Dunant 2013.

37. Brown Kevin, *The Pox – The life and death of a very social disease*, Sutton Publishing Limited, Gloucestershire 2006, p. 12.

38. Merians Linda Evi, *The Secret Malady: Venereal disease in eighteenth-century Britain and France*, University Press of Kentucky 1996, p. 2.

39. Brown 2006, p. 11.

40. The 'malady of Venus' is known as venereal disease in modern times.

41. Major R.H., *Classic Descriptions of Disease*, Springfield, USA: Charles C Thomas, 1932.

42. Cunningham Andrew, Grell Ole Peter, *The Four Horsemen of the Apocalypse*, Cambridge University Press, Cambridge 2000, p. 255.

43. Dunant 2013.

44. Arrizabalaga 1997, p. 34.

45. This fact is easily substanciated by the stark difference in birth rates between English upper- and working-class women. Parish records show that wealthy women usually gave birth annually while working-class women gave birth at noticeably longer intervals, generally about every three years. Historians attribute this dichotomy to the difference in upper- and lower-class infant feeding practices, as prolonged breast-feeding suppresses ovulation and is therefore a relatively reliable contraceptive. In pre-industrial England, it was not uncommon for wealthy women to have as many as eighteen children during the first twenty years of their marriages, a factor which must have weakened their health considerably. Upper-class demand for wet nurses at one time constituted a major industry in some rural counties. In seventeenth-century England wet nurses were often well known to the wealthy families who hired them, being former servants who had left the household to marry. In these cases wet nurses were trusted, reliable and infants were properly cared for. In most cases however, infants were raised far from their families for up to three years and in these cases there is evidence that as many as eighty percent of them died during infancy.

46. Shakespeare William *Measure for Measure*, 1.2.23. In: Fabricius Johannes, *Syphilis in Shakespeare's England*, Kingsley Press, Michigan 1994, p. 235.

47. Hayden 2003, p. 13.

48. Morton R.S., *Some early Aspects of Syphilis in Scotland*, British Journal of Venereal Diseases, 38 (1962), p. 179.

49. Thomas Jane Resh, *Behind the Mask: The Life of Queen Elizabeth I*, Clarion Books, UK 1998, p. 123.

50. Morton 1962, p.179.

51. Ibid.

52. By renowned Scottish archaeologist Sir Daniel Wilson.

53. Morton 1962, p. 179.

54. Ibid.

55. Brown 2006, p 55.

56. Dunant 2013.

57. Lowe K.J.P., *Church and Politics in Renaissance Italy: The Life and Career of Cardinal Francesco Soderini*, Cambridge University Press 2002.

58. This has culminated in the twenty-first century with what is sometimes described as the 'Michael Jackson Factor', in trying to improve on nature. However, 'nose jobs' are well documented in ancient Indian literature and date back to the second millennium BCE.

59. Reed C.S., *The codpiece: Social fashion or medical need?*, Occasional Medical History Series, In: Internal Medicine Journal 34:684-686, 2004, Sydney Australia.

60. Ibid., p. 685.

61. Cinnabar is the common ore of mercury. To produce quicksilver, or liquid mercury, crushed cinnabar ore is heated in rotary furnaces. Pure mercury separates from sulfur in this process and easily evaporates.

62. Reed 2004, p. 685.

63. Merians 1996, p. 5.

64. Morton 1962, p. 175.

65. Ibid.

66. Brown 2006, p. 14-15.

67. Fabricius Johannes, *Syphilis in Shakespeare's England*, Kingsley Press, Michigan 1994, p. 60-62.

68. Merians 1996, p. 20.

69. Stein 2009, p. 45.

70. Ibid., p. 41.

71. Ibid.

72. Ibid., p. 42.

73. Ibid.

74. Porter 1999, p. 175.

75. Brown 2006, p. 20.

76. Frith 2012.

77. Stein 2009, p.60.

78. Frith 2012.

79. Merians 1996, p. 22.

80. Ibid.

81. Ibid., p. 23.

82. Ibid., p. 21.

83. Storl Wolf L., *Healing Lyme Disease Naturally*, North Atlantic Books, California 2010, p. 255.

84. Siena Kevin Patrick, *Sins of the Flesh: Responding to sexual Disease in Early modern Europe*, Centre for Reformation and Renaissance Studies, Victoria University, Toronto Canada 2005, p. 65.

85. Ibid., p. 64.

86. Ibid.

87. Hayden 2003, p. XV.

88. Ibid.

89. Brown 2006, p 82.

90. Hayden 2003, p. 15.

91. Ibid., p. 14.
92. Quétel Claude, *History of Syphilis*, John Hopkins University Press, Baltimore 1990, p. 128-129.
93. Dunant 2013.
94. Leroux Gaston, *The Phantom of the Opera*, translated by Alexander Teixeira de Mattos, Harper Perennial, USA 1991, p.9.
95. Frith 2012
96. Mukherjee Siddhartha, *The Emperor of all Maladies*, Fourth Estate, London 2011, p. 86.

Chapter 15
Hysteria – the whimsical, wandering womb

1. Allen Prudence, *The Concept of Woman: The early Humanist Reformation 1250-1500*, Eerdmans Publishing 2005, p. 98.
2. Ibid., p. 99.
3. MacLean Ian, *The Renaissance Notion of Women: A Study in the Fortunes of Scholasticism and Medical Science in European Intellectual Life*, Cambridge University Press, 1983, p. 30.
4. King Helen, *Once upon a Text: Hysteria from Hippocrates*, In: Hysteria Beyond Freud, University of California Press 1993, p. 18.
5. Ibid., p. 25.
6. Not a single text of the Hippocratic corpus can be attributed with any certainty to the 'Father of Medicine'. Instead of a collection of genuine works, the *Hippocratic Corpus* is an assorted set of multi-author texts.
7. Meek Heather, *Of Wandering Wombs and Wrongs of Women: Evolving Conceptions of Hysteria in the Age of Reason*, In: English Studies in Canada, Volume 35, No 2-3, June/September 2009, p. 105-128.
8. Adams F., *On hysterical suffocation,* In: On the Causes and Symptoms of Acute Diseases, in book 2 of *The Extant Works of Aretaeus, the Cappadocian*, New Sydenham Society, London 1856, pp. 285-287.
9. King 1993, p. 25.
10. Hippocrates, *Aphorisms*, From the Latin Version of Verhoofd, by Elias Marks, M.D., Collins &Co. New York, 1817.
11. Padilla Mark William, *Rites of Passage in Ancient Greece: Literature, Religion, Society*, Bucknell University Press, 1999, p. 138.
12. The Greek word *hystera* means 'womb', Latinised into the word 'uterus', which is the anatomical name in English.
13. King 1993, p. 4.
14. Ibid., p. 8.
15. Ibid., p.5.
16. Ibid., p.19.
17. Ibid.
18. *Hysterike pnix* does however not have a place in Hippocratic medicine. In Hippocratic gynecology not all diseases described are named, and collections of symptoms are not fitted into pre-existing categories. Rather, it is conceded that individuals may suffer the same disease in different ways.
19. Adams 1856, pp. 285-287.
20. Hæger Knut, *The Illustrated History of Surgery*, revised by Sir Roy Calne, AB Nordbok, Gothenburg Sweden 2000, p. 67.

21. Ibid.
22. Cadden Joan, *The Meanings of Sex Difference in the Middle Ages: Medicine, Science and Culture*, In: Cambridge Studies in the History of Medicine, Cambridge University Press 1995, p. 15.
23. MacLean 1983, p. 30.
24. Ibid.
25. Stapelberg Monica-Maria, *Strange But True – a historical background to popular beliefs and traditions*, Crux Publishing, London 2014, p. 83.
26. Phillips Kate, *Capturing the Wandering Womb – Childbirth in Medieval Art*, In: The Haverford Journal, Vol. 3:1, 2007, pp. 40-55.
27. Pachter Henry, *Paracelsus: Magic into Science*, Henry Schuman Publishing, New York 1951, p. 212.
28. Stapelberg 2014, p. 83.
29. Achterberg Jeanne, *Woman as Healer – A panoramic survey of the healing activities of women from prehistoric times to the present*, Shambhala Publications, Boston 1990, p. 39.
30. Abbot Elisabeth, *A History of Celibacy*, Scribner, New York 2000, p. 54.
31. Heer F., *The Medieval World*, New American Library, New York 1961, p. 322.
32. Green Monica, *The Transmission of Ancient Theories of Female Physiology and Diseases Through the Early Middle Ages* (PhD thesis), Princeton University, New York 1985, 170-171.
33. Known as 'hypochromic anemia' in modern times.
34. King Helen, *The Disease of Virgins: Green Sickness, Chlorosis, and the Problems of Puberty*, Psychology Press, 2004, p. 15.
35. *Aristotle's Masterpiece*, Illustrated Edition, New York 1846, p. 45.
    Original manuscript viewed on: https://archive.org/details/8709661.nlm.nih.gov
1. Clark Andrew Sir, *Anaemia or Chlorosis of Girls, Occurring More Commonly between the advent of Menstruation and the Consummation of Womanhood*, In: Lancet 1887, Vol. 2, p. 1004.
2. 'The very pale colour of the urine and frequently also of the faeces, indicates that less colouring matter than usual is being furnished by haemoglobin and hence that fewer blood corpuscles are breaking down' (Stockman 1895, p. 1473) in other words the condition was seen as being linked to anaemia.
3. Lindemann Mary, *Medicine and Society in Early Modern Europe*, Cambridge University Press 1999, p. 34.
4. Stapelberg 2014, p. 72-86.
5. Lindemann 1999, p. 34.
6. Merskey Harold, Merskey Susan, *Hysteria or 'suffocation of the mother'*, In: Canadian Medical Association Journal, 1993, 148 (3), pp. 399- 405. p.402.
7. The full title of his treatise was: A briefe discourse of a disease called the suffocation of the mother: Written uppon occasion which hath beene of late taken thereby, to suspect possession of an evill spirit, or some such like supernaturall power. Wherein is declared that diverse strange actions and passions of the body of man, which in the common opinion, are imputed to the devil, have their true natural causes, and do accompanie this Disease.
8. Rosen Barbara, *Witchcraft in England 1558-1618*, University of Massachusetts Press 1969. p. 313.
9. Ibid.
10. Sharp Jane, *The Midwives Book or The Whole Art of Midwifery Discovered*, editor Elaine Hobby, Women Writers in English 1350-1850 Series, Oxford University Press 1999, p. 62.
11. Ibid., p. 97.

12.   Ibid., p. 98.

13.   Ibid., p. 99.

14.   *Aristotle's Masterpiece*, New York 1846, p. 93.

15.   Ibid., p. 97.

16.   MacLean 1983, p. 32.

17.   *Aristotle's Masterpiece*, New York 1846, p. 25.

18.   Ibid.

19.   Such differentiation was even applied to the creation of the soul, as the Church in medieval times decreed that God created the soul forty days after conception in the case of boys and eighty days after conception in the case of girls (Stapelberg 2011, p. 255).

20.   Lindemann 1999, p. 34.

21.   Meek 2009, p. 109.

22.   R. Brain, *The Concept of Hysteria in the Time of Harvey*, Proceedings of the Royal Society of Medicine, 1963, 56: 317-324.

23.   MacLean 1983, p. 40.

24.   Rousseau G. S., *A Strange Pathology: Hysteria in the Early Modern World, 1500-1800*, In: Hysteria beyond Freud, University of California Press 1993, p. 142.

25.   Mitchinson W., *Hysteria and Insanity in Women: A nineteenth century Canadian perspective*, In: Journal of Canadian Studies, 1986, 21 (3) 87-105, p. 90.

26.   Showalter Elaine, *Hysteria, Feminism and Gender*, In: Hysteria Beyond Freud, University of California Press 1993, p. 287.

27.   Adair Mark J, *Plato's View of the 'Wandering Uterus'*, In: *The Classical Journal* 91:2, 1996, p. 153.

Chapter 16
Women's woes – fertility, conception and menstruation

1.   Kudlein Fridolf, *The Seven Cells of the Uterus: the doctrine and its roots*, In: Bulletin of the History of Medicine 39 (1965): pp. 415-423.

1.   As the majority of people have always been right-handed, the left side of the body was considered the weaker side, associated with ill luck. This notion has left its mark on most western languages, which serves to explain why the Latin word *sinistra*, meaning 'on the left hand' became the English word 'sinister', describing all that is foreboding and ominous. In a similar context, the word 'awkward' meaning clumsy, originates from the Middle English word *awk*, which meant 'in the wrong direction'. The French word *gauche*, meaning left has a more negative connotation when used in English. Similarly, we state that someone is 'right', meaning the person to be 'correct'. (Stapelberg Monica-Maria, *Strange But True – a historical background to popular beliefs and traditions*, Crux Publishing, London 2014, p. 26-27).

2.   Allen Prudence, *The Concept of Woman: The Aristotelian Revolution 750 BC – AD 1250*, William Eerdmans Publishing 1997, p. 454.

3.   Pliny the Elder, *Natural History – A Selection*, translated by J.F. Healy, Penguin Books, London 1991, Vol.VII, v. 37, p.81.

4.   Allen 1997, p. 28.

5.   Cadden Joan, *Meanings of Sex Differences in the Middle Ages: Medicine, Science and Culture*, Cambridge 1995, p. 43.

6.   Simon Forman (1552 – 1611), functioned as an astrologer, occultist and herbalist in London during the reigns of Queen Elisabeth I and James I. He spent some time at

Oxford, studying medicine and astrology and later delved into the occult arts. In 1583 he started working as a physician and surgeon in London. After surviving an outbreak of the plague in the city during that year and again in 1594 his medical reputation began to spread and his astrological medical practice was thriving. Most of his consultations addressed medical issues, but others dealt with lost or stolen property, missing persons, or forthcoming journeys and voyages. Soon his success as a medical practitioner combined with magical practices attracted the attention of London's regulatory authorities and in 1593 he was called before the Barber–Surgeons and in 1595 before the College of Physicians. He confessed to having practiced medicine in England for sixteen years, and to have effected many cures although he had studied none of the orthodox medical authors. The college examined Forman on astrology and medicine and found him 'laughably ignorant, a conclusion which is difficult to reconcile with the scholarly pursuits recorded in his papers'. Forman continued to practice medicine until his death in 1611. He is known as one of the best-documented Elizabethans, probably because he wrote at length about himself and everything that interested him, leaving behind thousands of pages of unusual facts, including manuscripts dealing with his patients, as well as autobiographies, guides to astrology, plague tracts, notes on alchemy, medicine, mathematics, and magic. (*Oxford Dictionary of National Biography*).

7.   Kudlein 1965, pp. 415-423.
8.   Vicary Thomas, *The English Man's Treasure*, Imprinted at London By Thomas Creed, 1599, p.93-94.
9.   'Matrix' stands for womb.
10. Raynalde Thomas, Rösslin Eucharius, *The Birth of Mankind: Otherwise named the Woman's Book*, Editor Elaine Hobby, Translated by Richard Jonas, Ashgate Publishing 2009, pp. 35-36.
11. Stein Claudia, *Negotiating the French Pox in Early Modern Germany*, Ashgate Publishing 2009, p. 44.
12. Chauliac Guy de, *Inventarium Sive Chirurgica Magna*, edited by Michael McVaugh, In: Studies in Ancient Medicine, Brill Publishing 1997, p. 49.
13. King Helen, *Once upon a text*, In: Hysteria beyond Freud, by Gilman Sander L., King Helen, Porter Roy, Rousseau G. S., Showalter Elaine, University of California Press 1993 p. 43.
14. Woolley Benjamin, *The Herbalist – Nicholas Culpeper and the fight for medical freedom*, Harper Perennial, London 2005, p. 45.
15. Roach Mary, *Stiff: The Curious Lives of Human Cadavers*, W.W. Norton & Company, New York 2003, p. 214.
16. King 1993, p. 43.
17. Mortimer Ian, *The Time Traveller's Guide to Medieval England*, Vintage Books, London 2009, p. 55.
18. 'Mother' refers to 'womb'.
19. Sharp Jane, *The Midwives Book or The Whole Art of Midwifery Discovered*, editor Elaine Hobby, Women Writers in English 1350-1850 Series, Oxford University Press 1999, p. 62.
20. Phillips Kate, *Capturing the Wandering Womb, Childbirth in Medieval Art*, In: The Haverford Journal, 3, 2007, pp. 41.
21. *Aristotle's Masterpiece*, Illustrated Edition, New York 1846, p.11.
22. *Aristotle's Masterpiece* was first published in 1684, and remained in print until at least 1814.
23. *Aristotle's Masterpiece*, Illustrated Edition, New York 1846, p.11.
24. Ibid., p. 20.
25. Ibid., p. 15.

26. Woolley 2005, p. 183.
27. Quoted in Woolley 2005, p. 183.
28. Woolley 2005, p. 183.
29. King Helen, *The Disease of Virgins: Green Sickness, Chlorosis, and the Problems of Puberty*, Psychology Press, 2004, p. 62.
30. Ibid.
31. In *Natural History.*
32. Stapelberg 2014, p. 213.
33. Hindson Bethan, *Attitudes towards menstruation and menstrual blood in Elizabethan England*, In: Journal of Social History, Cengage Learning, University of Sheffield, volume 43, 2009, pp. 89-114.
34. Leviticus 15: 19-25.
35. Stapelberg 2014, p. 83.
36. In the biblical Old Testament Book of Leviticus it is stated that: 'If a woman have.... born a.... child: she shall be unclean.... She shall touch no hallowed thing, nor come into the sanctuary, until the days of her purifying be fulfilled....'(Leviticus 12: 2-5)
37. MacLean Ian, *The Renaissance Notion of Women: A Study in the Fortunes of Scholasticism and Medical Science in European Intellectual Life*, Cambridge University Press, 1983, p. 38.
38. Kassell Lauren, *Medicine and Magic in Elizabethan London: Simon Forman: Astrologer, Alchemist and Physician*, Oxford University Press 2005, p.188.
39. MacLean 1983, p. 38.
40. Raynalde Thomas, *The Birth of Mankind: Otherwise named the Woman's Book*, Editor Elaine Hobby, Translated by Richard Jonas, Ashgate Publishing 2009, p. 15.
41. MacLean 1983, p. 40.
42. McClive Cathy, *Menstrual Knowledge and Medical Practice in Early Modern France c.1555-1761*, In: Menstruation: A Cultural History, eds. Andrew Shail and Gillian Howie, Hampshire 2005, pp. 77-80.
43. Raynalde 2009, p. 57.
44. Ibid.
45. Gerard John, *The Herball Or Generall Historie of Plantes*, London, 1597, p. 185; and Turner William, *The first and seconde partes of the Herball of William Turner, corrected and enlarged with the thirde parte*, Cologne, 1568, p. 117.
46. Raynalde 2009, p. 57.
47. Hindson Bethan, *Attitudes towards menstruation and menstrual blood in Elizabethan England*, In: Journal of Social History, Cengage Learning, University of Sheffield, volume 43, 2009, pp. 89-114.
48. Furdell Elizabeth Lane, *The Royal Doctors: 1485-1714 – Medical Personnel at the Tudor and Stuart Courts*, University of Rochester Press 2001, p. 57.
49. Ibid., p. 58.
50. During centuries past, menopause came earlier to women. For instance, in the sixteenth century women usually went into menopause between the ages of forty-two and forty-five (Furdell 2001, p. 57).
51. Jorden Edward, *A briefe discourse of a disease called the suffocation of the mother*, Publisher John Windet, London 1603, Digitised 24 Aug 2011 by University of California, p. 17.
52. Raynalde 2009, p. 58.
53. Bowie Fiona, *Hildegard of Bingen and medieval women's sexuality*, In: Diskus 2:1, pp. 1-14, 1994.
54. Saunders J. B. and O'Malley D., *The Illustrations from the Works of Andreas Vesalius of Brussels*, Dover Publications, New York 1950, p. 172.

55. Ibid.
56. Raynalde 2009, p. XXIV, 65-73.
57. *The Midwives Book or the Whole Art of Midwifery Discovered*, published in 1671.
58. Sharp Jane, *The Midwives Book or The Whole Art of Midwifery Discovered*, editor Elaine Hobby, Women Writers in English 1350-1850 Series, Oxford University Press 1999, p. 62-63.
59. Jacobi Mary Putnam, *The question of rest for women during menstruation*, 1877, p. 64.
60. King 2004, p. 62.

Chapter 17
Women's woes continue – childbirth and 'with-women'

1. Furdell Elizabeth Lane, *The Royal Doctors: 1485-1714 – Medical Personnel at the Tudor and Stuart Courts*, University of Rochester Press 2001, p. 5.
2. It was not until the early eighteen hundreds that the term 'obstetrics' came into usage – probably, because the Latin term sounded more academic than Anglo-Saxon 'midwyf'. *Obstetrix,* the Latin word for 'midwife', is probably derived from *obstare,* to 'stand before', describing the midwife who stood in front of the labouring woman to receive the child.
3. Children were similarly of 'no interest to the medical profession at this time. They simply lived or died and were subjected to a variety of home remedies when they were ill' (Rhodes Philip, *An Outline History of Medicine*, Cambridge University Press 1986, p. 36).
4. MacLean Ian, *The Renaissance Notion of Women: A Study in the Fortunes of Scholasticism and Medical Science in European Intellectual Life*, Cambridge University Press, 1983, p. 41.
5. Woolley Benjamin, *The Herbalist – Nicholas Culpeper and the fight for medical freedom*, Harper Perennial, London 2005, p. 314.
6. Quoted in Woolley 2005, p. 314.
7. Like William Harvey.
8. Donnison Jean, *Midwives and Medical Men – A History of the Struggle for the Control of Childbirth*, Historical Publications, London 1999, p. 25.
9. 'Gossip' from the Old English *godsibb*, from God, and *sibb*, meaning 'relative'. A *godsibb* was a godmother, godfather or sponsor; literally someone 'related to one in God'. In Middle English the term *godsibb* came to mean 'any familiar acquaintance', especially women invited to attend a birth. Later, during the sixteenth century the term changed to 'gossip' and took on the meaning of a person, mostly a woman, attending a birth, but also delighting in idle talk. In later centuries the term was extended to also encompass the conversation of such a person, newsmonger, or tattler.
10. Donnison 1999, p. 25.
11. In many European countries painted wooden birth trays, known in Italian as *desco da parto were presented to the new mother.* These trays, depicting images of childbirth, first appeared around 1370 in Italy. Especially wealthy families commissioned ornately painted, gilded confinement scenes with appropriate religious or mythological themes. Immediately following childbirth, nourishing food would be presented to the mother on her *desco* da parto – later this birth tray would be hung in the bedroom as a decorative painting. Sometimes, birth trays were given to newlyweds as symbols of fertility – a clear message conveying the bride's maternal duty. But usually they were offered at the birth of a child, thus rewarding a healthy outcome. Poorer people also afforded desco da parto, or birth trays, by simply getting cheaper less ornate versions. Musacchio Jacqueline, *The Art and Ritual of Childbirth in Renaissance Italy,* Yale University Press, New Haven 1999.

12. The Christian practice of 'churching' refers to reintegrating the new mother into the religious community. Until the church ceremony of 'churching' or 'kirking', as it was referred to in Scotland, had been carried out, a woman after childbirth was looked upon as being unclean and believed to be a danger to her neighbours and the community at large (Stapelberg Monica-Maria, *Strange But True – a historical background to popular beliefs and traditions*, Crux Publishing, London 2014, p. 230.

13. Donnison 1999, p. 15.

14. Ibid.

15. The Latin term *cum mater* and the Spanish and Portuguese term *comadre*, have the same meaning: 'with woman'. The ancient Hebrews called her the 'wise woman' Similarly, she was known as *sage femme* in France, and as *weise Frau*, as well as *Hebamme*, or 'mother's helper', in Germany

16. Exodus 1:20

17. Similarly, Genesis 35:17, reports that when Rachel was in labour, the midwife said to her: 'Fear not, for now you will have another son'.

18. Donnison 1999, p. 14.

19. Ibid.

20. Porter Roy, *The Greatest Benefit to Mankind – A Medical History of Humanity from Antiquity to the Present*, Harper Collins Publishing, London 1999, p. 128.

21. For example, the town councils of Nürenberg in Germany and Mechelen in Flanders regularly called upon midwives to 'give opinions in cases of infanticides, suspected abortions, and examinations of female prisoners claiming they were pregnant'. In these countries 'ecclesiastical courts also called upon midwives to test virginity in annulment actions, for example or in cases of impotence' (Greilsammer Myriam, *The midwife, the priest, and the physician: the subjugation of midwives in the Low Countries at the end of the Middle Ages*, Journal of Medieval and Renaissance Studies, 21:2, 1991, p. 291-292).

22. Greilsammer Myriam, *The midwife, the priest, and the physician: the subjugation of midwives in the Low Countries at the end of the Middle Ages*, Journal of Medieval and Renaissance Studies, 21:2, 1991, p. 301.

23. Martin Luther, as was his manner, bluntly expressed this popularly held view 'If women die in childbirth that does no harm. It is what they were made for'. Pachter Henry, *Paracelsus: Magic into Science*, Henry Schuman Publishing, New York 1951, p. 212.

24. Donnison 1999, p. 16.

25. Ibid.

26. Bullough Vern L., *The Subordinate Sex*, University of Illinois Press, 1974, p. 119.

27. Already before the Papal Bull of 1484, Brussels was the first town in Europe, in 1424, 'to enact detailed regulations regarding the functions of midwives' (Greilshammer 1991, p. 296).

28. Porter 1999, p. 130.

29. Genesis 3:16.

30. Rhodes Philip, *An Outline History of Medicine*, Cambridge University Press 1986, p. 53.

31. Willughby Percivall, *Observations in Midwifery*, edited by Henry Blenkinsop, H.T. Crooke & Son, Warwick 1863, p. 13.

32. Although the Queen and her husband Prince Albert had already shown an interest in chloroform (discovered in 1831) in 1848, no anaesthetic was used in delivering her seventh child. But for the eighth delivery the Queen declared herself eager in trying the purported analgesic effects of chloroform – in spite of serious reservations regarding the use of anaesthesia in childbirth, from her physicians and ecclesiastic authorities representing the Church of England. The queen put herself in the care of English physician John Snow

(1813 – 1858), a pioneer in the use anaesthesia, as well as medical hygiene and generally considered one of the fathers of modern epidemiology due to his work in tracing the origin of the cholera outbreak in 1854 in London. Luckily there were no complications, an unnerving possibility, not only because this was a royal birth, but also because chloroform was a relatively new drug. Immediately there was an enormous public outcry, especially from various religious sources, stating that painful childbirth rendered any woman a better mother. However, in 1857, Snow repeated his administration of chloroform during Queen Victoria's ninth delivery, the birth of Princess Beatrice. Henceforth, chloroform became known as 'The Queen's Anaesthetic', grating guilt-free pain relief to hundreds of women during the Victorian age.

33. Donnison 1999, p. 14.
34. Greilshammer 1991, p. 291.
35. Raynalde Thomas, *The Birth of Mankind: Otherwise named The Woman's Book*, Editor Elaine Hobby, Translated by Richard Jonas, Ashgate Publishing 2009, p. XI.
36. Under King Henry VIII an Act was passed in 1512, for the regulation of physicians and surgeons. Although the Act 'did not mention midwives, they were licensed under the provisions (of the Act) soon afterwards, probably on the basis that midwifery, being a manual art, was considered part of surgery' (Donnison 1999, p. 19).
37. *The Rose-Garden for Pregnant Women and Midwives.*
38. Raynalde 2009, p. XXIII.
39. Amongst dozens of works of the same genre, the most renowned books on midwifery during the seventeenth century included Nicholas Culpeper's *Directory for Midwives* published in 1651; *The Midwives Book: or the Whole Art of Midwifery Discovered* in 1671 by British midwife Jane Sharp; *Observations in Midwifery*, written around 1670, by 'man-midwife' Percivall Willughby (his book presents a record of 150 case histories, only published in 1863); and *Aristotle's Masterpiece*, written by an unknown author claiming to be Aristotle. *Aristotle's Masterpiece* is a marriage and midwifery guide. It was first published in 1684, and remained popular in England through to the nineteenth century. All these works were written for midwives, male and female, as well as physicians.
40. Known in French as an *accoucheur*.
41. Green Monica, *Making Women's Medicine Masculine: The Rise of male Authority in Pre-Modern Gynaecology*, Oxford University Press, 2008, p. 139.
42. Donnison 1999, p. 21.
43. Kontoyannis Maria, Katsetos Christos, *Midwives in early modern Europe (1400-1800)*, Health Science Journal, Volume 5:1, 2011, pp: 31-36.
44. Willughby 1863, p. 21.
45. Ibid., pp. 94 and 164.
46. Ibid., p. 164.
47. Ibid.
48. Ibid., p. 165.
49. Rhodes 1986, p. 84.
50. Greilsammer 1991, p. 290.
51. Willughby 1863, p. 135.
52. MacDonald Helen, *Human Remains – Dissection and its Histories*, Yale University Press, London 2006, p. 20.
53. Ibid.
54. Loudon Irvine, *The Making of Man-Midwifery*, In: Bulletin of the History of Medicine, 1996, Volume 70:3, pp. 507-515.
55. Wilson Adrian, *The Making of Man-Midwifery: Childbirth in England 1660-1770*, Harvard

University Press, 1995.

56. It is interesting to note, that as a result of lying-in hospitals, around one million more deaths occurred in Britain and Ireland between 1730 and 1930 (due to infection), than would have occurred had home-births remained the norm (Sheldon D.C., *Man-midwifery history: 1730-1930*, In: Journal for Obstetrics and Gynaecology, 2012, 32:8, pp. 718-723).

57. Kontoyannis 2011, pp: 31-36.

58. Rhodes 1986, p. 69.

59. Donnison 1999, p. 53.

60. Loudon Irvine, *General practitioners and obstetrics: A brief history*, In: Journal of the Royal Society of Medicine Nov. 2008, 101:11, pp. 531-535.

61. Ibid.

62. Donnison 1999, p. 57.

63. Loudon 2008, pp. 531-535.

64. Loudon Irvine, *Death in Childbirth*, Clarendon Press, Oxford 1992, pp. 71–2.

65. Rhodes 1986, p. 85.

66. White Charles, *Treatise on the Management of Pregnant and Lying-In Women*, Edward and Charles Dilly Printers, London 1773, p. 52.

67. Ibid., p. 53.

68. Ibid., p. 54.

69. Radcliffe Walter, *Milestones in Midwifery*, Wright Publishing, London 1967, p. 80.

70. White 1773, p. 54.

71. Radcliffe 1967, p. 80.

72. At the time, Semmelweis worked at the Vienna General Hospital's obstetrical clinic. Such maternity institutions were generally set up in European countries to address the high rate of infantacide of illigitimate children. Here, at Vienna General Hospital's two obstetrical clinics, underprivileged women and prostitutes, in return for a free service, agreed to act as training subjects for doctors and midwives. Semmelweiss soon noticed a considerable fluctuation of mortality rates, due to puerperal fever, between the two clinics – the first clinic's doctor's wards had three times the mortality rates as the student midwives' wards in the second clinic. This troubled him gravely, and he began a meticulous process of elimination as to the cause of such a discrepancy. After some months, he established that the only difference between the two clinics was that the first clinic was a teaching facility for medical students, while the second clinic was for the instruction of student midwives only. Then a breakthrough occurred in 1847, when a collegue of his died after having been accidentally pricked with a student's scalpel. The collegue's autopsy indicated similar pathology to that of women dying from puerperal fever. Hence, Semmelweis concluded that the medical students carried 'cadaverous particles' on their unwashed hands from the autopsy room to the patients they examined in the first obstetrical clinic, hence causing infection. As the student midwives in the second clinic, were not engaged in autopsies and had no contact with corpses, this clinic had a much lower mortality rate.

73. Refer to: http://en.wikipedia.org/wiki/Ignaz_Semmelweis

74. Drife J., *The start of life: a history of obstetrics*, In: Postgraduate Medical Journal, 2002, Volume 78:919, pp. 311-315.

Chapter 18

Diagnosing death – a dire dilemma

1. Known as 'taphophobia' from Greek *taphos* meaning 'grave', and *phobia* from Greek *phobos* meaning 'fear'. In other words 'fear of the grave', or 'fear of being put into the grave while still alive'.
2. Until the 1950's, medical practitioners did not understand that cardiac arrest was wholly reversible.
3. In the past it was not uncommon in many European countries for live burials to be carried out as punishment for crimes such as infanticide, rape and even theft. This form of punishment is frequently recorded together with impalement in medieval German city statutes.
4. This was in part due to Hippocratic medical ethics, as well as his prohibition on treating incurable and dying patients.
5. Quote from Tebb William, *Premature burial, and how it may be prevented, with special reference to trance catalepsy, and other forms of suspended animation*, Second Edition by Walter R. Hadwen M.D., Swan Sonnenschein & Co.Limited, London 1905, p. 372.
6. Taylor Joseph, *The Danger Of Premature Interment – Proved From Many Remarkable Instances*, Simkin and Marshall, London 1816, p. 60.
7. Tebb 1905, p. 372.
8. Quote by Pliny from Tebb 1905, p. 9.
9. The 'Foramen of Winslow', the opening between the greater and lesser sacs of the peritoneum, is named after Jaques-Bénigne Winslow.
10. *The uncertainty of signs of death.*
11. Winslow Jacques-Bénigne, *The Uncertainty of the Signs of Death, and the Danger of Precipitate Interments and Dissections*, London 1746, p. 194.
12. Bondeson Jan, *Buried Alive – The Terrifying History Of Our Most Primal Fear*, Barnes and Noble Books, New York 2006, p. 13.
13. Brouardel P. and Benham Lucas, *Death and Sudden Death*, Baillière, Tindall & Co., London 1902, p. 18.
14. In 1816, René Laennec invented a rudimentary type of stethoscope. This device, made of wood, resembled the common ear trumpet and picked up internal sounds of the human body. The modern binaural stethoscope was first used in America in the 1850's.
15. Winslow 1746, p. 29.
16. This is a translation of his Latin thesis *Morte incertae signa*.
17. Winslow clearly stated that '…the Paleness of the Complexion, the Coldness of the Body, the Rigidity of the Extremities, and the Abolition of the external Senses, are very dubious and fallacious Signs' (Winslow 1746, p. 11).
18. Winslow suggested that the presumed corpse's gums be rubbed with acidic substances, and the body be '…stimulate(d) with Whips and Nettles', the intestines 'irritated' by '…Means of Clysters and Injections of Air or Smoke' as well as the limbs '…agitate(d) by violent Extensions and Inflexions', and the ears subjected to '…hideous Shrieks and excessive Noises', before being dissected (Winslow 1746, p. 21).
19. Winslow 1746, p. 23.
20. It was an old and deep-rooted notion in western culture that the corpse should never be left alone between death and burial. Family and friends of the deceased devised ways to ensure that death had indeed taken place and their loved-ones were not buried alive. This is partly how the custom of holding a wake originated. The 'death watch' or 'wake' as it is known today, was originally taken literally, the corpse carefully 'watched' for three days before burial. There was always the very real possibility that the person considered

dead could actually be in a swoon and 'wake' up at any time. (Stapelberg Monica-Maria, *Strange But True – a historical background to popular beliefs and traditions*, Crux Publishing, London 2014, p. 193).

21. 'Dissertation on the Uncertainty of the Signs of Death'.

22. Bruhier's books reformed burial practices, in the sense that it became accepted practice throughout Europe to wait at least twenty-four hours after death before burial took place. In addition his warnings regarding those who had 'died' as a result of drowning, freezing or apoplexy, were widely heeded by medical practitioners.

23. Bondeson 2006, p. 156.

24. Ibid., p. 32.

25. Ibid., p. 88.

26. Christoph Wilhelm Friedrich Hufeland (1762-1836) was a renowned, highly awarded and honoured German physician. Among his patients he counted German greats such as Wieland, Herder, Goethe and Schiller. In addition to a dedicated medical career, he was also a highly successful writer, authoring over four hundred publications, including themes discussing popular interests of the times: the role of electricity, its effect on living beings, and premature burial. His interest in live burial and 'diagnosing death' or determining the signs of death, were the subject of several publications, spanning almost two decades and ultimately leading to the creation of Germany's first waiting mortuary in Weimar in 1791.

27. Bondeson 2006, p. 91

28. *Der Spiegel* 1967, no.48, p.177.

29. In spite of such mortuaries mushrooming in numerous European countries, there is however not a single confirmed report of anyone ever having woken up or rung the bell rope, which had been placed in their 'dead' hands (Brouardel 1902, p.23).

30. *The Lancet*, 20 September, 1845, volume ii, p. 321.

31. The *British and Foreign Medico-Chirurgical Review*, 1855, volume XV. p. 75.

32. Tebb 1905, p. 341.

33. Huntsinger Wolf Elizabeth, *Georgetown Mysteries and Legends*, John F. Blair Publishing, 2007, p. 105.

34. Bateson's own dread and preoccupation of being buried alive prompted the designs of numerous other intricate alarm systems for use on his own coffin. He requested to be cremated after death, but fearing that his family would not carry out his last wishes, set himself alight, bringing about his own death in 1868.

35. Bondeson 2006, p. 127.

36. Various cases – just a few are named here – of premature burial appeared in American newspapers: 'A Dreadful Doom' appeared in *The Salt Lake Herald* on 22 Jan. 1891; 'Alive in Her Coffin' appeared in *The Roanoke Times* on 4 July 1893; 'A Man Buried Alive' appeared in *The New York Times* on 21 Feb. 1885.

37. Vadakan Vibul, *The Asphyxiating and Exsanguinating Death of President George Washington*, In: The Permanente Journal, Spring 2004, Volume 8, No. 2, p. 79.

38. Experiments, to determine death with certainty, performed at the Royal College of Surgery in London in the early 1800's, included thrusting a needle into the lifeless eyes of executed felons – this was done to elicit any effect, however minor, from the subject. 'Other investigations were undertaken in a more systematic way as College men sought to understand whether an absence of obvious animation was a sign that the life force had merely been suspended or was irretrievably extinguished' (MacDonald Helen, *Human Remains – Dissection and its Histories*, Yale University Press, London 2006, p. 15). In this context the College invited Professor Giovanni Aldini to perform galvanic experiments on the corpses of murderers. The professor preferred to work on his subjects immediately

after execution, believing that people who had recently died still retained their 'vital powers', hence could perhaps be revived and returned to life through galvanisation. Aldini's experiments were designed to benefit the British public, especially when people drowned. 'In contrast, those who had died of disease might have humors which would resist his experiments' (MacDonald 2006, p. 15). The College's experiments in animation of the dead also included stimulation of the heart of newly executed felons. One of the surgeons' greatest triumphs was when they succeeded in animating a heart, merely by the touch of a scalpel, to continue beating for four hours after the victim's execution (MacDonald 2006, p. 19).

39. Quain Richard (editor), *A Dictionary of Medicine*, Appleton & Company, New York 1884.

40. The *Lancet*, 1889, vol. I, p. 1173.

41. The *Lancet*, 22 December 1883, vol. I, p. 1078-80.

42. Tebb 1905, p. 47.

43. In his comprehensive book *Premature Burial And How It May Be Prevented*, English social reformer William Tebb, cited numerous cases where trances or 'lethargic stupor' almost led to premature burial – although unknowingly in many such cases it probably did. Tebb also gives the names of numerous well-known personages subject to such trance 'seizures': Statesman Benjamin Disraeli, who once fell into a week-long trance; philosopher and mystic Madame Blavatzky, who would have been buried alive, had not her assistant telegraphed to let her have time to awaken from her 'trance'; the mother of General Lee, Confederate general in the American Civil War – she was pronounced dead, and saved by the sexton who heard her crying out in her coffin (Tebb 1905, p. 45-46).

44. On 7 July 1867 the *Times* newspaper related the case of a young woman who had apparently died while having an epileptic seizure. During burial, while throwing shovelfuls of ground on the coffin, the gravedigger thought he heard a moaning from the tomb. The body was exhumed, exhibiting definite signs of life, but never fully recovered and died 'again' the next day (*Times*, 7 July 1867, p. 12, column 3). A similar story appeared in January 1889 in the London *Daily Telegraph*. The report concerned a man who had become intoxicated on potato brandy and had fallen into a profound sleep. Considered dead by family and friends he was duly buried. After the sexton heard moans from the grave, the man was exhumed. Unfortunately, he was found to be dead, but he had '… horribly mutilated his head in his frantic but futile efforts to burst his coffin open' (*Daily Telegraph* 18 January 1889) On August 19, 1895 the London *Star* newspaper reported a similar case: Muffled sounds were heard after lowering the coffin of a man into his grave. Once the coffin had been pulled up and opened the unfortunate occupant was indeed found to be alive, but died without uttering a word several days later, when a second funeral was held (*Star* newspaper August 19, 1895).

45. The *British Medical Journal*, October 31, 1885, p. 841.

46. 'Not even the most massive textbooks, like Professor Roy Porter's *The Greatest Benefit to Mankind*, contains a single word about the debate regarding the uncertainty of the signs of death that raged throughout the eighteenth and nineteenth centuries. A specialist book like *Death and the Enlightenment*, by Dr. J. McManners, briefly dismisses the eighteenth century fear of premature burial as a bizarre manifestation of French hypochondrial zeal' (Bondeson 2006, p. 14).

47. Zaner Richard W., *Death: Beyond Whole-Brain Criteria*, Kluwer Academic Publishers, Netherlands 1988, p. 52.

INDEX

W

X

Z

ALSO BY
MONICA-MARIA STAPELBERG

Strange but True:
A Historical Background to Popular Beliefs and Traditions

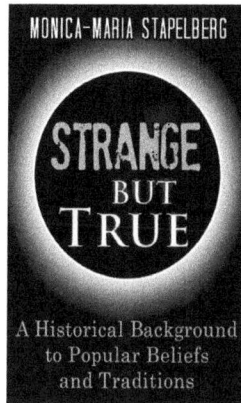

WHY DO WE:
- *Christen ships and sailing vessels or refer to them as 'she'?*
- *Avoid the number thirteen, breaking mirrors or walking under ladders?*
- *Use the phrase having a 'skeleton in the cupboard'?*
- *Dress baby boys in blue, speak of 'true blue' or 'blue-blooded'?*
- *Decorate the Christmas Tree or eat Easter Eggs?*
- *Kiss under the mistletoe or 'trick or treat' on Halloween?*

In this easy-to-read book – a revised and updated re-publication of her previous book, Curious and Curiouser! – author, lecturer and public speaker, Dr. Monica-Maria Stapelberg, shares the results of her many years of research to uncover the historical background behind numerous commonly-held beliefs and traditions. These range from general popular beliefs to the more specific and enlightening traditions of western culture. Strange but True also brings to light how many of our day-to-day words, phrases and actions are anchored in past ritual or sacrificial observances, or simply based on fearful superstitious notions. This book is a must read for a curious mind!

www.ingramcontent.com/pod-product-compliance
Lightning Source LLC
Chambersburg PA
CBHW071533200326
41519CB00021BB/6468